THE SCIENCE OF
CANCER TREATMENT

CANCER BIOLOGY AND MEDICINE
Series Editors M. J. Waring and B. A. J. Ponder

THE SCIENCE OF CANCER TREATMENT

Edited by

B. A. J. Ponder

Director, CRC Human Cancer Genetics Research Group,
Department of Pathology,
University of Cambridge, UK

and

M. J. Waring

Lecturer in Pharmacology,
University of Cambridge, UK

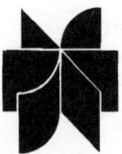

KLUWER ACADEMIC PUBLISHERS
DORDRECHT / BOSTON / LONDON

Distributors

for the United States and Canada: Kluwer Academic Publishers, PO Box 358,
Accord Station, Hingham, MA 02018–0358, USA
for all other countries: Kluwer Academic Publishers Group, Distribution Centre,
PO Box 322, 3300 AH Dordrecht, The Netherlands

British Library Cataloguing in Publication Data

The science of cancer treatment.
  1. Man. Cancer. Therapy
  I. Ponder, B. A. J. (Bruce Anthony John), *1944*– II. Waring, Michael, J.
  III. Series
  616.99406

ISBN-13: 978-94-010-6804-8   e-ISBN-13: 978-94-009-0709-6
DOI: 10.1007/978-94-009-0709-6

Copyright

Published in the United Kingdom by Kluwer Academic Publishers, PO Box 55,
Lancaster, UK.

Kluwer Academic Publishers BV incorporates the publishing programmes of D.
Reidel, Martinus Nijhoff, Dr W. Junk and MTP Press.

Typesetting by Witwell Ltd, Southport

Contents

List of Contributors

F. R. BALKWILL
Biological Therapy Department
Imperial Cancer Research Fund
PO Box 123, Lincoln's Inn Fields
London WC2A 3PX, UK

M. BAUM
Department of Surgery
Kings College School of Medicine and
   Surgery
Denmark Hill
London SE5 9NU, UK

R. H. J. BEGENT
Medical Concology Department
Cancer Research Campaign
   Laboratories
Charing Cross Hospital
Fulham Palace Road
London W6 8RF, UK

N. F. BOYD
Ontario Cancer Institute
500 Sherbourne St
Toronto
M4X 1K9, Canada

R. BROWN
CRC Department of Clinical
   Oncology
Alexander Stone Building
Garscube Estate, Switchback Road
Glasgow G61 1BD, UK

M. COUSINS
Ontario Cancer Institute
500 Sherbourne St
Toronto
M4X 1K9, Canada

H. EARL
Department of Radiotherapy and
   Oncology
University College Hospital
Gower Street
London WC1E 6AU, UK

A. HORWICH
Department of Radiotherapy and
   Oncology
Royal Marsden Hospital and Institute
   of Cancer Research
Down Rd, Sutton
Surrey SM2 5PT, UK

N. JAMES
Department of Clinical Oncology
Royal Postgraduate Medical School
Hammersmith Hospital
Ducane Road
London W12 0HS, UK

S. B. KAYE
CRC Department of Clinical
   Oncology
Alexander Stone Building
Garscube Estate, Switchback Road
Glasgow G61 1BD, UK

S. A. KELLY
Biological Therapy Department
Imperial Cancer Research Fund
PO Box 123, Lincoln's Inn Fields
London WC2A 3PX, UK

S. MALIK
Biological Therapy Department
Imperial Cancer Research Fund
PO Box 123, Lincoln's Inn Fields
London WC2A 3PX, UK

V. McGUIRE
Ontario Cancer Institute
500 Sherbourne St
Toronto
M4X 1K9
Canada

B. L. SAMUELS
Department of Medicine
University of Chicago
5841 South Maryland Avenue
Chicago
IL 60637, USA

R. L. SOUHAMI
Department of Oncology
University College and Middlesex
  School of Medicine
Mortimer Street
London W1N 8AA, UK

M. H. N. TATTERSALL
Department of Cancer Medicine
Blackburn Building
University of Sydney
NSW 2006
Australia

J. E. ULTMANN
Department of Medicine and the Cancer
  Research Center
University of Chicago
5841 South Maryland Avenue
Chicago
IL 60637, USA

J. WAXMAN
Department of Clinical Oncology
Royal Postgraduate Medical School
Hammersmith Hospital
Ducane Road
London W12 0HS, UK

Preface

Many of the most effective treatments for disease have been discovered empirically. Nowadays, however, we think that understanding the biology of a disease will lead us to design better treatments, and to improve the application of treatments we already have. To accomplish this, vast sums are expended on cancer research. Even so, to the casual observer of clinical oncology the proliferation of studies and trials of ever-different combinations of therapies looks like empiricism, at the best.

In the first part of this book, we have asked practising clinicians in different specialities to assess the contributions of biology and of empiricism to current approaches to treatment. In the second part, we have asked researchers in different areas of biology applied to cancer to assess the present and likely future impact of their type of biology on cancer treatment and control.

1
Surgery

M. BAUM

OBJECTIVES OF CANCER TREATMENT

The objectives of cancer treatment can be defined according to population requirements or according to the needs of the individual. As far as the population is concerned, Government authorities are entitled to expect that cancer treatment will lead to mortality reductions and cost containment. Furthermore, it is reasonable to expect that these mortality reductions will be concentrated amongst the most productive sections of society, so that the work force and the family are protected. As far as the individual is concerned, he or she is entitled to expect that the cancer treatment will either improve the length or quality of life. Regarding the objectives for the population at large, there is no good evidence that cancer treatment has achieved these goals. Viewed as a whole, there is no evidence of a reduction in mortality from the common solid tumours in Western cultures in spite of an enormous investment in high technology[1]. For example, we are familiar with the appalling increase in deaths from lung cancer, amongst men and women, almost entirely related to the adoption of smoking as a socially acceptable practice in the 1940s and the 1950s. At the same time, we have seen significant reductions in mortality from gastric cancer which are totally unrelated to therapy but are simply due to reduction in the incidence of the disease, perhaps as a result of improvements in social circumstances, or the removal of an as yet unidentified carcinogen from the environment. In contrast, mortality from breast cancer and colorectal cancer has remained relentlessly the same over the last four decades. In spite of these depressing statistics, most clinicians intuitively believe that their treatment helps the individual; otherwise we would all pack our bags and go home. When challenged, we will defend ourselves in terms like "all right, the treatment does not significantly prolong survival but it undoubtedly improves the quality of life." Yet, when we read publications concerning the treatment of cancer, it is exceptional to see any serious attempt to measure, or for that matter describe in any way, the impact of treatment on quality of survival. So why is it that surgeons, faced with patients with life-threatening cancers, persist in their treatments without attempting to appreciate the epistemology of their own subject?

1

ASSESSMENT OF MEDICAL TECHNOLOGY

Technology assessment in medicine is a growing subject, with its own academic departments in the United States of America, and yet very much a Cinderella subject in the United Kingdom. At a time of serious cost containment in the National Health Service, one would imagine that the Government agencies responsible would demand of the medical profession the highest quality of evidence in technology assessment before allowing the propagation of untested new medical technology. Yet, in the last couple of years, the Treasury was able to earmark £6 million for the purchase of a cyclotron for neutron therapy, an unproven and potentially hazardous treatment[2], and the Medical Research Council has seen fit to purchase a number of MR1 scanners at enormous expense with no evidence to date that the expected improvement in imaging will improve the length or quality of survival of patients suffering from cancer. At the same time, in the United States of America, the Institute of Medicine standing committee for the evaluation of medical technologies published a fascinating review on the subject in 1985[3]. In this review, they considered 28 topics ranging from internal mammary artery ligation for angina pectoris, through gastric freezing for the treatment of peptic ulceration, to hyperbaric oxygen for a variety of bizarre indications. They describe how many of these techniques were adopted uncritically, without proper scientific assessment, and have been abandoned following the reports on randomized clinical trials which, in most instances, demonstrated the futility of the procedures under study. An alternative way of looking at this subject is to consider the scientific philosophy that underlines the manner by which clinicians adopt or abandon medical treatments. These approaches can be lined up along a scientific spectrum from 'Aristotelian inductivism' at the primitive end to 20th century hypothetico-deductivism at the other extreme. Thus, we may start with anecdotal evidence or observational studies from personal case series at the left wing, passing through institutional case series judged against historical controls which may be accompanied by in-depth literature reviews by a single author parading his prejudices. Moving further to the right, there have been many attempts to establish comprehensive data bases upon which to judge therapeutic innovations or case-control studies which attempt to exclude random bias but unfortunately, by their very nature, cannot exclude systematic bias. Moving now to the extreme right wing of scientific validity, we have the randomized controlled trial which, more recently, has been strengthened by the new statistical device of overview analysis (meta analysis) of the results from all published or unpublished randomized trials addressing the same issue[4]. Somewhere hovering over all this activity are the fashionable consensus development conferences, which put together authoritative statements on treatment based on a mishmash of controlled and uncontrolled data whose final format is determined by the charisma of the various presenters rather than purely dispassionate assessment of evidence.

This author is a self-confessed Popperian who strongly believes that the logic of scientific discovery depends on our imaginative creation of hypotheses, coupled with the intellectual honesty involved in the design of experiments to refute those hypotheses[5]. A randomized controlled trial is the expression of science in medicine, and, if medicine is not a science, then we are nothing better than quacks[6]. Furthermore, whereas practitioners on the fringe use harmless placebos, our treatments are potentially toxic and often lethal. The other beauty of the scientific approach to medicine is that the very trials that are set up to refute our pet hypotheses generate biological fall-out, which can allow us to generate more attractive biological models, which then suggest alternative therapeutic strategies to be tested in the next generation of clinical trials. Thus, the modern scientific method constantly puts a limit on our ignorance whilst allowing us slowly step by step, to approximate to the truth.

Contrary to popular prejudice, the surgeons have been in the forefront of the adoption of the scientific method in the evaluation of their therapies. The successes of the scientific approach and the pitfalls of the non-scientific adoption of surgical technology have been beautifully described in the past by John Bunker and his colleagues; the reader's attention may be drawn to their work on the evaluation of shunts for portal hypertension, coronary artery by-pass grafts and total hip replacements[7].

MODELS OF DECISION-MAKING

Quality of evidence alone is not sufficient when doctors make a decision about treatment. From the physician's perspective, he also has to be assured of the availability of resources and he has to make beneficent calculations concerning his perception of the patient's needs and utilities. The patient approaches the doctor with a different set of priorities: hopes which may or may not be realistic; fears of certain therapies which again may or may not be realistic; a set of utility calculations, which may not be the same as the doctor's; and a wish to express his autonomy that may lead to the rejection of the doctor's best advice. However, it remains true that the most important factor in decision-making, both from the doctor's and patient's perspective, is the quality of evidence to support the view that the recommended treatment should at least improve the quality of the patient's life, even if it is unable to extend the duration of that life. Good quality of evidence depends on good science. Therefore, if surgery has any right to exist at all in the armamentarium of the clinical oncologist, it must be seen as applied biology. Good science and applied biology are not incompatible with compassion. On the contrary, the history of our subject is littered with the tragedies following the inductive application of new surgical technology in the absence of sound scientific justification[8]. To illustrate these points, it will be informative to concentrate on the history of the surgical management of breast cancer, showing how the shift from the naive inductivism of the late 19th century to the sophisticated scientific deductivism of the late 20th century contributed to improvements in the length and quality of survival for women suffering from this tragic disease.

The history of the treatment of breast cancer

Breast cancer has been recognized as a clinical entity from before the time of Hippocrates. An ancient Egyptian papyrus clearly described the disease and its demarcation from acute inflammatory mastitis. The ancient Egyptian physicians wisely advised a non-interventional approach. In fact, one of the greatest tragedies in the history of this subject has been the persistent error in confusing activity with progress. Mastectomy of a kind was introduced by the surgeons of the Greco-Roman period, but probably the first clearly-defined hypothesis concerning the nature of the disease and its appropriate treatment can be attributed to Galen. He preached that breast cancer was a systemic disorder due to the retention and excess of black bile (melancholia). As inductive support for this hypothesis, he pointed out that the disease was more common in postmenopausal women, who cease their monthly menstrual loss, and that the menstrual periods were a natural mechanism for clearing the body of excess black bile. The therapeutic implications, therefore, were self-evident, and women, for the next 1600 years, were treated by purgation and bleeding to rid the body of the putative excess of black bile[9]. Local therapy consisted predominantly of cautery and noxious topical applications for the management of offensive and bleeding ulcers. It goes without saying that nothing other than anecdotal support for these remedies existed in the literature. The first conceptual and, hence, therapeutic revolution dates from the time of Virchow in the 1860s. He demonstrated, by anatomical dissections of cadavers of women who had died of untreated advanced breast cancer, that the disease was commonly seen plugging the lymphatic channels and replacing the regional lymph nodes. He deduced, therefore, that the disease was not a systemic disorder but a localized abnormality, with the disease spreading along tissue planes via columns of cancer cells growing along the lymph channels. The cancer was then temporarily arrested in the lymph nodes which were thought to act as filter-traps. With exhaustion of the proximal lymph node barriers, the more distal lymph node barriers became infected and, ultimately, the disease gained access to the vital organs by a centrifugal extension of this process. The therapeutic consequences of this biological model were taken up by William Halsted in America, Wilhelm Meyer in German and Samson Handley in the United Kingdom, all within a few years of each other[10]. All three of these great and influential surgeons developed a radical type of mastectomy, which attempted to rid the body of the primary focus and all surgically accessible lymph node deposits, whilst avoiding cutting across infected lymphatic channels. There was never any *prima facie* evidence that the introduction of this radical approach improved on the more conservative type of surgery or, for that matter, systemic therapy prevalent until the 1880s[11]. On the contrary, publications exist demonstrating that, throughout the first thirty years of this century, the best result achieved by the radical approach was approximately a 10% ten-year survival which is almost identical to that achieved by Gross in Philadelphia in the 1880s[11]. In fairness to Halsted, it must be recognized that he successfully reduced the operative mortality and improved the local control of the disease. It also has to be remembered that the majority of the cases they were treating in that era would

4

be considered locally advanced today, and excluded from trials of primary local therapy. Surgeons became very frustrated with the failure of the Halsted radical mastectomy to cure breast cancer, but instead of questioning the underlying hypothetical model, improvements were sought by extending the concept to its logical conclusion, leading to the surgical barbarity of extended radical mastectomies and even forequarter amputations. Inevitably, there was a reaction against such barbarous treatment, and we should never forget the contributions of the great and distinguished British surgeon, Sir Geoffrey Keynes; in the face of all established surgical dogma, Keynes introduced a conservative mode of treatment for this disease in the early 1930s, eventually publishing an historical paper in the British Medical Journal demonstrating that the results of local excision plus radium needle insertion were equal to any published data advocating the use of the radical approach[12]. Perhaps as a result of the intervening war years, and Sir Geoffrey Keynes' retirement, this conservative approach never achieved popularity. On the contrary, Sir Stanford Cade, summing up a debate on the merits of the treatment of early breast cancer at the Royal Society of Medicine in 1947, sanctioned the radical mastectomy as the appropriate treatment for Stage I of the disease[13]. Thus we have the prospect of two great surgical names advocating diametrically opposite therapies. If the big men could not agree, what were the little men to do? As is the case throughout the history of our subject, the little men followed the dictates of the authority with the highest profile and the greatest charisma. This can hardly be considered science of any description, but more akin to the behaviour of the faithful within a religious cult. The appropriate scientific response to such a clash of convictions is neatly summed up in the words of Sir Karl Popper[5]:

"Instead of discussing the probability of the hypothesis, we should try to assess what trials it has withstood and how far it has been able to prove its fitness to survive."

Randomized controlled trials of loco-regional therapy

The first truly randomized trials for the treatment of early breast cancer can be credited to the Manchester Christie group, headed by Paterson and Russell[14]. Since then a host of complementary studies have been completed, with mature follow-up data available for between 10 and 30 years. These studies have compared, in a strictly scientific manner, treatments varying from extended radical mastectomy on the one hand to local excision, with or without radiotherapy, at the most conservative extreme. In retrospect, the trials of this period were really addressing themselves to two different questions. Firstly, would the use of radical radiotherapy provide the same degree of local control and the same cure rate as radical surgery? In other words, was radiotherapy as effective as surgery in ablating cancer from the regional nodes? The second set of trials was asking a more interesting biological question concerning the relevance of the regional lymph nodes in the putative immuno-surveillance of cancer[15]. Observed *in toto*, we can now say with the greatest of statistical confidence that, although the degree of local control varies directly with the magnitude of the treatment field, no important differences in survival have emerged within 10 years of treatment, irrespective of the magnitude of surgery employed. Biological extrapolations from these data might suggest one of two conclusions:

1. Untreated lymph node metastases do not act as a source of tertiary spread.
2. The metastasizing capacity of involved nodes is balanced by the immuno-surveillance mediated in some way by the intact uninvolved lymph nodes.

A very recent and surprising observation emerging from the most mature trials of early breast cancer concerns those studies where the only variable was whether the patient has post-operative radiotherapy or not. The long-term follow-up from these trials, individually or from a meta analysis, has demonstrated a small but significant excess mortality in those patients receiving routine post-operative radiotherapy who have survived beyond 10 years[16]. This excess mortality appears to be unrelated to deaths from breast cancer and is almost entirely ascribed to an excess of deaths from cardiovascular events, plus an excess of second primary cancers in sites remote from the original disease[17]. Biological speculation about these unanticipated events concerns the effect of radiotherapy on the vasculature of the myocardium and the putative immunosuppressive effect of inadvertently irradiating the thoracic duct and the recirculating pool of lymphocytes.

Whatever the explanation, these accumulated data support the concept of biological predeterminism, and further analysis of subgroups suggests that those patients with lymph nodes invaded by cancer at the time of diagnosis are those most often destined to die[18]. As a result of this experience, all but a few die-hards amongst surgeons and radiotherapists experienced a paradigm shift. The lymph node status of the patient is now looked upon as an expression, rather than a determinant, of prognosis. It is an amusing pastime to study the attitudes of the more conservative amongst the medical profession and their attempts to explain away the failures of the radical approach. It has been argued that if the patients were diagnosed early as a result of screening programmes, then the radical mastectomy would cure them all. Secondly, the failure of radical surgery and radical radiotherapy within randomized controlled trials represents the failure of the surgeons and radiotherapists to deliver the treatment correctly. The therapeutic inductivists still point to the uncontrolled data sets from the great radical surgeons and the centres of radiotherapeutic excellence. Finally, those women who have suffered radical mastectomy and are alive and well to tell their tale thirty years later are once again paraded as a living tribute to the perfection of the treatments they received. It is not unfair to say that this type of conceptual rationalization is no different from the logic adduced by proponents of fringe medicine[6].

The quality of life after the treatment of early breast cancer

It is a reasonable question for members of the lay public to ask whether there is life after mastectomy. The pioneering work of Peter Maguire has clearly demonstrated that about one-third of patients treated for breast cancer by some form of mastectomy will suffer serious and debilitating psycho-sexual morbidity[19]. Of course, the other side of the coin must not be overlooked. Seventy per cent of women provided with a modest amount of rehabilitation and prosthetic advice can enjoy a fulfilling and normal life by drawing on their natural reserves to cope with one of life's major crises. It is a reasonable assumption that the loss of the breast contributes the major component of the psychosexual morbidity associated with the treatment, but like all medical assumptions this needs challenging. In 1981, the Cancer Research Campaign launched a trial to compare mastectomy with breast conservation for women diagnosed as suffering from early breast cancer. The study was conducted with informed consent, and is unique in having built-in a formal assessment of the psychosexual morbidity in both arms of the trial. The results of this study are, to say the least, counter-intuitive, suggesting that the major contribution to the psychosexual morbidity is not so much the treatment as the diagnosis of the disease itself[20]. This should not suggest for a moment a return to the bad old days of radical mastectomy, but should redirect our attention to the development of counselling services, to enable women to come to terms with their diagnosis and the inevitable threat to their life that it poses.

Trials of adjuvant systemic therapy

If the majority of patients with early breast cancer and positive axillary nodes die, however perfect the loco-regional therapy, then surely they carry occult micrometastases present at the time of diagnosis. As that must be the case, then cure can only result from the addition of an effective systemic therapy. Experience with advanced breast cancer demonstrates an objective response rate of the order of 60% with prolonged cyclical combination therapy, which is twice that expected with an endocrine approach. *Ipso facto*, node-positive patients should be cured by adjuvant systemic chemotherapy. So compelling were these arguments and so beautiful the new hypothesis, that many medical oncologists felt it unethical to do randomized trials and, like all inductivists, soon found sufficient corroborative evidence to satisfy themselves. Such individuals are as guilty as those who uncritically accepted the Halstedian dogma seventy years ago, particularly since some of these chemotherapeutic excesses can be considered the medical equivalent of a forequarter amputation! A recent review of the results of randomized controlled trials of adjuvant chemotherapy has arrived at the following general conclusions[21]:

1. Whatever combination regimen is used, there is likely to be a significant delay in the time to first relapse.

2. Although many individual trials have yet to show an improvement in crude survival, a statistical overview of all the available data suggests that a 30% reduction in the risk of dying over the first five years may be achieved following the treatment of premenopausal women with node-positive disease. The benefits for postmenopausal women are marginal.

What, therefore, are the biological implications of these results? Firstly, there is little doubt that the natural history of early breast cancer has been perturbed, lending support to the deterministic model. Whether this perturbation will translate itself into a useful therapeutic advantage for groups other than premenopausal node-positive patients remains to be seen. Secondly, the intriguing difference between the behaviour of pre- and postmenopausal women deserves some explanation. The chemotherapy lobby is not short of inductivists and much support has been generated for the concept that the effect of adjuvant systemic chemotherapy is dose related[22]. Postmenopausal women seem incapable of tolerating the maximum (optimum?) doses prescribed. This suggestion requires further exploration, with trials of high-dose *versus* low-dose chemotherapy. To accept the suggestion without prospective studies is to be guilty of a tautology, yet, at the same time, if older women were incapable of tolerating high-dose chemotherapy, then this surely is an inherent defect of the treatment unless one is prepared to push the drugs beyond the tolerance of the patient, surely a dangerous and inhumane policy. An alternative explanation for this differential effect might be that the cytotoxic drugs are mediating their effect by what might be termed chemical castration. This hypothesis has already won some support, following studies of ovarian and pituitary function in women receiving adjuvant chemotherapy[23]. It follows, therefore, that to test the hypothesis generated by the trials of adjuvant chemotherapy, one should conduct trials of adjuvant endocrine therapy investigating prophylactic castration and the use of adjuvant tamoxifen.

Trials of prophylactic castration following local treatment for cancer are not new but have suffered in the past from inadequate sample size leaving uncertainty as to its potential benefit. This subject has recently been reviewed, suggesting that such an approach might indeed produce results of the same order achieved by polychemotherapy for premenopausal women, but at the great expense of inducing a premature menopause in young women already facing up to the threat of loss of a breast[24]. For the purpose of this paper, though, it is better to concentrate on the trial of tamoxifen therapy, which can be judged to have had the most profound effect on our biological thinking about the disease. The Nolvadex Adjuvant Trial Organisation (NATO) launched a study in 1977 to investigate whether the anti-oestrogen tamoxifen (Nolvadex) would have any benefit for women undergoing mastectomy for early breast cancer[25]. Approximately 1300 patients were recruited over a period of two and a half years. These consisted of premenopausal node-positive and negative cases. Following local therapy, women were randomized to the group receiving tamoxifen, 10 mg twice daily for two years, or to an untreated control group. A second-order hypothesis suggested that the women most likely to benefit were those whose primary tumour was rich in oestradiol receptor (E2R). Therefore, as a parallel study, attempts were made to collect samples of the tumours from all patients entered into the trial. However, for logistic reasons, this was only possible in about 50% of the cases. The published data have demonstrated a significantly prolonged disease-free interval in the treated group as a whole, which has recently been translated into a 30% reduction in the risk of dying within the first five years following treatment[26]. (Support for the fact that this result was not a statistical fluke has emerged from the statistical overview conducted by Mr Richard Peto and his colleagues[27].) Paradoxically, a Cox's multivariant regression analysis within the NATO trial has failed to demonstrate any interaction between the treatment and subgroups divided according to menopausal, nodal or E2R status[28]. (This observation has again been supported by the same meta analysis of all trials of similar design[29].)

Biological insights gained from trials of adjuvant tamoxifen

If the survival advantage of patients treated for two years with tamoxifen persists long term, this would suggest that the anti-oestrogen has a tumoricidal capacity against the putative micrometastases present at the time of diagnosis. This in itself would be interesting, suggesting that subclinical tumour deposits are biologically different from overt metastatic disease. Of potentially greater interest is the suggestion that the oestrogen-receptor status of the primary tumour does not predict the likelihood of response to adjuvant tamoxifen. As such a conclusion fails to reinforce popular prejudice, there would naturally be the temptation to ignore or reject these data. It has already been suggested that the measurement of E2R in a multicentre trial with inter- and intra-laboratory variation will produce many false negative results. This, indeed, may be the case, but it remains unquestionable that the assay of E2R in this study has told us something of biological relevance about the primary cancers, as there is a powerful correlation between the E2R status and prognosis, irrespective of primary or adjuvant therapy[30]. Rather than ignore these data out-of-hand, I believe it will be more fruitful to try to reconcile the findings within a modified hypothesis that can explain previous observations about the behaviour of breast cancer whilst, at the same time, incorporating the new and apparently inconsistent observation. There is little doubt that the major pathway mediating the antitumour effect of tamoxifen in advanced breast cancer is via the oestradiol receptor; but the observations from the NATO trial raise the question as to whether tamoxifen exerts some of its effect on microscopic foci of the disease by another pathway, perhaps via the ubiquitous tamoxifen-binding protein, which is unrelated to E2R[31]. Furthermore, tamoxifen in sufficiently high concentrations can inhibit the growth of both oestrogen-receptor-positive and oestrogen-receptor-negative human breast cancer cell lines[32].

Exciting new discoveries concerning the nature of oncogenes and the relationship between oncogenic sequences in the cellular genome, and the production of specific growth factors or the expression of growth factor receptors, could easily be incorporated with these observations into a new biological model concerning the nature of breast cancer[33]. If tamoxifen can inhibit the cellular cascade of biochemical reactions which are a consequence of the activation of the epidermal growth factor receptor, then this might suggest that the oestradiol receptor status of breast cancer is merely an epiphenomenon of cellular differentiation, indirectly reflecting the rate of inappropriate growth factor activation. Thus, the E2R serves as a prognostic indicator, reflecting the growth rate of the cancer rather than simply an expression of endocrine sensitivity. According to this model, the oestrogen receptor could act as an amplifying mechanism concentrating the tamoxifen within the cancer cell, where it can act as an antigrowth factor. This would then explain the apparent selectivity of tamoxifen for advanced breast cancer amongst the oestrogen-receptor-positive cells, whilst at the same time explaining why it retains modest activity against microscopic deposits of oestrogen-receptor-negative cancer cells. Further support for the idea that the E2R is an indirect expression of the rate of growth factor production comes from the following observations. E2R-positive cancers are predominantly well differentiated on histological grading[34]. The E2R status of breast cancers is inversely correlated with the rate of replication of cells *in vitro*[35]. Growth factors are known to attract monocytes potently[36] and a monocytosis is a recognized response to an actively growing tumour, so that a heavy stromal round cell infiltrate is associated with a negative E2R status[37]. In addition, two recent pieces of work have shown an inverse correlation between the oestrogen receptor content of a breast cancer and the expression of epidermal growth factor (EGF) receptors using specific monoclonal antibodies raised against EGF receptors[38,39].

To summarize, therefore, at one extreme we might have a breast cancer with a very high expression of EGF receptors, where the rate of replication and protein synthesis does not allow sufficient time or supply of substrates for the assembly of E2R, whilst, at the other extreme of EGF receptor expression, E2R assembly proceeds to completion. This then raises the intriguing possibility that tamoxifen may slow the tumour via an anti growth factor pathway until E2R is reassembled, and the cancer cell becomes redifferentiated, as a result of which the tamoxifen is further concentrated so as to exhibit its secondary effect along the classical pathway.

Even now the model is incomplete. Micrometastases of cancer cells do not exist *in vacuo* but are inevitably in close opposition to the stromal cells of the host and the ubiquitous lymphocytes. Stromal cells, lymphocytes and cancer cells constantly exchange messages and many of these biological regulators have been identified. Of particular interest in contemporary biology are the growth stimulatory and inhibitory polypeptides. These autocrine and paracrine substances can be produced by cancer cells as well as stromal cells. As far as epithelial cells are concerned, the stimulatory growth factors are the epidermal growth factors, EGF, and the closely related transforming growth factor alpha (TGFα). As regards inhibitory growth factors, the relevant one appears to be transforming growth factor beta (TGFβ). Epithelial cells are exquisitely sensitive to minute quantities of TGFβ. The work from Marc Lippman's laboratory has already focused attention on the ability of breast cancer cells to produce TGFβ under the stimulus of tamoxifen, which can have an autocrine effect on the oestrogen-receptor-positive cell and a paracrine effect on adjacent oestrogen-receptor-negative cells[40]. However, of potentially greater importance is some recent work conducted in our laboratory in collaboration with Michael Sporn's unit at the National Cancer Institute in Washington. These *in vitro* studies have demonstrated unequivocally that cultures of human fetal fibroblasts can be induced to synthesize increased levels of TGFβ by the triphenylethylene group of drugs, including tamoxifen[41]. This effect is not seen in the presence of any other steroid molecule. Whether this is of relevance *in vivo* remains to be seen, but the intriguing possibility emerges that the most successful treatment for breast cancer discovered this century exerts its effect not by directly killing the cancer cell but by indirectly instructing the host cells to produce tumoricidal growth-inhibitory substances.

CONCLUSIONS

Looking back over the last 100 years of progress in the management of breast cancer, it is reasonable to conclude that the subject stagnated until about 20 years ago, when surgery became a biological science with the introduction of the randomized controlled trial. Since then, there has been a hypothetico-deductive cascade which has led to the abandonment of the classic radical mastectomy and the widespread adoption of more conservative treatments which may in themselves not prolong survival but are likely, with further refinement, to contribute to improvement in the quality of life. At the same time, the paradigm shift in our biological models of the disease has contributed to the development of adjuvant systemic therapy which has led to a significant improvement in duration of survival. These trials of adjuvant therapy themselves have generated biological insight which may one day improve our understanding of the disease and suggest a new class of biological response modifiers aimed at redressing the balance between stimulatory and inhibitory growth factors in the microenvironment of the micrometastases. If this short history does not define surgical oncology as the scientific application of biology, then nothing else will convince the reader. Finally, if challenged at a consensus development conference as to what is the treatment of choice for patients with breast cancer, then this author would have to agree with Richard Gelber and Aaron Goldhirsch that the treatment of choice would be randomization within a clinical trial[42]. Only this strategy can look after the interest of the individual whilst demonstrating concern for the population at large and the generations of cancer sufferers yet to come.

References

1. Breslow, L. and Cumberland, W. G. (1988). Progress and objectives in cancer control. *J. Am. Med. Assoc.*, **259/11**, 1690–1694
2. Timmins, N. (1988). Controversy grows over cancer machine scheme. Article in *The Independent Newspaper*, 6 October, page 2
3. Committee for Evaluating Medical Technologies (1985). *Assessing Medical Technologies.* (Washington DC: National Academy Press)
4. Early Breast Cancer Trialists Collaboratives Group (1988). The effects of adjuvant tamoxifen and of cytotoxic therapy on mortality in early breast cancer: an overview of 61 randomized trials among 28,896 women. *N. Engl. J. Med.*, **319**, 1681–1692
5. Popper, K. R. (1959). *The Logic of Scientific Discovery.* (London: Hutchinson)
6. Baum, M. (1983). Quack cancer cures or scientific remedies? *Clin. Oncol.*, **9**, 275–280
7. Bunker, J. P., Hinkley, D. and McDermott, W. V. (1978). Surgical innovation and its evaluation. *Science*, **200**, 937–941

8. Barnes, B. (1977). Discarded operations: surgical innovation by trial and error. In Bunker, J. P., Barnes, B. A., Mosteller, F. (eds.) *Costs, Risks and Benefits of Surgery*, pp. 109–123. (New York: Oxford University Press)

9. De Moulin, D. (1983). *A Short History of Cancer*. (Lancaster: Martinus Nyhoff Publishers)

10. Halsted, W. S. (1898). The radical operation for the cure of carcinoma of the breast. *Johns Hopkins Hosp. Rep.*, **28**, 557

11. Gross, S. W. (1880). *A Practical Treatise of Tumours of the Mammary Gland*. (New York: Appleton)

12. Keynes, G. (1937). Conservative treatment of cancer of the breast. *Br. Med. J.*, **2**, 643–647

13. Cade, Sir S. (1948). Discussion: the treatment of cancer of the breast. *Proc. R. Soc. Med.*, **41**, 129

14. Paterson, R. P. and Russell, M. H. (1959). Clinical trials in disease. *J. Fac. Radiol.*, **10**, 130

15. Berstock, D. A., Houghton, J., Haybittle, J. and Baum, M. (1985). The role of radiotherapy following total mastectomy for patients with early breast cancer. *World J. Surg.*, **9**, 667–670

16. Cuzick, J., Stewart, H., Peto, R., Baum, M., Lythgoe, J. P., Ribeiro, G., Scheurlen, H. and Wallgren, A. (1987). Overview of randomized trials of postoperative adjuvant radiotherapy in breast cancer. *Cancer Treat. Rep.*, **71**, 15–29

17. Haybittle, J. L., Brinkley, D., Houghton, J., A'Hern, R. P. and Baum, M. (1989). Post-operative radiotherapy and late mortality: evidence from the CRC (King's/Cambridge) trial for early breast cancer. *Br. Med. J.*, **298**, 1611–1614

18. Fisher, B. (1970). In *Current Dilemmas in the Primary Therapy of Invasive Breast Cancer. A Critical Appraisal. Current Problems in Surgery*. (Chicago: Year Book Publishers)

19. Maguire, P. (1982). Psychiatric morbidity associated with mastectomy. In Baum, M., Kay, R. and Scheurlen, H. (eds.) *Birkhauser Clinical Trial in Early Breast Cancer* (2nd Heidelberg symposium), pp. 373–380

20. Fallowfield, L., Baum, M. and Maguire, G. P. (1988). The effects of breast conservation on the psychological morbidity associated with the diagnosis and treatment of early breast cancer. *Br. Med. J.*, **293**, 1331–1334

21. Goldhirsch, A., Gelber, R. D. and Davis, B. W. (1986). Adjuvant chemotherapy trials in breast cancer: an appraisal and lessons for patient care outside the trials. In *Breast Disease*, Chap. 10, pp. 123–138. (Edinburgh: Churchill Livingstone)

22. Bonadonna, G. and Valagusa, P. (1981). Dose–response effect on adjuvant chemotherapy in breast cancer. *N. Engl. J. Med.*, **30**, 10–15

23. Rose, D. P. and Davis, T. E. (1977). Ovarian function in patients receiving adjuvant chemotherapy for breast cancer. *Lancet*, **1**, 1174

24. Cole, M. P. (1970). Prophylactic compared with therapeutic X-ray artifical menopause. *2nd Tenovus Workshop on Breast Cancer*, pp. 2–11. (Cardiff: Alpha-Omega)

25. Nolvadex Adjuvant Trial Organisation (NATO) (1983). Controlled trial of tamoxifen as single adjuvant agent in management of early breast cancer. (1983). Interim analysis at 4 years by NATO. *Lancet*, **1**, 257–261

26. Nolvadex Adjuvant Trial Organisation (NATO) (1985). Controlled trial of tamoxifen as single adjuvant agent in management of early breast cancer. (1985). Analysis at 6 years by NATO. *Lancet*, **1**, 836–840

27. Early Breast Cancer Trialists Collaborative Group (1988). The effects of adjuvant tamoxifen and of cytotoxic therapy on mortality in early breast cancer: an overview of 61 randomized trials among 28,896 women. *N. Engl. J. Med.*, **319**, 1681–1692

28. Nolvadex Adjuvant Trial Organisation (NATO) (1985). Six year results of a controlled trial of tamoxifen as single adjuvant agent in management of early breast cancer. *World J. Surg.*, **9**, 756–764

29. Overview of adjuvant trials – JNCI Supplement: 1989 in press.

30. Nolvadex Adjuvant Trial Organisation (1988). Analysis at eight years of a controlled trial of tamoxifen as a single adjuvant agent in the management of early breast cancer. *Br. J. Cancer*, **57**, 608–611

31. Kon, O. L. (1983). An antiestrogen-binding protein in human tissues. *J. Biol. Chem.*, **258**, 3173

32. Lippman, M. E. (1975). Oestrogen responsive human breast cancer in long term tissue culture. *Nature (London)*, **256**, 592–593

33. Dunn, A. R. (1986). Viral and Cellular oncogenes: a molecular basis for breast and other

cancers. In Forbes, J. F. (ed.) *Breast Disease*, Chap. 5, pp. 59–68. (Edinburgh: Churchill Livingstone)

34. Fisher, B., Redmond, C. and Fisher, E. R. (1980). The contribution of recent NSABP trials of primary breast cancer therapy to an understanding of tumour biology. *Cancer,* **46**, 1009

35. Meyer, J. S., Rao, B. R., Stevens, S. C. and White, W. L. (1977). Low incidence of oestrogen receptor in breast carcinoma with rapid rates of cellular replication. *Cancer,* **40**, 2290

36. Waterfield, M. D., Scrace, G. T., Whittle, N. *et al.* (1983). Platelet derived growth factor is structurally related to the putative transforming protein p28 of simian sarcoma virus. *Nature (London),* **304**, 34

37. Steele, R. J. C. (1983). Clinical, histological and immunological studies in human breast cancer. *MD Thesis*, University of Edinburgh

38. Sainsbury, J. R. C., Farndon, J. R., Sherbet, G. V. and Harris, A. L. (1985). Epidermal-growth factor receptors and oestrogen receptors in human breast cancer. *Lancet,* **1**, 364–366

39. Trivedi, D. (1986). Antigenic profile of human breast tumours. *PhD Thesis*, University of London

40. Knabbe, C., Lippman, M. E. and Wakefield, L. (1987). Evidence that factor beta is a hormonally regulated negative growth factor in human breast cancer cells. *Cell,* **48**, 417–428

41. Coletta, A. A., Wakefield, L. M., Howell, F. V., Ebbs, S. R., Sporn, M. and Baum, M. (1989). Oestrogen receptor independent synthesis of transforming growth factor beta 1 induced by triphenylethylenes. *J. Molec. Endocrinol.* (in press)

42. Gelber, R. D. and Goldhirsch, A. (1988). Can a clinical trial be the treatment of choice for patients with cancer? *J. Natl. Cancer Inst.,* **80**, 886–887

2
Radiotherapy and its relationship to radiobiology

A. HORWICH

INTRODUCTION

Radiotherapy has been used to treat cancer since the beginning of this century. Clinical experience has indicated its capacity to damage normal as well as malignant tissue and thus developments have been aimed at improving the selectivity of its biological effects. The detailed observations of Regaud on the irradiated ram's testis were among the first to illustrate selectivity since greater radiation toxicity was seen in spermatogonia than in spermatozoa[1]. This was attributed to the increased radiation sensitivity of cycling cells. Regaud became director of the Radium Institute in Paris and subsequently proposed that radiation of cancers be protracted in order to exploit their greater degree of proliferation[2].

In the 1920s Coutard transformed this concept into fractionated radiotherapy and reported successful treatments of head and neck cancer[3]. Studies of the parameters of fractionated ratiotherapy were developed further in the 1940s and 1950s, especially by Paterson[4,5] and McWhirter[6] in Manchester, and by Baclesse[7] in Paris. It was apparent that protraction of radiation treatment reduced the biological effects of irradiation and, following a study of dose/time characteristics in the treatment of skin tumours, Strandqvist[8] illustrated the isoeffective dose/time relationship to be linear on a log/log plot (Figure 2.1). His graph was used to adjust fractionated treatment schedules for different overall treatment times.

Radiotherapy is conventionally administered in 15–35 fractions, delivering one fraction per day and 3–5 fractions per week. The overall radical treatment course lasts between 3–7 weeks. The biological basis of fractionated radiotherapy has been ascribed to four principles known as the 'Rs' of radiobiology.

1. Repair of sublethal damage[9].
2. Repopulation by tumour stem cells[10].
3. Reoxygenation[11].
4. Reassortment of the cell cycle distribution[12].

15

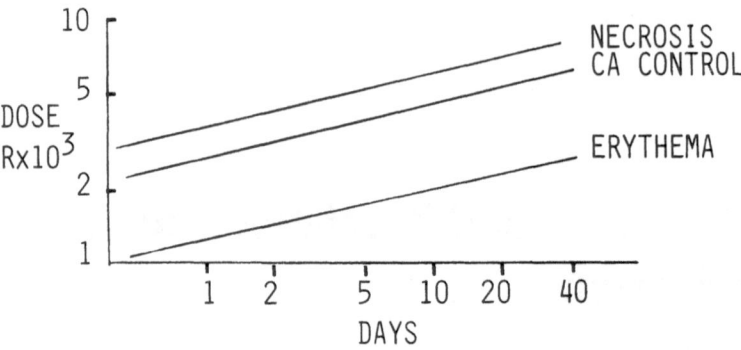

Figure 2.1 A 'Strandqvist' plot of log radiation dose against log overall treatment time for 3 different biological isoeffects in the radiotherapy of skin tumours

Differences between the magnitude and kinetics of these processes comparing tumour and normal tissue contribute to the therapeutic ratio of radiotherapy. Repair of radiation damage between fractions and repopulation between fractions reduce the cytotoxicity of radiotherapy, whereas reoxygenation and cell cycle reassortment increase cytotoxicity[13].

In the first half of the century, radiotherapy was effectively limited by machine technology to the treatment of superficial tumours or tumours accessible to interstitial implantation of radioactive sources. The development of higher energy X-ray machines avoided the severe skin reactions which had previously been the major dose-limiting toxicity. In the 1950s, telecobalt (cobalt-60) units and subsequently linear accelerators were developed which allowed the homogeneous irradiation of deep-seated tumours using a variety of multi-beam techniques[14].

Recent developments in tumour imaging and localization by computer tomographic (CT) scanning have enabled further improvements in the precision of radiotherapy, and integration of planning computers allows optimization of technique in the individual by planning directly on the digitalized CT image (Figure 2.2). The concepts underlying current radiotherapy assume a homogeneous irradiation of a block of tissue which inevitably contains some normal tissues. The argument for homogeneity of radiation distribution is based simply on the concept that overdosed tissue will contribute to severe toxicity and underdosed tissue to poor tumour control and, in practice, doses within the 'target' area should be within 5% of the modal dose.

This chapter will examine ideas underlying current radiotherapeutic practice and research, especially those relating to fractionation of radiotherapy, and the possibility will be explored of optimizing fractionation based on individual biological characterization of the tumour to be treated.

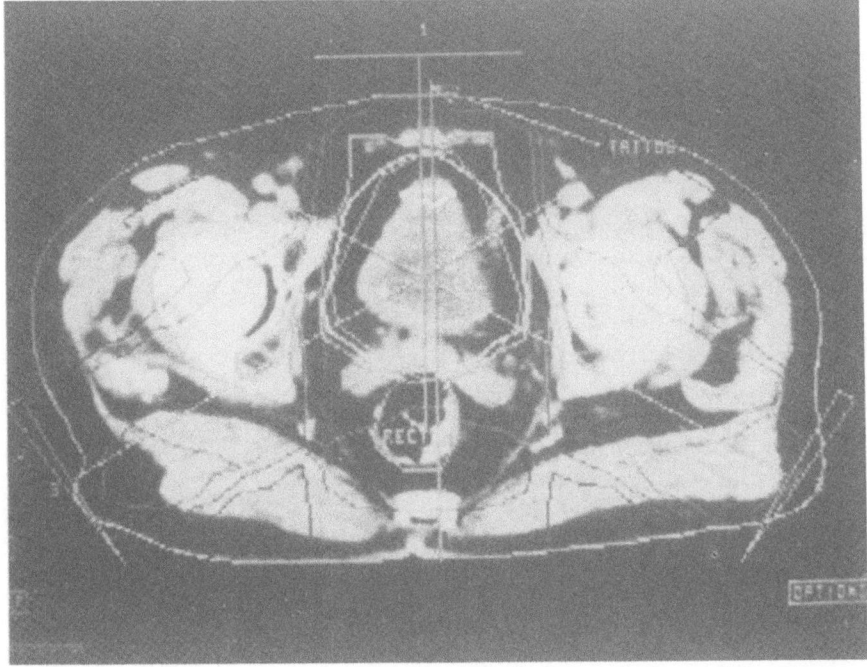

Figure 2.2 Radiation plan for three field treatment of bladder cancer. The radiation isodose distribution is calculated using body outline and tissue photon density information from computer tomographic scanning and displayed directly on the axial image

CELLULAR RADIOSENSITIVITY

The cell survival curve

Typical cell survival curves for human tumour cell lines are illustrated in Figure 2.3a. They illustrate the relationship between the dose of radiotherapy administered in a single fraction and the proportion of surviving clonogenic tumour cells. Since conventional doses of radiotherapy are of the order of 2 Gy per fraction, it can be seen that the shape of the shouldered region of survival curve is important in determining radiation cytotoxicity. A number of models have been proposed to explain this shape of curve. The multi-target model suggested that each cell contained a number of targets which all needed to be inactivated to cause cytotoxicity. The cell survival curve would be described by the formula:

$$S = 1 - (1 - \exp(-D/D_0))^n$$

where D is the dose, n is the extrapolation on the Y axis and D_0 is the dose required on the exponential part of the curve to reduce survival to e^{-1}. This model implied no cytotoxicity at low radiation doses and thus a zero initial slope on the cell survival curve. Also the high-dose region of the curve should

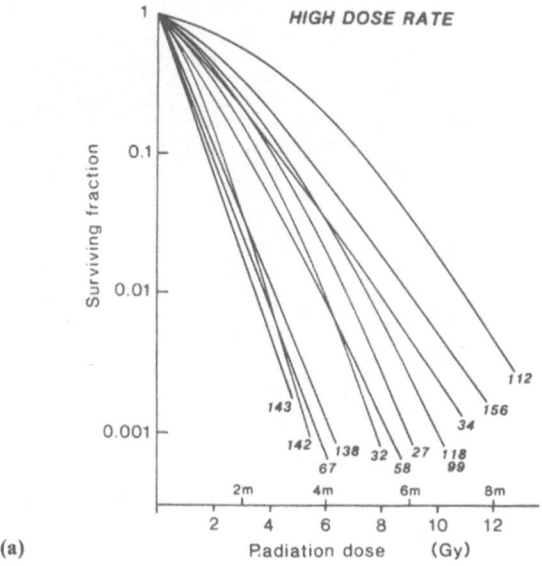

(a)

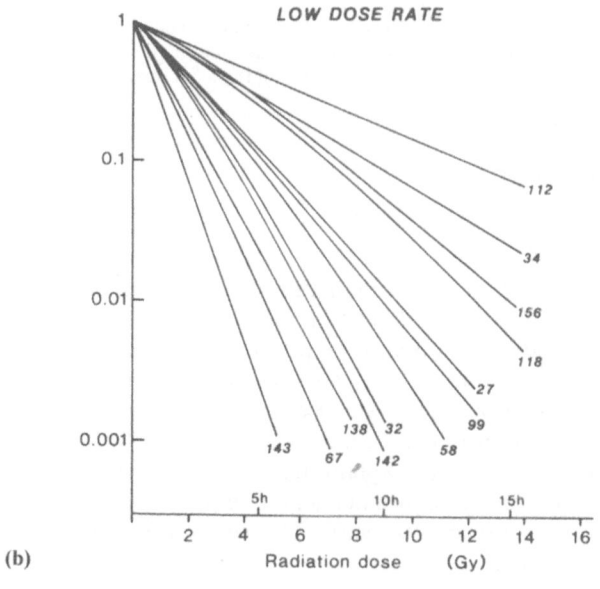

(b)

Figure 2.3 Cell survival curves for 12 human tumour cell lines irradiated at high dose rate (150 cGy/min) or at low dose rate (approximately 1.6 cGy/min). The duration of exposure is marked on the abscissa. Lines 34 and 118 = melanoma, 32 and 58 = pancreas, 99 = breast, 156 = cervix, 67 and 112 = bladder, 27 = teratoma, 138, 142 and 143 = neuroblastoma. (Data from Steel *et al.*, 1987)[21]

be exponential. In practice, very few cell survival curves have this shape and the model has been modified by addition of a single-hit cytotoxicity component.

Recently the linear quadratic model has been extensively employed to describe cell survival relationships. The cell survival formula is as follows:

$$S = \exp(-\alpha D - \beta D^2)$$

This was originally based on a molecular model of cytotoxicity which proposed that the DNA double-strand break was a critical cellular lesion which could arise either by a single particle track affecting both DNA strands or by random single-strand damage occasionally producing lesions close enough to lead to the critical double-strand break[15]. Microdosimetric assessments raise considerable doubts about the probability of these single-strand interactions at conventional doses[16]. However, the linear quadratic model has proved extremely useful in defining the implications of fraction size for dose response and in particular the α/β ratio is used to describe the shape of the shoulder region. The ratio indicates for a particular survival curve the dose at which the α component and β component of cell killing are equal.

A number of other cell survival models are of great theoretical interest in stimulating research on the nature of the initial shoulder region and these include repair saturation models[17], the lethal/potentially lethal dynamic model of Curtis[18] and the 'incomplete repair' model[19] which adds a time constant for repair of damage to the linear quadratic acute cell survival.

The results of single fraction irradiation are amplified if the same pattern of cell survival is repeated up to 35 times during a course of radical radiotherapy. In their early studies of repeated radiation fractions, Elkind and Sutton[9] found that survival fitted the assumption that the shoulder was reproduced with each fraction. This has similarly been demonstrated *in vivo* in a study of radiation effects on mouse skin[20].

Assessment of cellular recovery from radiation damage

A simple method of studying recovery from radiation damage is to reduce the dose rate of irradiation from the conventional range of 100–300 cGy per minute down to the range of 1–10 cGy per minute. This allows the process of radiation recovery to occur during radiation yet, with moderate irradiation doses, the overall treatment time is not long enough to allow other radiobiological factors, such as reassortment or repopulation, to influence survival. The half-time of radiation recovery is of the order of 1 hour, whereas, for most human cells, reassortment would take at least 6–12 h and repopulation more than 1 day. Figure 2.3b illustrates the effect on human tumour cell survival curves of reducing radiation dose rate to approximately 2 cGy per minute[21]. The survival curves represent a linear extrapolation of the initial slope of the high dose rate curves. The curves illustrate first that there is a major difference in radiosensitivity between different human tumour cell lines, and, secondly, that this difference is maintained and even amplified when full recovery from radiation damage is allowed. The low-dose-rate plots represent the α component of cell killing on the linear quadratic model[21].

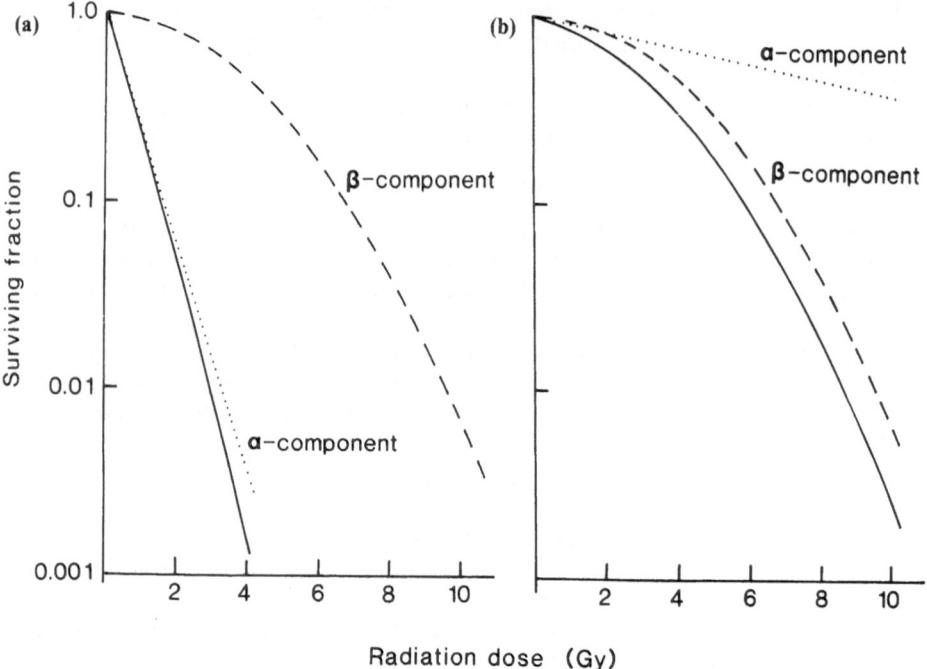

Figure 2.4 Cell survival curves for a radiosensitive (a) and radioresistant (b) cell population. The curves can be modelled using a linear quadratic formula (see text) where $S = \exp(-\alpha D - \beta D^2)$ and the figure illustrates that profound differences in the apparent shape of the low-dose region of the survival curve can be accounted for entirely by differences in the α component since the β component is identical in the two figures

Other manifestations of cellular recovery include:

1. *Sublethal damage repair:* This is usually demonstrated by the increase in survival obtained when a particular dose of radiotherapy is divided into 2 fractions separated by at least 6 hours thus allowing reconstruction of the shoulder on the survival curve.

2. *Potentially lethal damage repair:* This represents the variation in recovery which can be achieved by manipulating the postirradiation cellular environment *in vitro*. This is usually assessed by leaving cells in stationary phase tissue culture following radiotherapy. The effect is not usually seen in rapidly multiplying cells and it is likely that this component of damage is fixed following mitosis.

In the linear quadratic model, the β component represents the capacity of the cell to recover from radiation damage; however, it is extremely difficult to measure this accurately from a single acute cell survival curve since the pattern at low radiation doses is so heavily dominated by the α component. This is illustrated in Figure 2.4a and 2.4b where the solid lines represent survival curves which have identical β components and, thus, where their

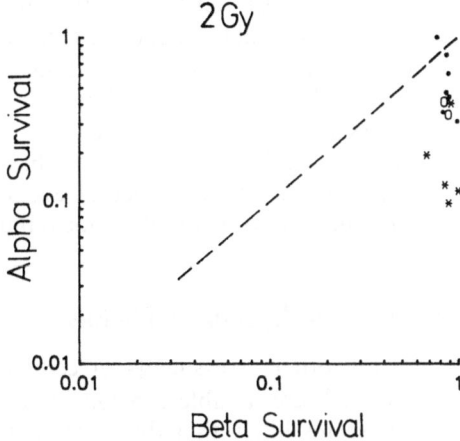

Figure 2.5 The relative contribution of the α and β components of cytotoxicity in radiation-resistant gliomas (•) and radiation-sensitive medulloblastomas (O) and neuroblastomas (*) illustrating that variation in human tumour sensitivity is due to the α component

dramatic change in survival pattern is entirely due to the α components. A more accurate measure of the β component can be obtained by measuring the recovery ratio in split-dose experiments at different levels of cell survival. Reformulation of the linear quadratic equation would predict that:

$$\text{recovery ratio} = e^{2\beta d^2}$$

and thus a plot of log recovery ratio against $2d^2$ gives a straight line with a slope of β[22].

Differences in human tumour radiosensitivity

A range of human tumour radiosensitivity is demonstrated in Figure 2.3. Analogy with the genetically-determined radiosensitivity syndrome ataxia telangiectasia might suggest that the explanation for the extreme radiosensitivity of certain tumours is that they are recovery deficient. The sensitivity of ataxia lymphocytes and skin fibroblasts[23] has been mirrored by disastrous effects of therapeutic radiation[24]. The lack of radiation recovery has been demonstrated both by assessments of potentially lethal damage repair and by low-dose-rate experiments[25].

On the other hand, when analysing the relative contributions of α and β cell kill in a range of human tumour cell lines, it has not been found that radioresistant cells have a greater recovery capacity than radiation-sensitive cells. On the contrary, as shown in Figure 2.5, differences in human tumour radiosensitivity appear to be determined entirely by the initial slope (the α component) which dose-rate studies suggest is not repaired[22].

This observation stimulates the hypothesis that differences in human tumour radiosensitivity are due to the extent of the initial radiation damage.

It seems likely that the lesion required for cytotoxicity is a type of DNA double-strand break[26-28]. The overall frequency of DNA double-strand break induction has been correlated with cytotoxicity under different radiation conditions[29] and it has been known for some time that cell death following exposure to X-rays is associated with loss of chromosome fragments[30,31]. However, the majority of radiation-induced double-strand breaks are repaired, and it seems, therefore, that the lethal event must follow from something more specific, such as, for example, a local multiply-damaged site within the genome[28].

Modification of radiosensitivity by repair inhibitors

Low-dose-rate studies and other assessments of cellular recovery indicate that most human tumour cells are capable of a considerable amount of repair of radiation damage. It seems likely that this is mediated via DNA repair enzymes. Conceptually, a range of inhibitors may interfere with different aspects of the repair process; however, in practice, inhibitors are rarely very specific. Inhibitors which have been studied in conjunction with irradiation include:

1. Inhibitors of DNA precursor production, e.g. deoxyadenosine, hydroxyurea.
2. Inhibitors of DNA polymerization, e.g. cytosine arabinoside, aphidicolin and dideoxythymidine.
3. Inhibitors of topoisomerase-2, e.g. novobiocin.
4. Inhibitors of ADP-ribosyltransferase, e.g. 3-aminobenzamide.
5. Inhibitors of mitotic delay, e.g. caffeine.

At present, these agents remain tools for the investigation of the mechanisms of radiation cytotoxicity[32]. Their usefulness in cancer treatment will depend entirely on defining situations where a greater inhibition of recovery is achieved in tumour than in associated normal tissue. That the agents may have some tissue-specific properties is suggested by studies indicating a variation in sensitization in different cell lines. For example, 3-aminobenzamide

Table 2.1 Dose enhancement ratios* for HX156 cells at high and low dose rate

Inhibitor	Concentration† (μmol/L)	Dose enhancement ratio at	
		150 cGy/min	3.2 cGy/min
Aphidicolin	1	0.95	0.96
3-Aminobenzamide	7000	1.15	1.16
Novobiocin	500	1.05	1.08
Hydroxyurea	125	1.14	1.14
Caffeine	2500	1.11	1.22
β ara A	80	1.06	1.17

*Determined at a surviving fraction of 0.01
†Add 2 h prior to irradiation and remove 24 h afterwards

was used to inhibit radiation recovery in four tumour cell lines, one deriving from germ cell tumour, one from neuroblastoma, one from carcinoma of the cervix and one from large cell lung cancer[33]. The germ cell tumour was sensitized to the greatest degree with a Dose Enhancement Ratio of 1.27; the cervix and neuroblastoma line also showed enhanced radiosensitivity with a DER of 1.18 whereas the lung carcinoma line was not sensitized. The cervix cell line has been studied with a range of inhibitors and it can be seen from Table 2.1 that the majority of them enhanced radiation cytotoxicity at both high and low dose rate. Modelling has revealed that the inhibitors usually increase the α parameter of the linear quadratic equation[34].

Relevance of cell survival curves to clinical radiotherapy

The relevance of *in vitro* cell survival to clinical radiotherapy has been studied by comparing a clinical ranking of the radiosensitivity of a range of tumours of different histologies with steepness of the initial part of the *in vitro* cell survival curve, expressed either as the α component of cell killing or as the surviving fraction at 2 Gy (SF2). The initial report that *in vitro* radiosensitivity was an important determinant of clinical local control of tumours treated with ionizing radiation was by Fertil and Malaise[35] and this was confirmed by Deacon *et al.* in 1984[36]. A weakness of these analyses was that tumours were not studied individually for their *in vitro* and *in vivo* radiosensitivity, but were grouped into broad categories of clinical radiosensitivity, and, within groups, the mean value of various measures of radiosensitivity was used to establish the correlation. The broad range of sensitivity within even one histological subtype of cancer weakens the clinical classification of radiation response: however, extension of these observations to large numbers of cell lines has tended to confirm that the extremes of clinical radiosensitivity and radiation resistance are reflected appropriately by the initial slope of the *in vitro* cell survival curve[37]. These tumours are lymphomas and neuroblastomas at the sensitive end of the range and melanomas and glioblastomas at the resistant end. The common epithelial tumours are not discriminated easily from one another and it may be that factors other than intrinsic cellular radiosensitivity influence the clinical response.

RADIOSENSITIVITY OF NORMAL TISSUE AND THE RATIONALE FOR HYPERFRACTIONATED RADIOTHERAPY

Normal tissue damage from radiotherapy may be 'early', appearing during or shortly after treatment; or may be 'late', not appearing until 6 months to many years later. The kinetics of radiation injury are related to cellular proliferation rate. Intestinal mucosa has a high labelling index and a short cell cycle time and exhibits early expression of radiation damage, whereas renal tissue has a low labelling index and damage is expressed late. Within the same organ, different cellular compartments may express damage at different times.

Acute toxicity results from cell depletion in a rapidly proliferating tissue. Examples include skin desquamation and mucositis. Early reactions usually resolve within weeks; however, major acute toxicity can lead to secondary chronic damage.

Dose–response curves for early effects tend to be linear and thus relatively independent of fraction size. Using the linear quadratic formula (see page 19), the α/β for acute reactions is approximately 10 (i.e. the dose at which $\alpha = \beta$ cell killing is 10 Gy).

Late normal tissue reactions occur in slowly proliferating tissues such as spinal cord, kidney, lung and bladder. This form of damage is usually irreversible and even progressive and may be life threatening. Thus, late normal tissue reactions are usually dose limiting in clinical practice. Dose–response curves usually have a pronounced shoulder, described using the linear quadratic model as an α/β of 2–4.

Most tumours appear to respond to radiation as if they were acute-reacting tissues. The implications of the differently shaped cell survival curves are that, for a given overall treatment time, tumour control will be determined by dose independently of fraction size, whereas late normal tissue damage will be influenced by both total dose and dose per fraction. Less normal tissue damage occurs with smaller doses per fraction since each dose is within the shouldered region of the curve and so causes relatively little cytotoxicity. This theory is supported by extensive evidence that at total doses isoeffective for acute radiation damage an increase in dose per fraction leads to an increased incidence of late normal tissue damage[38–41]. The corollary is that, if a small dose per fraction is used, there will be a reduction in late normal tissue damage at total doses which give equivalent tumour control. This concept provides the basis for hyperfractionated radiotherapy, since the principles may be extended to allow an increase in total dose and thus an increase in tumour control at a dose isoeffective for late normal tissue damage. The use of small fraction sizes implies that the total number of fractions will be increased and, in order to avoid increasing the overall treatment time, more than 1 fraction per day is employed[42,43].

A clinical example of this form of altered fractionation is the trial of radical radiotherapy of carcinoma of the bladder reported by Edsmyr et al.[44]. This prospective randomized trial compares a standard treatment of 64 Gy in 32 fractions over 8½ weeks with hyperfractionated radiotherapy to a dose of 84 Gy in 84 fractions, giving 3 fractions per day with a minimum interval of 4 hours between fractions. One hundred and sixty-eight patients were randomized and analysis revealed a significantly higher local control rate at 6 months for patients treated by hyperfractionation (65% versus 36% ($p<0.001$)). A higher incidence of late complications in the patients treated by hyperfractionation has been ascribed to the improved survival in this group.

A trial of hyperfractionation in squamous carcinoma of the oropharynx has been conducted by the EORTC[45]. Conventional radiotherapy was to a dose of 70 Gy in 2 Gy fractions and this was compared with 2 fractions of 1.15 Gy per day to a total dose of 80.5 Gy. Preliminary analysis has revealed that the 3-year actuarial local control rate was higher in patients treated with hyperfractionated radiotherapy (72% versus 65%). The improvement was only significant in patients with a high performance index[46].

TUMOUR PROLIFERATION RATES

As discussed in the preceding section, radiation resistance in acutely responding normal tissues and in tumours is a consequence of stem cell proliferation.
It has been postulated that this may be an important cause of treatment
failure during the protracted irradiation of human tumours. Simple measurement of volume doubling time might suggest that tumour growth is too slow
to influence response to a 6-week course of radical radiotherapy: however, cell
kinetic studies have demonstrated that tumour stem cells proliferate rapidly
and the apparent slow growth of human tumours is caused by cell loss[47]. Data
on human tumours have been limited during the time that cell cycle parameters were studied using incorporation of tritiated thymidine as a measure
of DNA synthesis. Recently, non-toxic techniques for labelling of tumour
DNA *in vivo* have been developed, based on uptake of halogenated pyrimidines, such as bromodeoxyuridine[48] or iododeoxyuridine[49]. Studies in a range
of tumour types have suggested that the potential doubling time of tumour
stem cells is usually between 3 and 10 days, and, at the shorter end of this
range, it can be calculated that there will be significant tumour cell proliferation during protracted radiotherapy. Furthermore, the initial fractions of
radiotherapy treatment or prior cytotoxic chemotherapy might stimulate
tumour stem cells to divide even more rapidly (accelerated repopulation).
This has been demonstrated in animal tumours[50,51] and may also occur in
normal tissue[52,53]. Retrospective analysis of the results of clinical radiotherapy
has suggested that accelerated repopulation may occur during standard radiation treatment, since the dose needed for local control appears to rise progres-
sively when the overall duration of treatment is greater than approximately 28
days[54].

Clinical data supporting the idea that protracted treatments are a cause of
radiation failure are scanty. Analyses of split-course treatment, where a $2\frac{1}{2}$
week break was inserted, suggest lower control rates than are obtained with
continuous fractionated treatment[55]. Similarly, a retrospective analysis of
radiotherapy for carcinoma of the larynx emphasized the importance of
overall treatment time for local control[56]. In a review of the clinical contexts
in which accelerated treatment may be relevant, published data on both
tumour proliferation parameters and time to clinical recurrence were
analysed[57]. The conclusion was that squamous carcinomas of the head and
neck and cervix, poorly differentiated bladder carcinomas and colorectal
carcinomas may have potential stem cell doubling times of only 3–4 days and
should, thus, benefit from accelerated fractionation.

Accelerated fractionation

This technique is designed to reduce the overall treatment time and the pure
concept would imply no alteration in total dose. Fraction size remains small
in order to avoid increase in late normal tissue damage and therefore acceleration is achieved by giving more than one standard fraction size per day. As
with other techniques using more than one fraction per day, it is important to

maintain at least 6 hours between fractions to allow the full expression of sublethal damage repair. Nevertheless, an increase in acute radiation reactions is to be expected and this increased biological effect is theoretically parallelled by an increased antitumour effect. The probability of late radiation injury is not affected by reducing the overall treatment time. However, as previously discussed, a very severe acute reaction can lead to chronic effects and these may be life threatening[58].

There are a variety of techniques of accelerated fractionation. The 'concomitant boost' technique maintains a standard fractionation schedule to a large target volume and, during part of the treatment course, a second fraction is given to a small boost volume. The rapid acceleration of head and neck cancer radiotherapy was found to generate such severe acute reactions that a prolonged gap in treatment was necessary and overall treatment time was not reduced significantly[59]. Usually, treatment was interrupted after a dose of 48 Gy in 10 days but, more recently, a planned gap of treatment after 24 Gy and 5 days has allowed early resumption and completion of the accelerated schedule. A similar approach has been followed by the Royal Marsden Hospital Urological Oncology Group in the radical radiotherapy of bladder cancer where the standard schedule of 64 Gy and 32 fractions over $6\frac{1}{2}$ weeks is being compared in a randomized trial with the same dose administered in the same number of fractions over 26 days.

A third approach has been to accelerate treatment greatly so that the entire radical radiotherapy course is completed within 12 days. There is compromise of both dose and fraction size. This approach has been pioneered at Mount Vernon Hospital and is termed CHART (continuous hyperfractionated accelerated radiation therapy). Three fractions per day of 1.5 Gy are given, a minimum of 6 h between fractions; 36 fractions are administered over a 12-day period with treatment continued through the weekend[60,61]. The regimen has been explored in both head and neck cancer and in non-small-cell lung cancer. Toxicity to oral and oesophageal mucosa was severe: however, the reports of efficacy in this single-arm study are very encouraging and tumour control rates are higher than obtained in recent historical matched control series.

On the other hand, accelerated fractionation has not proved useful for treatment of primary brain tumours[62]. This randomized EORTC study evaluated a dose of 60 Gy given in 2 treatment courses each of 30 Gy in 15 fractions over 5 days. A 2-week rest was inserted to avoid severe skin reactions, so the overall treatment time was 4 weeks compared with the conventional 6 weeks.

TUMOUR HYPOXIA

In vitro studies illustrate that cells irradiated under hypoxic conditions are approximately 3 times more resistant to ionizing radiation than oxygenated cells. Histological studies of human tumours revealed hypoxic tissue at a distance of 150 μm from blood vessels[63], and it was postulated that, adjacent to frankly necrotic areas, there may be pools of radiation-resistant but viable tumour cells. There is abundant biological evidence for hypoxic radiation resistance in animal tumours[64]. Attempts to measure oxygenation of human tumours have been hampered by the problem that invasive techniques may cause artifactual changes in oxygen levels secondary to tissue damage. Nevertheless, microelectrode measurements have demonstrated reduced oxygenation within tumours and the extent of hypoxia has been correlated with radiation resistance[65].

Indirect clinical evidence for the importance of tumour oxygenation comes from hyperbaric oxygen trials in advanced head and neck cancer where significant benefit accrued to patients treated with this technique compared with those treated in air[66].

The difficulties of treating patients with hyperbaric oxygen stimulated the development of chemical radiosensitizers of hypoxic cells[67,68]. Early studies with misonidazole compared tumour growth delay following radiation with or without radiosensitizer in patients with multiple subcutaneous nodules[69,70]. The results were strongly suggestive of sensitization. Unfortunately, very extensive clinical testing of both metronidazole and misonidazole in prospective randomized clinical trials of fractionated radiotherapy has failed to show a benefit from radiosensitizer except in a Danish study of head and neck cancer, where subgroup analysis revealed benefit to patients with supraglottic and pharyngeal carcinomas[71].

Two drugs from the new generation of hypoxic cell radiosensitizers are currently under clinical evaluation. SR-2508 suffers the same dose-limiting toxicity as misonidazole, namely peripheral neuropathy, although at higher doses[72]. R0-03-8799 does not cause peripheral neuropathy, and the dose-limiting toxicity is to the central nervous system. A particular advantage of this drug appears to be an ability to concentrate within tumours, which is possibly related to local pH[60]. SR-2508 is being investigated predominantly in head and neck cancer whereas R0-03-8799 is being studied in advanced carcinoma of the cervix.

If human tumours do contain significant numbers of hypoxic cells, there seems little doubt that response to a single fraction of radiotherapy will be compromised. A very small proportion of hypoxic cells within a tumour may become increasingly important after repeated treatments since it may be expected that initial fractions will selectively destroy well-oxygenated cells and the remaining hypoxic fraction may become the major population for subsequent fractions. On the other hand, once destroyed cells cease utilizing oxygen, this may become available to previously hypoxic areas of the tumour, a process termed reoxygenation. In animal tumours, this process takes 1–3 days, but the kinetics of reoxygenation in human tumours are unknown. The longer the time period between fractions of radiotherapy, the more likely that reoxygenation will occur. In theory, this may be a disadvantage of accelerated fractionation regimens.

PREDICTIVE TESTING FOR RADIATION RESPONSE

Current management strategies are based predominantly on the stage and histology of the tumour and on the performance status of the patient. Thus for example management of a patient with a localized muscle-invasive carcinoma of the bladder may be by radical radiotherapy to a dose of 64 Gy in 32 fractions over 6½ weeks, or may be by combined radiotherapy and cystectomy. New approaches to the same clinical presentation include initial combination chemotherapy followed by either radical radiotherapy or cystectomy. The treatment decision is based on past experience of efficacy and toxicity in patients with the same stage of tumour. The radiobiological parameters affecting radiation response which have been described earlier in this chapter are not taken into account in the management decision. The challenge to the field of predictive testing is to develop rapid assays of these biological parameters so that the result can be available before a management decision is made, in practice within approximately 2 weeks. Predictive tests differ from prognostic information because they are applied specifically to a particular clinical management decision.

A number of predictive tests based on radiobiological parameters are currently being evaluated. In principle, these evaluations seek, first, to compare the test results with the radiation response, secondly, to determine whether the test contributes information which remains significant when analysed with other prognostic factors by multiple factor regression analysis, and, thirdly, to determine the ability to respond to the test information by successful adjustment of management.

An important theoretical problem of predictive testing is that the critical cell for analysis is the tumour stem cell, yet the requirements for a rapid test do not allow sufficient time for clonogenic types of assay. Tests are therefore carried out on a mixture of clonogenic and non-clonogenic tumour cells and may not reflect the status of the stem cell.

Radiosensitivity testing

Clonogenic cell survival assays have proved unreliable when applied to primary human tumour cultures. The assay has been more successful when modified to prevent artefacts caused by cell clumping[73,74]. The poor plating efficiency of most human tumours, and thus the long time required for the assay, mean that this approach is in any case unlikely to provide a useful predictive test.

Non-clonogenic assays in mass culture have the advantage of speed. For radiosensitivity testing, duplicate cultures are irradiated at graded doses and an assay of cell number is performed 3–14 days later.

A major problem of this approach is that it requires the growth of pure populations of tumour cells from the mixed cellular population of a clinical biopsy sample. Culture systems for primary human cultures are required which retard proliferation of stromal fibroblasts and of any normal epithelial cells which may be contained in the biopsy. A test which is currently undergoing evaluation is based on cell culture in plates coated with 'cell adhesion matrix' which has been reported to promote cell attachment and growth[75]. Cytogenetic studies have tended to confirm that this system grows tumour cells. Cytotoxic treatment is carried out 1 day after establishment of the cultures, and, 2 weeks later, the total number of cells remaining in culture is assessed by crystal violet staining. In practice, the assays are carried out at a range of dilutions to avoid artefacts due to overcrowding of cultures. This assay has been investigated most extensively at the M.D. Anderson Hospital. Results have been expressed in terms of the surviving fraction at 2 Gy. A broad range of surviving fractions is seen within each histological type of tumour studied. For example, in 16 biopsies from melanoma, surviving fraction at 2 Gy (SF2) ranged from 23% to over 80%. Melanoma biopsies consistently had a higher SF2 than biopsies from squamous cancers of the head and neck or from Ewings sarcoma[76]. A current study will correlate the measured SF2 using this technique with the risk of recurrence after radical ratiotherapy of squamous tumours of the head and neck.

An alternative method of assessing numbers of residual viable cells is by their ability to reduce a tetrazolium dye (MTT) to an insoluble formazan product, a reaction associated with a change of colour from yellow to blue[77,78]. The test assays mitochondrial function. Studies on cell lines indicate that, in radiosensitivity testing, the results are very similar to those from clonogenic assays[79].

The potential sensitivity of measurement of survival fraction at 2 Gy can be judged from an extrapolation of the range of results to a 30-fraction regimen. Thus, if SF2 ranges from 35% to 65% in different tumours, the dose required to leave 1 surviving cell would range from 40 Gy to almost 100 Gy. Clearly this calculation should not be applied in isolation from other radiobiological factors: even so, the test would be useful if it merely produced an accurate ranking of individual tumour radiosensitivities.

The micronucleus assay

The micronucleus assay of radiation effect has the advantage that it does not require cell culture. Micronuclei derive from chromosomal breaks. An acentric fragment lags behind the segregating chromosomes during mitosis and is therefore left in the cytoplasm of the daughter cell. It is visible by light microscopy after the first postirradiation cell division. The presence of a micronucleus in a cell indicates severe radiation toxicity[31]. The assay shows a good correlation with cell survival curves. Unfortunately, this is a difficult technique to assess *in vivo* since the proportion of cells demonstrating micronuclei depends on factors other than cellular radiosensitivity. For example, cells which are not cycling will not express micronuclei, whereas proliferating normal cells will. The technique has been used to predict radiation response in rectal carcinomas[80].

Tumour cell proliferation

Most information on the cell kinetics of human tumours has been based on tritiated thymidine labelling and autoradiography[10]. The potential hazard from administration of this radioactive material to patients has limited the widespread assessment of individual tumours with this technique. As discussed previously (p. 25), low doses of the halogenated pyrimidines are not toxic and they can be used instead of tritiated thymidine as a measure of DNA metabolism[81]. The incorporation of these agents can be measured with a monoclonal antibody[82], the result being assessed either by flow cytometry or on tissue sections. The tissue section technique allows an experienced pathologist to ensure that he is counting only tumour cells to produce a labelling index. A possible advantage of flow cytometry is that the technique can be modified to allow assessment not only of the labelling index but also of the duration of S phase[83], thus allowing calculation of the potential doubling time[10]. The potential doubling time for a range of human tumours has been found to be in the range of 2–20 days[84].

An alternative method of assessing cellular proliferation employs an antibody to a proliferation-dependent antigen. The Ki-67 antibody recognizes a nuclear antigen present throughout the cell cycle but not in cells that are out of cycle[85]. It may be considered to identify the growth fraction of tumours. Ki-67 indices for a range of human tumours have been analysed[86-88]. This form of labelling may provide information independent of conventional histological parameters such as cell type or tumour differentiation. Certainly, a wide range of staining is seen. In breast cancer, the Ki-67 index has ranged from less than 1% to 60% in different tumours.

Tumour hypoxia

For reasons discussed above, the ideal assessment of tumour metabolism should be non-invasive. A difficulty for predictive testing is that it is important to recognize even a minor proportion of hypoxic cells within a tumour (less than 10%). Techniques currently being assessed include nuclear magnetic resonance spectroscopy[89,90]. Alternatively, uptake of oxygen-15 can be measured using positron emission tomography (PET)[91]. Neither of these techniques has yet been investigated extensively in patients. They have a potential, not only for measuring the hypoxic fraction of tumours prior to

Table 2.2 Predictive testing: clinical response

Assay	Result	Possible clinical responses
Proliferation	Rapid	Accelerated fractionation
	Slow	Protracted fractionation
Radiosensitivity	Sensitive	Hyperfractionation
		Reduce total dose
	Resistant	Surgery
		Neutrons
		Chemical sensitization
		Increase dose
Metabolism	Hypoxic	Hyperbaric oxygen
		Hypoxic cell radiosensitizer
		Debulking surgery

treatment, but also for monitoring patterns of reoxygenation between fractions of radiotherapy.

Clinical response to predictive testing

If rapid reliable radiobiological information is available on individual tumours, patients could be stratified in studies which would test the appropriate response to the information (Table 2.2): thus, for example, patients with rapidly proliferating tumours may be treated successfully if radiotherapy is accelerated. Patients with radiosensitive tumours may be treated more successfully by reducing the individual radiation fraction size thus allowing a higher dose of radiotherapy to be delivered (hyperfractionation). On the other hand, tumours with low radiosensitivity may be more appropriately treated by an alternative modality, such as surgery. Alternatively, it may be appropriate to try to improve tumour radiosensitivity by concomitant treatment with DNA repair inhibitors or other chemical radiosensitizers. Tumours with large hypoxic fractions or with impaired reoxygenation between fractions would be appropriate for the study of hypoxic cell radiosensitizers.

References

1. Regaud, C. and Blanc, J. (1906). Actions des rayons X sur les diverses generations de la lignee spermatique: extreme sensibilite des spermatogonies a ces rayons. *C. R. Soc. Biol.*, **61**, 163–165.
2. Regaud, C. (1922). Distribution chronologique rationelle d'un traitement de cancer epithelial par les radiations. *C. R. Soc. Biol.*, **86**, 1085–1088
3. Coutard, H. (1932). Roentgentherapy of epitheliomas of the tonsillar region, hypopharynx and larynx from 1920–1926. *Am. J. Roentgenol.*, **28**, 313–331
4. Paterson, R. (1936). The radical x-ray treatment of the carcinomata. *Br. J. Radiol.*, **9**, 671–679
5. Paterson, R. (1952). Studies in optimum dosage. *Br. J. Radiol.*, **25**, 505–516
6. McWhirter, R. (1936). *13th Annual Report of the British Empire Cancer Campaign*, pp. 131–144 (London)
7. Baclesse, F. (1951). Roentgentherapy of carcinoma of the larynx. *J. Fac. Radiol.*, **3**, 3–12
8. Strandqvist, M. (1944). Studien uber die Kumulative Wirkung der Roentgenstrahlen bei Fraktionierung. *Acta Radiol. Suppl.*, **55**, 1–300
9. Elkind, M. M. and Sutton, H. (1960). Radiation response of mammalian cells grown in culture. I. Repair of x-ray damage in surviving Chinese hamster cells. *Radiat. Res.*, **13**, 556–593
10. Steel, G. G. (1977). *Growth Kinetics of Tumours*. (Oxford: Clarendon Press)
11. Thomlinson, R. H. (1968). Changes of oxygenation in tumors in relation to irradiation. *Front. Radiat. Ther. Oncol.*, **3**, 109–121
12. Sinclair, W. K. and Morton, R. A. (1966). X-ray sensitivity during the cell generation cycle of cultured Chinese hamster cells. *Radiat. Res.*, **29**, 450–474
13. Hall, E. J. (1988). *Radiobiology for the Radiologist*. (USA: Harper & Row)
14. Dobbs, J. and Barrett, A. (1985). *Practical Radiotherapy Planning*. (London: Edward Arnold)
15. Chadwick, K. H. and Leenhouts, H. P. (1981). *The Molecular Theory of Radiation Biology*. (Berlin: Springer-Verlag)
16. Goodhead, D. T. (1982). An assessment of the role of microdosimetry in radiobiology. *Radiat. Res.*, **91**, 45–76

17. Alper, T. (1979). *Cellular Radiobiology*. (Cambridge: Cambridge University Press)
18. Curtis, S. B. (1986). Lethal and potentially lethal lesions induced by radiation – a unified repair model. *Radiat. Res.*, **106**, 252–270
19. Thames, H. D. (1985). An "incomplete-repair" model for survival after fractionated and continuous irradiations. *Int. J. Radiat. Biol.*, **47**, 319–339
20. Joiner, M. C. and Denekamp, J. (1986). Evidence for a constant repair capacity over 20 fractions. *Int. J. Radiat. Biol.*, **49**, 143–150
21. Steel, G. G., Deacon, J. M., Duchesne, G. M., Horwich, A., Kelland, L. R. and Peacock, J. H. (1988). The dose-rate effect in human tumour cells. *Radiother. Oncol.*, **9**, 299–310
22. Peacock, J. H., Cassoni, A. M. and McMillan, T. J. (1988). Radiosensitive human tumour cell lines may not be recovery deficient. *Int. J. Radiat. Biol.*, **54**, 945–953
23. Paterson, M. C. and Smith, P. J. (1979). Ataxia-telangiectasia: A inherited human disorder involving hypersensitivity to ionizing radiation and related DNA damaging chemicals. *Annu. Rev. Genet.*, **13**, 192–318
24. Cunliffe, P. N., Mann, J. R., Cameron, A. H., Roberts, K. D. and Ward, H. W. C. (1975). Radiosensitivity in ataxia-telangiectasia. *Br. J. Radiol.*, **48**, 374–376
25. Cox, R. (1982). A cellular description of the repair defect in ataxia telangiectasia. In Bridges, B. A. and Harnden, D. G. (eds.) *Ataxia Telangiectasia: A Molecular Link between Cancer, Neuropathology and Immune Deficiency*, pp. 141–154. (Chichester, New York: Wiley)
26. Frankenberg, D., Frankenberg-Schwager, M. and Harbich, P. (1984). Split-dose recovery is due to the repair of DNA double-strand breaks. *Int. J. Radiat. Biol.*, **46**, 541–553
27. Kemp, L. M., Sedgwick, S. G. and Jeggo, P. A. (1985). X-ray sensitive mutants of Chinese hamster ovary cells defective in double-strand break rejoining. *Mutat. Res.*, **132**, 189–196
28. Ward, J. F. (1986). Mechanisms of DNA repair and their potential modification for radiotherapy. *Int. J. Radiat. Oncol. Biol. Phys.*, **12**, 1027–1032
29. Radford, I. (1985). The level of induced DNA double-strand breakage correlates with cell killing after X irradiation. *Int. J. Radiat. Biol.*, **48**, 45–54
30. Grote, S. J., Joshi, G. P., Revell, S. H. and Shaw, C. A. (1981). Observations of radiation-induced chromosome fragment loss in live mammalian cells in culture, and its effect on colony-forming ability. *Int. J. Radiat. Biol.*, **39**, 395–408
31. Joshi, G. P., Nelson, W. J., Revell, S. H. and Shaw, C. A. (1982). X-ray induced chromosome damage in live mammalian cells and improved measurements of its effects on their colony-forming ability. *Int. J. Radiat. Biol.*, **41**, 161–181
32. Collins, A. (1987). Cellular responses to ionizing radiation: effects of interrupting DNA repair with chemical agents. *Int. J. Radiat. Biol.*, **51**, 971–983
33. Kelland, L. R., Burgess, L. and Steel, G. (1988). Differential radiosensitization by the poly (ADP-ribose transferase inhibitor 3-aminobenzamide in human tumor cells of varying radio-sensitivity. *Int. J. Radiat. Biol. Phys.*, **14**, 1239–1246
34. Kelland, L. R. and Steel, G. G. (1988). Modification of radiation dose-rate sparing effects in a human carcinoma of the cervix cell line by inhibitors of DNA repair. *Int. J. Radiat. Biol.*, **54**, 229–244
35. Fertil, B. and Malaise, E. P. (1981). Inherent cellular radiosensitivity as a basic concept for human tumor radiotherapy. *Int. J. Radiat. Oncol. Biol. Phys.*, **7**, 621–629
36. Deacon, J., Peckham, M. J. and Steel, G. G. (1984). The radioresponsiveness of human tumours and the initial slope of the cell survival curve. *Radiother. Oncol.*, **2**, 317–323
37. Malaise, E. P., Fertil, B., Deschavanne, P. J., Chavaudra, N. and Brock, W. A. (1987). Initial slope of radiation survival curves is characteristic of the origin of primary and established cultures of human tumor cells and fibroblasts. *Radiat. Res.*, **111**, 319–333
38. Withers, H. R., Thames, H. D. and Peters, L. J. (1982). Differences in the fractionation response of acutely and late-responding tissues. In Kaercher, K. H., Kogelnick, H. D. and Reinartz, G. (eds.) *Progress in Radio-oncology*, vol. 2, pp. 287–296. (New York: Raven Press)
39. Fowler, J. F. (1984). Review: total doses in fractionated radiotherapy – implications of new radiobiological data. *Int. J. Radiat. Biol.*, **46**, 103–120
40. Turesson, I. and Notter, G. (1984). The influence of fraction size in radiotherapy on the late normal tissue reaction. 2. Comparison of the effects of daily and twice-a-week fractionation on human skin. *Int. J. Radiat. Oncol. Biol. Phys.* **10**, 599–606
41. Cox, J. D. (1985). Large-dose fractionation. *Cancer*, **55**, 2105–2111

42. Thames, H. D., Withers, H. R., Peters, L. J. and Fletcher, G. H. (1982). Changes in early and late radiation responses with altered dose fractionation: implications for dose-survival relationships. *Int. J. Radiat. Oncol. Biol. Phys.*, **8**, 219–226
43. Thames, H. D., Peters, L. J., Withers, H. R. and Fletcher, G. H. (1983). Accelerated fractionation vs. hyperfractionation: rationales for several treatments per day. *Int. J. Radiat. Oncol. Biol. Phys.*, **9**, 127–138
44. Edsmyr, F., Andersson, I., Esposti, P. L., Littbrand, B. and Nilsson, B. (1985). Irradiation therapy with multiple small fractions per day in urinary bladder cancer. *Radiother. Oncol.*, **4**, 197–203
45. Horiot, J. C., van den Bogaert, W., de Pauw, M., van Glabbeke, M., Gonzales, D. G. and van der Schueren, E. (1985). EORTC prospective trials of altered fractionation using multiple fractions per day (MFD). In *Proceedings 16th Int. Congress of Radiology.* p. 95. (Honolulu, Hawaii)
46. Withers, H. R. and Horiot, J. C. (1988). Hyperfractionation. In Withers, H. R. and Peters, L. J. (eds.) *Innovations in Radiation Oncology*, pp. 223–230. (Berlin, Heidelberg, New York, London, Paris, Tokyo: Springer-Verlag)
47. Steel, G. G. (1967). Cell loss as a factor in the growth rate of human tumours. *Eur. J. Cancer*, **3**, 381–387
48. Wilson, G. W., McNally, N. J., Dische, S., Saunders, M. I., Des Rochers, C., Lewis, A. A. and Bennett, M. H. (1988). Measurement of cell kinetics in human tumours in vivo using bromodeoxyuridine incorporation and flow cytometry. *Br. J. Cancer*, **58**, 423–431
49. Begg, A. C., Moonen, L., Hofland, I., Dessing, M. and Bartelink, H. (1988). Human tumour cell kinetics using a monoclonal antibody against iododeoxyuridine: Intratumour sampling variations. *Radiother. Oncol.*, **11**, 337–347
50. Hermens, A. F. and Barendsen, G. W. (1969). Changes of cell proliferation characteristics in a rat rhabdomyosarcoma before and after x-irradiation. *Eur. J. Cancer*, **5**, 173
51. Stephens, T. C. and Steel, G. G. (1980). Regeneration of tumors after cytotoxic treatment. In Meyn, R. E. and Withers, H. R. (eds.) *Radiation Biology in Cancer Research*, pp. 385–395
52. Denekamp, J. (1973). Changes in the rate of repopulation during multifractionation irradiation of mouse skin. *Br. J. Radiol.*, **46**, 381–387
53. Archambeau, J. O., Hauser, D. and Shymko, R. M. (1989). Swine basal cell proliferation during a course of daily irradiation, five days a week for six weeks (6000 RAD). *Int. J. Radiat. Oncol. Biol. Phys.*, **15**, 1383–1388
54. Withers, H. R., Taylor, J. M. G. and Maciejewski, B. (1988). The hazard of accelerated tumor clonogen repopulation during radiotherapy. *Acta Oncologica*, **27**, 131–146
55. Parsons, J. T. (1984). Results of twice-a-day irradiation of squamous cell carcinomas of the head and neck. *Int. J. Radiat. Oncol. Biol. Phys.*, **10**, 2041–2051
56. Maciejewski, B., Preuss-Bayer, G. and Trott, K. (1983). The influence of the number of fractions and of overall treatment time on local control and late complication rate in squamous cell carcinoma of the larynx. *Int. J. Radiat. Oncol. Biol. Phys.*, **9**, 321–328
57. Trott, K. R. and Kummermehr, J. (1985). What is known about tumor proliferation rates to choose between accelerated fractionation or hyperfractionation? *Radiother. Oncol.*, **3**, 1–9
58. Peracchia, G. and Salti, C. (1981). Radiotherapy with thrice-a-day fractionation in a short overall time. *Int. J. Radiat. Oncol. Biol. Phys.*, **7**, 99–104
59. van den Bogaert, W., van der Schueren, E., Horiot, J-C. *et al.* (1986). Early results of the EORTC randomized clinical trial on multiple fractions per day (MFD) and misonidazole in advanced head and neck cancer. *Int. J. Radiat. Oncol. Biol. Phys.*, **12**, 587–591
60. Saunders, M. I., Dische, S., Anderson, P. J., Tothill, M., Stratford, M. R. L. and Minchinton, A. I. (1984). The clinical testing of Ro 03-8799: pharmacokinetics, toxicology, tissue and tumour concentrations. *Int. J. Radiat. Oncol. Biol. Phys.*, **10**, 1759–1763
61. Dische, S. and Saunders, M. I. (1989). Continuous hyperfractionated, accelerated radiotherapy (CHART). *Br. J. Cancer*, **59**, 325–326
62. van der Schueren, E., Ang, K. K., Horiot, J. C., Gonzalez, D. G., Glabbeke, M. V. and De Pauw, M. (1985). Concentrated radiotherapy schedules: role of repair and repopulation. In *Proceedings of the XVI International Congress of Radiology*, July 8–12, pp. 99–103. (Hawaii)
63. Thomlinson, R. H. and Gray, L. H. (1955). The histological structure of some human lung cancers and the possible implications for radiotherapy. *Br. J. Cancer*, **9**, 539–549

64. Moulder, J. E. and Rockwell, S. (1984). Hypoxic fractions of solid tumors: experimental techniques, methods of analysis and a survey of existing data. *Int. J. Radiat. Oncol. Biol. Phys.*, **10**, 695–712

65. Gatenby, R. A., Kessler, H. B., Rosenblum, J. S., Coia, J. A., Moldofsky, P. J., Hartz, W. H. and Broder, G. J. (1988). Oxygen distribution in squamous cell carcinoma metastases: Relationship to outcome of radiation therapy. *Int. J. Radiat. Oncol. Biol. Phys.*, **14**, 831–838

66. Henk, J. M. (1986). Late results of a trial of hyperbaric oxygen and radiotherapy in head and neck cancer: A rationale for hypoxic cell sensitizers? *Int. J. Radiat. Oncol. Biol. Phys.*, **12**, 1339–1341

67. Adams, G. E. and Dewey, D. L. (1963). Hydrated electrons and radiobiological sensitization. *Biochem. Biophys. Res. Commun.*, **12**, 473–477

68. Adams, G. E., Flockhart, I. R., Smithen, C. E., Stratford, I. J., Wardman, P. and Watts, M. E. (1976). Electron-affinic sensitization. 7. A correlation between structure, one-electron reduction potentials and efficiencies of nitroimidazoles as hypoxic cell radiosensitizers. *Radiat. Res.*, **67**, 9–20

69. Dawes, P. J. D. K., Peckham, M. J. and Steel, G. G. (1978). The response of human tumour metastases to radiation and misonidazole. *Br. J. Cancer*, **37**, 290–296

70. Ash, D. V., Peckham, M. J. and Steel, G. (1979). The quantitative response of human tumours to radiation and misonidazole. *Br. J. Cancer*, **40**, 883–889

71. Overgaard, J., Hansen, H. S., Jorgensen, K. and Hansen, M. H. (1986). Primary radiotherapy of larynx and pharynx carcinoma – an analysis of some factors influencing local control and survival. *Int. J. Radiat. Oncol. Biol. Phys.*, **12**, 515–521

72. Coleman, C. N. (1984). Initial report of the phase I trial of the hypoxic cell radiosensitizer SR 2508. *Int. J. Radiat. Oncol. Biol. Phys.*, **10**, 1749–1753

73. Courtenay, V. D. and Mills, J. (1978). An in vitro colony assay for human tumours grown in immune-suppressed mice and treated in vivo with cytotoxic agents. *Br. J. Cancer*, **37**, 261–268

74. Rofstad, E. K., Wahl, A. and Brustad, T. (1987). Radiation sensitivity in vitro of cells isolated from human tumor surgical specimens. *Cancer Res.*, **47**, 106–110

75. Baker, F., Spitzer, G., Ajani, J., Brock, W., Lukeman, J., Pathek, S., Tomasovic, B., Thielvoldt, D., Williams, M., Vines, C. and Tofilon, P. (1986). Drug and radiation sensitivity measurements of successful primary monolayer culturing of human tumor cells using cell-adhesive matrix and supplemented medium. *Cancer Res.*, **46**, 1263–1274

76. Brock, W. A., Maor, M. H. and Peters, L. J. (1985). Predictors of tumour response to therapy. *Radiat. Res.*, **104**, 290–296

77. Mossman, T. (1983). Rapid colorimetric assay for cellular growth and survival: Application to proliferation and cytotoxic assays. *J. Immunol. Meth.*, **65**, 55–63

78. Carmichael, J., DeGraff, W. B., Gazdar, A. F., Minna, J. D. and Mitchell, J. B. (1987). Evaluation of a tetrazolium-based semiautomatic colorimetric assay: Assessment of radiosensitivity. *Cancer Res.*, **47**, 943–946

79. Wasserman, T. H. and Twentyman, P. R. (1988). Use of a colorimetric (MTT) assay in determining the radiosensitivity of solid murine tumours. *Int. J. Radiat. Oncol. Biol. Phys.*, **15**, 699–702

80. Streffer, C., Beuningen, D., Gross, E., Schabronath, J., Eigler, F. W. and Rebman, A. (1986). Predictive assays for the therapy of rectum carcinoma. *Radiother. Oncol.*, **5**, 303–310

81. Dolbeare, F., Gratzner, H., Pallavicini, M. G., Vanderlaan, M. and Gray, J. W. (1983). Flow cytometric measurement of total DNA content and incorporated bromodeoxyuridine. *Proc. Natl. Acad. Sci. (USA)*, **80**, 5573–5577

82. Gratzner, H. G. (1982). Monoclonal antibody to 5-bromo-and 5-iododeoxyuridine: A new reagent for detection of DNA replication. *Science*, **218**, 474–475

83. Begg, A. C., McNally, N. J., Schrieve, D. C. and Karcher, H. (1985). A method to measure the duration of DNA synthesis and the potential doubling time from a single sample. · *Cytometry*, **6**, 620–626

84. Wilson, G. W., McNally, N. J., Dische, S., Saunders, M. I., Des Rochers, C., Lewis, A. A. and Bennett, M. H. (1988). Measurement of cell kinetics in human tumours in vivo using bromodeoxyuridine incorporation and flow cytometry. *Br. J. Cancer*, **58**, 423–431

85. Gerdes, J., Schwab, U., Lemke, H. and Stein, H. (1983). Production of a mouse monoclonal antibody reactive with human nuclear antigen associated with cell proliferation. *Int. J.*

Cancer, **31**, 13-16

86. McGurrin, J. F., Doria, M. I., Dawson, P. J., Karrison, T., Stein, H. O. and Franklin, W. A. (1987). Assessment of tumour cell kinetics by immunohistochemistry in carcinoma of breast. *Cancer,* **59**, 1744-1750

87. Burger, P. C., Shibata, T. and Kleihues, P. (1986). The use of the monoclonal antibody Ki-67 in the identification of proliferating cells. *Am. J. Surg. Pathol.,* **10**, 611-617

88. Gatter, K. C., Dunnill, M. S., Gerdes, J., Stein, H. and Mason, D. Y. (1986). New approach to assessing lung tumours in man. *J. Clin. Pathol.,* **39**, 590-593

89. Griffiths, J. R., Cady, E., Edwards, R. H. T., McCready, V. R., Wilkie, D. R. and Wiltshaw, E. (1983). ^{31}P-NMR studies of a human tumor in situ. *Lancet,* **1**, 1435-1436

90. Okunieff, P. G., Koutcher, J. A., Gerwick, L., McFarland, E., Hitzig, B., Urano, M., Brady, T., Neuringer, L. and Suit, H. D. (1986). Tumour size dependent changes in a murine fibrosarcoma: Use of in vivo^{31} PNMR for non-invasive evaluation of tumour metabolic status. *Int. J. Radiat. Biol. Oncol. Phys.,* **12**, 793-799

91. Ito, M., Lammertsma, A. A., Wise, R. J. S., Bernardi, S., Frackowiak, R. S. J., Heather, J. D., McKenzie, C. G., Thomas, D. G. T. and Jones, T. (1982). Measurement of regional cerebral blood flow and oxygen utilization in patients with cerebral tumors using ^{15}O and positron emission tomography: Analytical techniques and preliminary results. *Neuroradiology,* **23**, 63-74

3
The evolution of current chemotherapy regimens

M.H.N. TATTERSALL

INTRODUCTION

A wide variety of factors have influenced the development of modern cancer chemotherapy. At differing times over the past 40 years during which chemotherapy has evolved, the influence of pharmacological considerations (pharmacokinetic and drug distribution data), of knowledge of tumour biology (particularly information on cell cycle kinetics and tumour cell heterogeneity), and clinical research (both formal clinical trials and serendipity) have dominated the development and direction of cancer chemotherapy. In addition, success in treating particular cancers has led to the application of the successful strategy and/or recipe in other tumour types, sometimes with impressive results. The importance of experimental chemotherapy studied with transplanted animal tumours must also be acknowledged, not only in providing a means for screening drugs for potential anticancer activity, but also for demonstrating that, with many tumours, cure is possible using appropriately selected and scheduled chemical treatment.

There is currently no satisfactory classification of drugs used in cancer control. From a historical perspective, the origins and subsequent development of endocrine approaches to cancer treatment have been rather separate from those which pertain to 'cytotoxic' drugs. The former treatments have been based on the hormonal sensitivity of tumours of particular tissues, while the latter have until recently been based on enlightened empiricisms and on the use of transplanted animal tumours as a screening system. Only in the past few years have these two branches of cancer chemotherapy become interactive, not merely in the laboratory where the new biological products do not fit comfortably into a single category, but also in the management of several cancers where combined endocrine and cytotoxic treatments have been utilized.

LESSONS FROM LEUKAEMIA, LYMPHOMA AND CHILDHOOD CANCERS

Recognition of the fact and possible causes of failure of cancer chemotherapy has also played a part in the development of current approaches to the treatment of cancer, especially the use of combination chemotherapy and the development of combined modality treatments. Combination cancer chemotherapy evolved during the 1960s, particularly in the management of acute leukaemia and Hodgkin's disease. Intermittent treatment with maximally tolerated doses of drugs having differing toxicities to normal tissues, with judicious breaks to allow normal tissues to recover, was found to be an effective strategy for improving the tumour response rate and survival prospects of patients with leukaemia and lymphoma. Other types of cancer seen in childhood were subsequently found to benefit from this aggressive treatment approach, and this led to the integration of chemotherapy with surgery and/or radiotherapy in the curative treatment strategy for Wilms' tumour, embryonal sarcomas and neuroblastoma. The central nervous system in children with leukaemia was soon recognized as a common site of relapse, and the notion of sanctuary sites where cancer cells might escape exposure to therapeutic drug concentrations was advanced. In turn, this led to the investigation of intrathecal treatment, and of cranial (spinal) radiation as a means of treating the CNS, initially for overt CNS leukaemia, and later as an 'adjuvant' in children at high risk of developing the disease.

These successful developments of chemotherapy in leukaemia, lymphoma and childhood cancers were then applied to the treatment of cancer in adults. It soon became apparent that the outcome of cancer chemotherapy in adults was usually less successful, with intrinsic tumour insensitivity and/or acquired drug resistance posing frequent problems. During the past 15 years, the optimism for aggressive high-dose multidrug multimodality treatment approaches, which have proved so successful in treating leukaemia, lymphoma and types of childhood cancer, has waned in the face of results from trials where such approaches were found not to be appropriate or necessarily effective in many cancer types seen in adults. In 1989, cancer chemotherapy applied to adult tumour types is more influenced by a reappraisal of the goals of treatment and determination of appropriate end-points by which to measure the impact of therapy.

Recognition and definition of the obstacles to successful chemotherapy in adult types of cancer has exposed the need for improved communication between the basic cancer biologists and cancer clinicians. New tumour screens are needed in order to identify drugs active against slow-growing adult cancer types, and reliable prognostic factors, including those based on specific tumour characteristics, are required to individualize treatment. The optimal means whereby modalities may be integrated in curative and palliative treatment of different cancer types is now recognized as a reasonable topic for clinical research, as is the appropriate evaluation of new biological treatments with, for example, growth factors and their analogues, lymphokines, and the like.

NEW DRUGS AND THEIR EVALUATION AS ANTICANCER AGENTS

The identification of potential anticancer drugs has relied on serendipity and the application of a transplanted animal tumour screen. The most widely used tumour screens have been the P388 and L1210 murine lymphoma lines. Latterly, concern has grown that screening with more slowly growing tumours might identify drugs with an improved chance of activity in adult cancer types, and has led to the use of some murine solid tumours and of human tumours growing as xenografts in immune-deprived animals. The outcome of these new 'screens' is being assessed.

The identification of appropriate tumour models to screen new endocrine agents and new biologicals is being pursued, but their role in selecting which drugs should be investigated clinically remains controversial.

Evaluation of anticancer drugs

Historically, the sequence of phase I, II and III clinical trials has been rigorously applied in the U.S., but more loosely adhered to in the British and European anticancer drug evaluation programs. A phase I trial of an anticancer drug has as its endpoint the determination of the maximally tolerated dose (MTD) of the new drug according to the specified administration schedule. In a phase II trial, the antitumour effects of the drug at the MTD are determined in a variety of tumour types utilizing the endpoint of tumour response. In a phase III trial, the new drug is incorporated into treatment of particular tumour types, and the efficacy is sometimes determined by comparison with the best existing 'standard treatment' in randomized trials. This sequence of clinical evaluation of new anticancer drugs is now being challenged. On the one hand, it may not be necessary or appropriate to determine the MTD of a new drug, particularly if the proposed mechanism of antitumour action is completely unrelated to its toxic effects on normal tissues. Secondly, knowledge of the specific drug target in tumour cells may be a valid basis for selecting patients and tumour types for phase II and III trials. Thirdly, the endpoint of tumour response (shrinkage) may not be the only reasonable yard stick by which to measure treatment efficacy: such other indicators as effect on immune function, metastatic ability, tumour cell cycle pattern etc., may be equally, or even more, relevant.

Cancer patients and their availability for clinical research

The evolution of cancer chemotherapy has been greatly influenced by the attitude of the medical profession and the community in general to 'experimental' treatment and participation in clinical trials. Historically, the first patients in whom cancer chemotherapy was investigated were children and young adults with leukaemia and advanced lymphoma. For these patients, it was recognized that local treatment (surgery or radiotherapy) was not beneficial, and that drug treatment offered the only real chance of benefit. Success in treatment of some of these patients during the 1960s led to trials of chemotherapy in other advanced cancer types, and impressive results with childhood cancers led naturally to the integration of chemotherapy with surgery and radiotherapy in curative treatment approaches for less advanced disease.

Adjuvant radiotherapy and chemotherapy (CNS prophylaxis) was then found to delay relapse in childhood acute lymphoblastic leukaemia, and the use of adjuvant chemotherapy after local treatment in apparently localized drug-sensitive childhood cancers was found generally to improve the outcome compared with a 'wait and see' policy. These results paved the way for the evaluation of combination chemotherapy as a modality for treatment of common types of adult cancers, initially in advanced stages of disease, and later as adjuvant treatment in patients with 'high-risk' local disease. These clinical trials established that, while some common cancers in adults were sensitive to chemotherapy, complete tumour regression was rare, and many tumour types were refractory to standard chemotherapy. These findings led to the evaluation of 'high-dose' chemotherapy regimes, and to regional chemotherapy undertaken with the goal of achieving higher drug concentrations in tumours than were likely with intravenous treatment. These strategies have continued to merit study in drug-sensitive tumours but with the drug-resistant tumours they have been largely abandoned.

Overcoming drug resistance

The observation that in drug-sensitive adult cancers complete tumour regression was rare, and that the average duration of tumour response was usually measured in months, directed attention to means of minimizing the prospect of drug resistance and to developing strategies of alternating 'non-cross-resistant' chemotherapy regimens. The Goldie–Coldman model of drug resistance has been influential in the development of current combination chemotherapy schedules[1], and this model has drawn support from experimental chemotherapy in transplanted animal tumours. The concept of utilizing chemotherapy as the initial treatment for patients with locally advanced drug-sensitive tumours (so-called neoadjuvant treatment) evolved during the 1980s with the goal of enhancing the efficacy of subsequent local treatment as well as improving systemic disease control[2]. Preliminary evidence that this strategy was not influencing long-term disease control has directed attention to defining the causes of treatment failure and finding means of improving local control by concurrent chemotherapy and local treatment.

Adjuvant chemotherapy

The place of adjuvant chemotherapy in common types of cancer in adults has been investigated in randomized controlled trials over the past 15 years. The basic strategy has been to apply, as an adjuvant after local treatment, the favoured combination chemotherapy programme which causes tumour response in advanced disease. The earliest adjuvant chemotherapy studies in adults were based on the observation of circulating tumour cells immediately after surgery. Hence perioperative chemotherapy was investigated. Later it was appreciated that microscopic metastases commonly existed at the time of initial presentation and surgery; thereafter adjuvant chemotherapy was continued for a 'reasonable' time.

In germ cell tumours, the value of monitoring tumour markers to determine the duration of treatment became established, but where such markers of residual but clinically undetected disease were not available, adjuvant treatment was initially applied based on 'maintenance' programmes for the treatment of leukaemia. More recently, prospective comparison of different durations of adjuvant treatment has been undertaken. In breast cancer, adjuvant cytotoxic and endocrine treatments have been recognized as modestly effective[3], and, in other adult tumour types, adjuvant therapies continue to be investigated. The importance of proper design of trials and the need for large numbers of patients is now widely accepted, while the use of meta analysis to identify any biologically and clinically significant outcomes of adjuvant treatment has been promoted[4].

Combination chemotherapy – theory and practice

The success of empirical combination chemotherapy developed during the 1960s in curative treatment of leukaemia and lymphoma, and later of some drug-sensitive adult tumour types, led to the promulgation of various *post hoc* principles of designing multidrug therapy regimens. The guiding criterion was to combine drugs known to be active as single agents, in the doses and schedules at which their single agent activity was already proved. Pragmatically, this led to the incorporation of drugs with different modes of toxicity towards normal tissue. The cell cycle, and biochemical consequences of drug action, were also thought to be important, and, thus, combining drugs with differing mechanisms of action and sites of action in the mitotic cycle were favoured considerations. Later, as attention turned towards the importance of drug resistance and its mechanisms, the role of 'non-cross-resistant' drug combinations was investigated. Unfortunately, the latter clinical studies only loosely explored non-cross-resistance, and, perhaps for that reason, the concept has recently been brought into question.

It is now fashionable to question some of the old criteria for selecting drugs for combination chemotherapy, and several groups are combining drugs with similar mechanisms of action but differing mechanisms of resistance (e.g. multiple alkylating agents or multiple antifolates). As yet, the value of these new approaches is not established.

Lessons from treatment of transplanted animal tumours

There has been some contribution from experimental combination chemotherapy of transplanted animal tumours, and from studies of multidrug therapy *in vitro*. These laboratory controlled studies have not always been rigorous in their design or the use of such terms as synergism. Nevertheless, the supra-additive antitumour effects of some multidrug combinations observed *in vitro* and *in vivo* have led to the same cocktails being utilized clinically. During the early 1980s, the interaction of methotrexate and fluorouracil, drugs used frequently in clinical combination chemotherapy, was the subject of detailed laboratory studies[5]. The importance of drug sequence was established *in vitro* and in some transplanted animal tumours. The biochemical basis for the supra-additive drug effects *in vitro* was identified, and several clinical trials utilizing the 'optimal sequence' were commenced. Subsequently, further laboratory studies have highlighted the differences between conditions *in vitro* and those in tumour-bearing mice, compared with those in humans, and the clinical trials have not demonstrated a major effect of methotrexate/ fluorouracil sequence in clinical cancer chemotherapy.

The dogma that combination chemotherapy is always the optimal approach to drug treatment has been questioned in recent years, particularly when the goal of treatment is palliation and not necessarily maximal tumour response. Under these circumstances, the trade-off of increased toxicity must be balanced against the improved response, and, under some circumstances, sequential drug use may be preferable to combination chemotherapy applied at the outset of treatment.

PROSPECTS FOR THE FUTURE

The development of new biological therapies whose toxicity may not be directly related to their therapeutic activity necessitates the development of new methods of drug screening and evaluation. Similarly, the possibility that new drugs may promote cell differentiation rather than cell death requires the introduction of new criteria for assessing the effects of treatment.

It seems certain that, in the short-term, combination chemotherapy and multimodality therapies will continue to be the most widely used forms of treatment in cancer management. However, the incorporation of different endpoints, such as quality of life and patient preference, will complicate the evolution of new regimens for drug treatment.

References

1. Goldie, J. M. and Coldman, R. J. (1979). A mathematical model for relating the drug sensitivity of tumours to the spontaneous mutation rate. *Cancer Treat. Rep.,* **63**, 1727–1733
2. Frei, E. (1982). Clinical cancer research: an embattled species. *Cancer,* **50**, 1979–1992
3. Early Breast Cancer Trialists Cooperative Group, (1988). Effects of adjuvant tamoxifen and of cytotoxic therapy on mortality in early breast cancer: an overview of 61 randomized trials among 28,896 women. *N. Engl. J. Med.,* **319**, 1681–1691
4. Sacks, H. S., Berrier, J., Reitman, D., Ancona-Berk, V. A. and Chalmers, T. C. (1987). Meta-analyses of randomized controlled trials. *N. Engl. J. Med.,* **316**, 450–455
5. Bertino, J. R. (1983). Sequential methotrexate fluorouracil. *Semin. Oncol.,* **10**, Suppl. June.

4
New endocrine therapies for cancer

J. WAXMAN AND N. JAMES

INTRODUCTION

The last decade has seen a change in our approach to the management of patients with cancer. The biochemical basis for the action of many established hormonal agents has become clarified and, as a result of this clarification, there have been rational pharmacological developments. These developments have the aim of producing therapies for cancer that are entirely specific in their activity and lack the side-effects of conventional treatment. This has led to a substantial gain for the patient, not necessarily in terms of increased expectation of cure, but rather in the improved quality of life which has resulted from the use of these new therapies. In recent years, our ideas as to the nature of hormones have changed. The view that a hormone is a systemically acting substance produced in a distant endocrine gland has had to be revised as a result of the discovery of local feedback loops involving growth factors acting in a stimulatory or inhibitory fashion to control cell growth and division. This chapter reviews some of the advances during the past decade in the endocrine therapy of cancer and in our understanding of the biological basis of hormone-dependent malignancies.

PROSTATIC CANCER

Clinical aspects

Gonadotrophin releasing hormone agonists were introduced as alternative treatments for prostatic cancer in the early part of this decade. They provide a medical alternative to orchidectomy without the cardiovascular toxicity of oestrogen therapy. This group of compounds is conventionally thought to act by down-regulation of the pituitary–gonadal axis. A single dose of a gonadotrophin releasing hormone agonist causes supraphysiological release of luteinizing hormone and follicle stimulating hormones from the pituitary, but the repeated administration leads to decreased synthesis and secretion. This is because the conformational change conferred by the amino acid substitution leads to an increased resistance to the action of the pituitary arylamidases

Table 4.1 Leuprolide vs. diethylstilboestrol: long-term follow-up[2]

	Leuprolide	*DES*
Median time to treatment failure (weeks)	51	49
Median duration of survival (weeks)	146	136
Side-effects		
Gynaecomastia	3	49
CVS	10	33
G-1	10	20

DES, diethylstilboestrol; CVS, cardiovascular toxicity, such as heart attacks and strokes

Table 4.2 'Total' androgen ablation for prostatic cancer

Patients:	215 with stage D2 prostatic cancer
Treatment:	205 gonadotrophin releasing hormone analogue and flutamide
	10 orchidectomy and flutamide
Initial response:	CR 26.1%
	PR 30.7%
Median duration of survival:	38.5 months

F. Labrie: Unpublished data July 1988

which degrade endogenous gonadotrophin releasing hormone. This results in an increased pituitary half-life of the agonist and down-regulation of the receptor after initial stimulation[1].

These agonist compounds were initially applied as five or six times daily nasal spray insufflations or daily subcutaneous injection, and response rates equivalent to conventional therapies were obtained. Subsequently, the activity of these compounds was compared in randomized prospective trials with diethylstilboestrol and orchidectomy and an equivalence was found in initial response rate, remission duration and median survival. Most important, all of the side-effects of this group of compounds were found to be much less severe than those seen with oestrogen therapy; they are described in Table 4.1.

It has been suggested[2] that the use of an antiandrogen in combination with a gonadotrophin releasing hormone agonist will provide an advantage to the patient with prostatic cancer in terms of improved initial response rate, duration of remission, and survival. The rationale for this lies in the belief that, in a disease that is androgen dependent, it is important to eliminate all sources of androgen production. Although 95% of serum testosterone is testicular in origin and 5% adrenal, in the prostate, because of local concentrating mechanisms, a much higher proportion of androgens are of adrenal origin. The clinical results of the Canadian studies supporting this hypothesis are represented in Table 4.2. The National Cancer Institute Urological

Table 4.3 NCI intergroup study 0036: 3rd analysis

	Leuprolide	*Leuprolide + flutamide*
Patients	301	304
Complete response	7.1%	7.9%
Partial response	28.2%	35.7%
Median time to progression	13.8 months	16.5 months (p=0.01)
Median survival	28.3 months	>30 months (p=0.01)

E. David Crawford: Unpublished data July 1988

Study Group have investigated this hypothesis in a randomized trial and the results of their study are shown in Table 4.3. It can be seen that there is no significant difference in initial response rate between therapy with single-agent gonadotrophin releasing hormone agonist and combination therapy using agonist plus flutamide which is a pure androgen receptor blocker. However, the median duration of response was slightly increased and the median duration of survival appears marginally greater in the combination therapy group. This study represents a partial vindication of Professor Labrie's claims (see Table 4.2); however, the advantage of combination therapy is modest and the use of flutamide may be associated with side-effects. Gonadotrophin releasing hormone agonist therapy as originally applied is impracticable in an elderly population, and, for this reason, more convenient routes of administration have been investigated. Depot preparations effective in producing sustained release of agonists over prolonged periods of time have recently been developed. There are a number of different depot vehicles, but lactide–glycolide copolymer produces the most consistent and reliable release characteristics which vary according to the ratio of lactide and glycolide within the preparation and its coating. Initial reports have described the successful use of a depot preparation designed to be implanted on a monthly basis. Although this represents an advance, such treatment is still far from ideal. More recently, a preparation leading to effective testosterone suppression if applied on a two-monthly basis has entered into limited clinical study and has been found to be effective[3]. In a small group of patients treated at the Hammersmith Hospital, a new depot, consisting of 10 mg buserelin in the same copolymer base has been given three-monthly to four patients who have been treated for a mean period of fifteen months. During this period of follow-up, all patients maintained castrate levels of testosterone. Thus, it would seem that, in the future, we will be able to offer optimal medical treatment for prostatic cancer in the form of gonadotrophin releasing hormone agonist given three-monthly by depot injection. This offers a real advance to our patients who no longer need to contemplate the increased risk of cardiovascular death from oestrogen therapy or the emotional disadvantages of orchidectomy.

Laboratory developments

Prostatic cancer is the second most common malignancy among men in the Western World. Despite the importance of this disease as a clinical entity, laboratory investigations into the significance of cellular oncogenes have been limited to a few studies. Levels of c-myc RNA were assessed by densitometric scanning of northern blots of RNA from prostatic cancer and benign hypertrophy. Levels were twice as high in the cancer specimens as in benign hypertrophy, but there was no correlation between c-myc RNA levels and tumour stage and grade[4]. The ras oncogene product p21 was assayed by an immunocytochemical method in benign hypertrophy, normal prostatic tissue and malignant prostate. There was no staining in normal and hypertrophic prostatic tissue but material from the prostatic tumours of 23 out of 29 patients stained positively for p21. This staining correlated with histological grade and was positive in all seventeen undifferentiated tumours but in only six of twelve differentiated tumours[5]. Different probes have been used to assess oncogene expression in human prostatic cancer cell lines. Many oncogenes were found to be expressed, the most common of which were Ha-ras, Ki-ras, N-ras, c-myc, c-fos, c-myb, c-fms and c-sis. Short-term cultures were established of the androgen-sensitive PC82 cell line. Androgen was withdrawn from the culture medium and oncogene mRNA levels assayed. It was found that there was a ten-fold reduction in c-fos mRNA over a two-week period and a two-fold reduction in Ha-ras mRNA levels without any change in c-myc expression[6]. Although these findings may represent a non-specific change, it is just possible that androgens induce the expression of specific cellular oncogenes and that these oncogenes are the primary genetic elements that control proliferation.

We have investigated the possibility that, in prostatic cancer, gonadotrophin releasing hormone agonists act at the level of the tumour rather than indirectly through suppression of serum testosterone levels. Gonadotrophin releasing hormone agonist binding has been examined in two human prostatic cancer cell lines. LNCaP is a human hormone-sensitive line derived from a lymph node metastasis and DU145 is a human hormone-insensitive cell line derived from a brain secondary. These cell lines were established in culture and the binding of gonadotrophin releasing hormone assessed by Scatchard analysis. The DU145 cell line had a binding constant of 10^{-5}M and the LNCaP line had a binding constant of 10^{-8}M. The binding in the hormone-insensitive cell line was almost completely abolished by protease substrate which indicates that the binding is non-specific. Protease substrate had no effect upon binding in the human hormone-sensitive cell line. Cell culture media were assayed for the presence of gonadotrophin-like peptide using a radioimmunoassay. Culture media contained a gonadotrophin releasing hormone-like peptide at a concentration of 70 pg/ml. Growth stimulatory experiments were carried out with the LNCaP cell line and it was found that gonadotrophin releasing hormone agonists had a direct stimulatory effect on cell growth that was dependent upon their concentration within the culture media[7]. A novel antibody directed against the bovine pituitary gonadotrophin releasing hormone receptor was applied to human

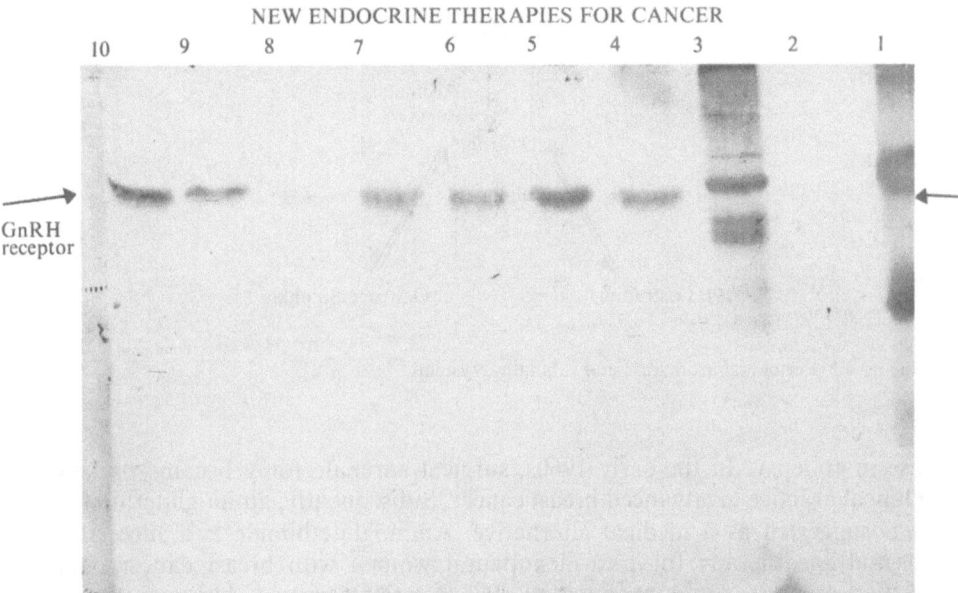

Figure 4.1 Western immunoblotting in benign and malignant prostatic tumours
1. Protein markers. 2. Negative control (hypothalamus). 3. Positive control (pituitary). 4–10.
Prostatic specimens

prostatic tumours and Western immunoblotting performed. Western immunoblotting was positive in these tumours with variable staining in different specimens (Figure 4.1). These data support the possibility that gonadotrophin releasing hormone and its receptor may be involved in an autocrine loop and that they are implicated in the hormonal regulation of human prostatic cancer.

BREAST CANCER

Clinical aspects

Many of the treatments used in the management of breast cancer have a variety of effects and side-effects. Understanding the biochemical nature of the action of these compounds has led to pharmacological refinements such that agents entirely specific in their effect have recently entered phase I and II clinical studies.

Aromatase inhibitors

Aminoglutethimide was introduced into clinical practice as an anti-epileptic drug. It soon became apparent that this compound had side-effects which led to many patients developing hypoadrenalism and so it was withdrawn from

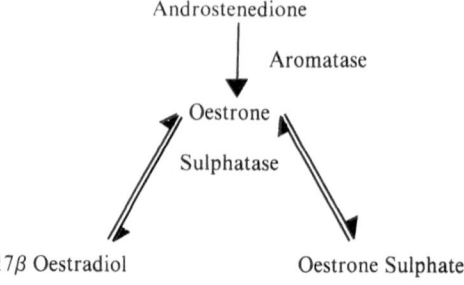

Figure 4.2 Peripheral aromatase and sulphatase systems

use in epilepsy. In the early 1960s, surgical adrenalectomy became part of clinical practice in advanced breast cancer. Subsequently, aminoglutethimide was suggested as a medical alternative. Aminoglutethimide is a successful second-line therapy for post-menopausal women with breast cancer, and responses are seen in approximately 30% of patients treated. Although, in the initial stages of treatment with aminoglutethimide, there is an inhibition of adrenal steroidogenesis, due to hepatic enzyme induction, these effects are temporary and the most important inhibitory effect of aminoglutethimide is on the peripheral aromatase system of enzymes. This system is responsible for the hydroxylation of androstenedione, which is the main adrenal androgenic steroid. The sulphatase system converts oestrone, the product of this reaction, to 17 β-oestradiol and oestrone sulphate (Figure 4.2). This reaction takes place in fat, skeletal muscle and liver. In the dosages conventionally used, aminoglutethimide has significant side-effects in 40 to 60% of patients and these include nausea, vomiting, skin rashes and lethargy. Less commonly, bone marrow toxicity is reported. Because of these side-effects, agents that are more specific in their effects are required. A series of compounds having structural similarities to androstenedione have been investigated as agents to inhibit the aromatase system. In preclinical studies, one of the most successful is a compound called 4-OH-androstenedione. This compound was found to inhibit ovarian steroidogenesis, androstenedione aromatization in tumours and lead to the regression of breast cancers in experimental animal models[8]. The first clinical trials were published in the middle of this decade and responses were reported in three out of eleven patients treated. These responses were without the toxicity of aminoglutethimide. The studies have been expanded[9] and the agent, which was initially formulated as an intra-muscular preparation, can now be given orally. Over one hundred patients have been treated and a response rate equivalent to aminoglutethimide without the side-effects of aminoglutethimide has been described (R. C. Coombes, personal communication). There have been significant problems in the manufacture of aromatase inhibitors, however, and it is hoped that, in the future, when the production problems have been sorted out, this compound will offer a real improvement in the quality of life for women with breast cancer.

Tamoxifen analogues

Tamoxifen has a major role as a first-line endocrine agent for the treatment of breast cancer both in premenopausal and postmenopausal groups of patients. Two important clinical studies have demonstrated the additional value of tamoxifen in an adjuvant setting, where it provides an advantage both in terms of disease-free interval and overall survival for women with breast cancer[10] (see also Chapter 10). Tamoxifen, although safe, is not a perfect compound. A very small percentage of patients treated with it will develop abdominal pain, and, very rarely, retinal degeneration is reported. Tamoxifen is a partial oestrogen agonist, and, in approximately 10% of patients with breast cancer metastatic to bone, the drug may cause tumour flare with increased bone pain and hypercalcaemia. As a result, attempts have been made to develop pure oestrogen antagonists without stimulatory effect. Additional urgency surrounds the need to develop these compounds. This is because an increased incidence of endometrial cancer has been reported in women having breast cancer treated with tamoxifen, again thought to be due to the partial oestrogen agonist effects of tamoxifen[11]. A number of compounds have been investigated; amongst the most successful is toremifene, a triphenyl ethylene anti-oestrogen which was first synthesized in the early 1980s. Animal and cell culture studies have shown this compound to have similar antineoplastic effects to tamoxifen. Toremifene binds specifically and with high affinity to oestrogen receptors, and this binding is competitive with oestradiol. Testing in animals, measuring uterine weight after treatment, shows a dose-dependent inhibition of growth. Toremifene has an inhibitory dose-dependent effect upon the growth of MCF7 cells in culture. In addition, toremifene inhibits the growth of dimethylbenzanthracene-induced mammary carcinomas in rats, both decreasing the number of new tumours formed and inhibiting existing tumour development[12]. A number of limited clinical studies have now appeared showing responses in four out of eight and three out of twelve patients with locally advanced or recurrent breast cancer who had previously failed to respond to endocrine treatments. All responses occurred in postmenopausal women[13]. This compound has not been investigated in premenopausal patients. Virtually no side-effects from treatment have been reported.

If it can be confirmed that toremifene is safe and without any stimulatory effect, it may be that this compound will offer an advance over conventional hormonal treatment using tamoxifen.

Laboratory developments

Growth factors

The c-Neu oncogene was identified following transfection assays with DNA from chemically-induced central nervous system tumours in rats. It encodes a 185 000 Da protein, p185. c-Neu is structurally related to c-ErbB-1, which partly encodes the epidermal growth factor (EGF) receptor. The human homologue of c-Neu is termed c-ErbB-2. This encodes a 190 000 Da protein with tyrosine kinase activity. Overexpression of the c-ErbB-2 protein, and point mutations within the molecule, have been reported in breast, bladder and brain tumours. EGF receptor status of breast tumours has been found to relate to prognosis. This correlation is independent of oestrogen receptor status and is of particular interest because it may be a better prognostic indicator than the oestrogen receptor itself[14]. This is because a significant proportion of oestrogen receptor-positive patients fail to respond to endocrine therapy and a proportion of receptor-negative patients do respond. It is hoped that EGF receptor status may take over from oestrogen receptor status as a predictor for response to hormonal therapies.

Transforming growth factor alpha (TGFα) and its mRNA can be demonstrated at high concentrations in culture media and MCF-7 cells respectively when growth has been stimulated with 17β-oestradiol. This finding in cell lines has been confirmed in biopsy material, where TGFα mRNA was found to be present more frequently in oestrogen receptor-negative than in oestrogen receptor-positive tumours. As TGFα is one of the ligands for the epidermal growth factor receptor, it is of great interest that there is a strong correlation between the presence of TGFα mRNA and epidermal growth factor receptor positivity, implicating this receptor and one of its ligands in an autocrine loop[15].

Another growth factor, insulin-like growth factor-1 (IGF-1), is produced by breast cancer cells. The addition of 17β-oestradiol to MCF-7 cells grown in culture results in a five-fold increase in the local concentration of this insulin-like growth factor. The increase can be limited by anti-oestrogens. This result in a hormone-dependent cell line is in marked contrast to hormone-independent lines where the addition of 17β-oestradiol fails to alter insulin-like growth factor-1 production[16].

EGF, TGFα and IGF-1 are all stimulatory to cell growth, and this is in contrast to transforming growth factor beta (TGFβ) which is one of the most extensively investigated inhibitory growth factors. Its production is stimulated by anti-oestrogens and inhibited by oestrogens. The growth of a variant MCF-7 cell line which is oestrogen receptor positive but hormone independent can be inhibited by transforming growth factor beta. This line expresses TGFβ mRNA[17]. This suggests that in this cell line hormone independence has two components, a permanent setting of proliferative signals to 'on' coupled with an inability to respond to 'off' signals.

Steroid hormone receptor structure and function

One of the most interesting observations in recent years in breast cancer has been the revelation of the homology between steroid receptor genes, the oncogene v-erbA, and its cellular homologue c-erbA. The c-erbA gene has been cloned and its protein product found to be the thyroid hormone receptor. There are significant structural homologies between this oncogene and the steroid hormone receptor genes[18]. These homologies occur in the DNA-binding section of the oncoprotein, suggesting that there has been mechanistic conservation during the evolution of these proteins.

OVARIAN MALIGNANCY

Clinical aspects

The last decade has seen the development of complicated cytotoxic chemo-therapy programmes for the treatment of ovarian cancer. With their investigation has come the realization that, despite initial hopes, there is no long-term advantage, in terms of increased patient survival, in using combination therapies compared with single-agent regimens.

As a result of this therapeutic disappointment, new treatments have been actively sought. It has been found that there is a substantial hormonal basis to ovarian malignancy. Endocrine changes are found on presentation and can be used to predict relapse prior to its clinical manifestation. Abnormal serum levels of pituitary gonadotrophins and ovarian steroid secretion have been described in ovarian epithelial malignancy compared with matched controls. Hormonal treatments, such as tamoxifen, have been used to treat patients with ovarian cancer to little effect. The gonadotrophin releasing hormone agonists have also been applied as treatments for recurrent ovarian cancer. The first report of the effect of this group of compounds was of the use of decaptyl to treat a 78-year-old woman with pelvic nodal metastases. Her case was reported in 1986. Since that time, more patients have been treated with the same analogue and, in a recent update, responses (described according to criteria defined by the Union Internationale contre le Cancer) were reported in six out of thirty-four patients[19]. All of these patients had had previous cytotoxic chemotherapy. The biochemical basis for response is unclear. The effect of the agonists may be direct, at the level of the tumour itself, for the presence of hormonal receptors in ovarian cancer is well described. In epithelial ovarian cancer cells, receptors for the steroid hormones, oestradiol and progesterone, as well as for luteinizing hormone (LH) have been identified. Response may relate to changes in serum LH levels which follow the use of agonist, or to any secondary change in sex hormone or steroid levels.

Laboratory developments

The existence of Mullerian inhibiting substance was first postulated in the early part of the century to explain the phenomenon of the freemartin calf, the masculinized female of a dizygotic twin pair. Mullerian inhibitory substance is produced early in foetal life by the testis and causes a regression of the Mullerian duct system which, in the normal female, develops into the lower genital tract. This peptide is present in the foetal and new-born calf testis in significant amounts and its production decreases during the early weeks of infant life. Bovine testis has been used as a source of this peptide hormone which has been purified and its structure identified as a glyco-protein dimer linked by disulphide bonds. The gene for the glycoprotein has been cloned and contains 640 base pairs. It displays striking structural homology with the gene for TGFα[20]. There has been interest in the possible use of this compound for treating gynaecological tumours. Colony-forming assays were performed on twenty-eight gynaecological tumours, eleven of which showed more than 60% inhibition of colony growth by Mullerian inhibiting substance[21]. It may be that these effects are non-specific because a melanoma and adenocarcinoma of pulmonary origin were also subject to growth inhibition by this substance. Alternatively, it may just be true that this compound is important, and if so, its role will be established when significant amounts of purified, cloned, Mullerian inhibiting substance become available for clinical trial.

CARCINOID TUMOURS

Clinical advances

Somatostatin is a tetradecapeptide synthesized widely throughout the central nervous system and gastrointestinal tract. It has been described as a pan-endocrine bleach. Its many effects include the inhibition of growth hormone release, decreased pancreatic exocrine and endocrine function, and decreased gastric acid secretion. It was suggested that somatostatin might have a role in the treatment of patients with acromegaly; however, the plasma half-life of somatostatin is three minutes and, because of this, treatment could only be given as a continuous infusion which would be impractical. In 1980, Bauer and colleagues synthesized a synthetic analogue of somatostatin termed SMS201995 (sandostatin) which retained all of the endocrine features of the parent molecule but had a much longer half-life (Figure 4.3). This octapeptide has been used to treat a number of endocrine malignancies besides acromegaly and these include glucagonomas, vipomas, carcinoid tumours and insulinomas. Sandostatin is given by subcutaneous injection and its use results in marked relief of the symptoms caused by the secretory products of the tumours. As a result, the watery diarrhoea of vipomas and the hypo-glycaemia of insulinomas resolves. One of the most dramatic effects of treatment is the relief of the 5-hydroxytryptamine-like effects that are found in patients with metastatic carcinoid[22]. A number of studies have been under-taken to investigate whether somatostatin analogues have the potential to cause any regression of human tumours. The consensus view is that there is no effect; however, it may be that a partial or minimal response may be obtained using somatostatin analogues in combination with interferon.

SOMATOSTATIN

H-Ala-Gly-Cys-Lys-Asn-Phe-Phe-Trp-Lys-Thr-Lys-Thr-Phe-Thr-Ser-Cys-OH

SMS 201 995

H-D-Phe-Cys-Phe-D-Trp-Lys-Thr-Cys-Thr-ol,acetate

Figure 4.3 The structure of somatostatin and its long acting analogue SMS 201 995

CONCLUSIONS

Although clinical advances over the last decade have not led to any substantial change in the prospects of cure, there is no doubt that the wider application of the newer therapies will improve the quality of life for people with cancer. Developments in molecular biology have revealed the possibility of our eventually understanding the biological basis of cancer, and never has this possibility seemed more likely. It is to be hoped that, in the next decade of scientific endeavour, this once-impossible insight will dawn.

References

1. Waxman, J. H. (1987). Gonadotrophin hormone releasing analogues open new doors in cancer treatment. *Br. Med. J.,* **295**, 1084–1085
2. Labrie, F., Dupont, A., Belanger, A., Giguere, M., Lacoursiere, Y., Emond, J., Monfette, G. and Bergeron, V. (1985). Combination therapy with flutamide and castration (LHRH agonist or orchiectomy) in advanced prostate cancer: A marked improvement in response and survival. *J. Steroid Biochem.,* **23**, 833–841
3. Waxman, J. H., Sandow, J., Abel, P., Farah, N., O'Donoghue, E. P. N., Fleming, J., Cox, J., Sikora, K. and Williams, G. (1989). Two-monthly depot gonadotrophin releasing hormone agonist (Buserelin) for treatment of prostatic cancer. *Acta Endocrinol.,* **120**, 315–318
4. Fleming, W. H., Hamel, A., MacDonald, R., Ramsey, E., Pettigrew, N. M., Johnston, B., Dodd, J. G. and Matusik, R. J. (1986). Expression of the c-myc protooncogene in human prostatic carcinoma and benign prostatic hyperplasia. *Cancer Res.,* **46**, 1535–1538
5. Viola, M. V., Fromowitz, F., Oravez, S., Deb, S., Finkel, G., Lundy, J., Hand, P., Thor, A. and Schlom, J. (1986). Expression of ras oncogene p21 in prostate cancer. *N. Engl. J. Med.,* **314**, 133–137
6. Rijinders, A. W. M., van der Korput, J. A. G. M., van Steenbrugge, G. J., Romijn, J. C. and Trapman, J. (1985). Expression of cellular oncogenes in human prostatic carcinoma cell lines. *Biochem. Biophys. Res. Commun.,* **132**, **2**, 548–554
7. Qayum, A., Scaletsky, R. and Waxman, J. (1990). Autocrine stimulation by gonadotrophin-releasing hormone-like factors of human hormone-responsive prostate cancer cells in culture. In Newling, D. W. (ed.) *Prostate Cancer and Testicular Cancer EORTC Genito-Urinary Group Monograph 7.* (New York: Alan R. Liss) (in press)
8. Brodie, A. M. H. and Longcope, C. (1980). Inhibition of peripheral aromatization by aromatase inhibitors, 4-hydroxy- and 4-acetoxy-androstene-3,17-dione. *Endocrinology,* **106**, **1**, 19–21
9. Dowsett, M., Goss, P. E., Powles, T. J., Hutchinson, G., Brodie, A. M. H., Jeffcoate, S. L. and Coombes, R. C. (1987). Use of the aromatase inhibitor 4-hydroxyandrostenedione in postmenopausal breast cancer: optimization of therapeutic dose and route. *Cancer Res.,* **47**, 1957–1961
10. Breast Cancer Trials Committee (MRC) Edinburgh (1987). Adjuvant tamoxifen in the management of operable breast cancer: the Scottish trial. *Lancet,* **2**, 171–175
11. Fornander, T., Cedermark, B., Mattsson, A., Skoog, L., Theve, T., Askergren, J., Rutqvist, L. E., Glas, U., Silfversward, C., Somell, A., Wilking, N. and Hjalmar, M. (1989). Adjuvant tamoxifen in early breast cancer: occurrence of new primary cancers. *Lancet,* **1** 117–119
12. Kallio, S., Kangas, L., Blanco, G., Johansson, R., Karjalainen, A., Perila, M., Piippo, I., Sundquist, H., Sodervall, M. and Toivola, R. (1986). A new triphenylethylene compound, Fc-1157a. I. Hormonal effects. *Cancer Chemother. Pharmacol.,* **17**, 103–108
13. Valavaara, R., Pyrhonen, S., Heikkinen, M., Rissanen, P., Blanco, G., Nordman, E., Taskinen, P. and Hajba, A. (1985). FC 1157a in the treatment of advanced breast cancer. Phase II Clinical investigation. Abstract 661 in 3rd ECCO meeting, June 16–20, Stockholm
14. Berger, M. S., Locher, G. W., Saurer, S., Gullick, W. J., Waterfield, M. D., Groner, B. and Hynes, N. E. (1988). C-erbB2 gene amplification and protein expression in human breast

carcinoma correlates with nodal status and nuclear grading. *Cancer Res.,* **48**, 1238–1242

15. Salamon, D. S., Zweibel, J. A., Baro, M., Losoonczy, I., Fehnel, P. and Kidwell, W. R. (1984). Presence of transforming growth factors in human breast cancer cells. *Cancer Res.,* **44**, 4069–77

16. Huff, K. K., Krabbe, C., Kaufman, D., Gabbary, K. H. and Dixon, R. B. (1986). Hormonal regulation of insulin-like growth factor I (IGF-1) Secretion from MCF-7 human breast cancer cells. *Proc. Endocr. Soc. Analieus C A*, Abstr. 205

17. Krabbe, C., Huff, K., Wakefield, L., Lippman, M. E. and Dixon, R. B. (1987). Evidence that TGFB is a hormonally regulated negative growth factor in human breast cancer cells. *Cell,* **48**, 417

18. Green, S., Walter, P., Kumar, V., Krust, A., Bornert, J., Argos, P. and Chambon, P. (1986). Human oestrogen receptor cDNA sequence, expression and homology to v-erb-A. *Nature (London)* **320**, 134–139

19. Parmar, H., Rustin, G., Lightman, S., Phillips, R., Hanham, J. and Schally, A. (1988). Response to D-Trp-6-luteinising hormone releasing hormone (decapeptyl) microcapsules in advanced ovarian cancer. *Br. Med. J.,* **296**, 1229.

20. Cate, R. L., Mattaliano, R. J., Hession, C., Tizard, R., Farber, N. M., Cheung, A., Ninfa, E. G., Frey, A. Z., Gash, D. J., Chow, E. P., Fisher, R. A., Bertonis, J. M., Torres, G., Wallner, B. P., Ramachandran, K. L., Ragin, R. C., Manganaro, T. F., MacLaughlin, D. T. and Donahoe, P. K. (1986). Isolation of the bovine and human genes for mullerian inhibiting substance and expression of the human gene in animal cells. *Cell,* **45**, 685–698

21. Fuller, A. F., Krane, I. M., Budzik, G. P. and Donahoe, P. K. (1985). Mullerian inhibiting substance reduction of colony growth of human gynecologic cancers in a stem cell assay. *Gynecol. Oncol.,* **22**, 135–148

22. Bloom, S. R. and Polak, J. M. (1987). Somatostatin. *Br. Med. J.,* **295**, 288–290

5
Drug resistance and the problem of treatment failure

R. BROWN AND S.B. KAYE

WHAT DO WE MEAN BY TREATMENT FAILURE?

Although the use of chemotherapy as a major form of treatment for malignant disease is in its infancy, its introduction 40 years ago has led to significant advances in treatment of certain forms of cancer. However, for many types of cancer, the spectre of treatment failure is all too familiar. Cancer treatment frequently involves a combination of local therapy, i.e. surgery and/or radiotherapy, and systemic therapy, i.e. chemotherapy and/or hormone therapy. Treatment failure, the failure of systemic therapy to control tumour growth, appears in a variety of ways. These range from rapid tumour growth with little evidence of impact of any treatment leading to death within months, to a much more prolonged natural history in which systemic treatment may initially appear effective, but in which disease relapse may occur years later. This chapter will focus on failure of cytotoxic drug therapy, and, in particular, on the role of cellular drug resistance. This frequent and frustrating problem is attracting increasing attention from many research groups. Their aim is to acquire a better insight into the mechanisms involved, as a result of which rational strategies aimed at circumvention of resistance can be developed.

Cytotoxic drug resistance appears to take two main clinical forms. Firstly, several types of cancer appear to respond only infrequently to initial treatment with cytotoxic drugs (in perhaps 15% to 20% of cases). This has been termed *intrinsic drug resistance*, and examples include colorectal cancer, non-small-cell lung cancer, renal cancer, sarcoma and melanoma. Secondly, other cancer types do respond frequently to initial treatment with many agents (in at least 50% to 70% of cases) only for the cancer to regrow in the majority of cases, in the face of further chemotherapy, generally proving fatal. This is termed *acquired drug resistance* and examples include small-cell lung cancer, breast cancer, ovarian cancer, cervical cancer, bladder cancer and head and neck cancer. Are intrinsic and acquired cytotoxic drug resistance fundamentally different biological processes? Insufficient data exist at present to answer this question, but it appears probable that common mechanisms can give rise to drug resistance in different tumour types. This question will be discussed further in the next section.

Three categories of agents can be defined on the basis that, at present, they are reckoned to be most active against the tumours listed above: (a) natural products, particularly adriamycin; (b) cisplatin and other alkylating agents; (c) antimetabolites, e.g. methotrexate and 5-fluorouracil.

(a) Adriamycin is amongst the most widely used of cytotoxic agents, particularly in breast cancer and small-cell lung cancer, which together probably account for a large proportion of the chemotherapy used in 1988. In both these tumours, adriamycin is one of the most active single agents; indeed in breast cancer treatment with full-dose adriamycin may be as effective as any drug combination[1]. Similarly, in sarcoma, adriamycin is the standard therapeutic agent by which other drug schedules are currently being judged[2]. Although cardiac toxicity becomes a problem after a certain cumulative dose has been given, in practice, the utility of adriamycin is not severely limited by this but by the development of resistance.

(b) Cisplatin is now recognized as rivalling adriamycin in the breadth of its activity against common epithelial cancers. It has had major impact in the treatment of testicular and ovarian cancer[3], but it is also amongst the most active agents for treatment of squamous cell cancers, such as non-small-cell lung cancer, cervical cancer, bladder cancer and head and neck cancer.

(c) Two of the most widely used antimetabolites in solid tumours are methotrexate and 5-fluorouracil. Methotrexate is among the most active drugs in head and neck and bladder cancer, while 5-fluorouracil is the most active agent (albeit with a response rate of only 15% to 20%) in colorectal cancer[4].

Given this well-documented level of antitumour activity, why is it that the drugs fail, either initially or after initial response, to produce objective shrinkage of tumours? One possibility is that a resistant subpopulation of cells is present in the tumour at the time of treatment and this dominates the clinical effects of therapy. Before discussing in some detail how this might arise, it is important to recognize that other clinical factors may apply. Failure to respond to treatment could be the result of inadequate exposure of tumour cells to the drug concerned. This could be caused by inadequate dosage, perhaps because of the patient's poor general condition or because of excessive systemic toxicity. Inadequate drug exposure of the tumour cells could also arise due to their localization in sites such as brain, testis, or the necrotic centre of large tumour masses[5]. Other factors relating to the host, rather than the tumour, include changes in metabolic profiles, such as liver function, which will determine rates of drug activation or inactivation in certain cases. Overall, these factors may give rise to so-called pharmacological resistance, and manoeuvres to overcome this include the use of high-dose chemotherapy and cytotoxic drug targeting, both of which will be discussed in detail in other chapters.

Finally, the proliferative state of the tumour cells at the time of drug exposure may have some bearing on the efficacy of chemotherapy[6]. It has been suggested that drug resistance can occur if an inadequate proportion of tumour cells are in the appropriate phase of the cell cycle during drug administration. However, the clinical data in support of this hypothesis are unconvincing. Furthermore, although it might be expected that, in general, the most rapidly dividing tumour cells would be the most sensitive, in practice, it is a common clinical observation that tumours with apparently very short doubling times may be quite refractory to treatment. Thus, kinetic factors, while probably affecting drug sensitivity to some degree, are unlikely to be of prime importance in the development of drug resistance.

WHAT MECHANISMS OF DRUG RESISTANCE HAVE SO FAR BEEN IDENTIFIED?

Mechanisms of drug resistance have been intensively studied in cells selected in tissue culture that are resistant to various therapeutic agents[7-9]. These resistant cell lines have allowed the genetic and molecular basis of some types of drug resistance to be elucidated and have led to the development of molecular tools for the analysis of treatment failure in human cancer. In this section, we will describe the main types of mechanisms so far identified which can lead to the various forms of drug resistance to commonly used therapeutic agents, such as adriamycin, cisplatin and some antimetabolites. In later sections, we will discuss the evidence for and against these alterations occurring in human tumours which fail to respond to treatment and the implications for treatment approaches that could overcome resistance in tumours.

Alteration in drug transport

One mechanism of drug resistance involves the flux of the cytotoxic drug across the plasma membrane. If a transport mechanism common to several drugs is affected, the cells will become cross-resistant to these drugs. Biedler and Riehm[10] were the first to show that cell lines made resistant to a single chemotherapeutic agent by stepwise incubation in increasing amounts of the drug could also be resistant to other structurally unrelated cytotoxic compounds. This phenomenon of broad resistance was termed 'pleiotropic or multi-drug resistance' or 'MDR'. In their studies, they showed that cells made resistant to dactinomycin were cross-resistant to structurally dissimilar drugs including daunomycin and vinblastine. Ling and his colleagues[11] showed that MDR was associated with decreased intracellular drug accumulation and they were the first to identify the presence of an approximately 170 000 Dalton plasma membrane-associated glycoprotein (P-glycoprotein) in their MDR cells that was undetectable in the parental drug-sensitive cells. Furthermore, Ling's group demonstrated that membrane P-glycoprotein content correlated both with the degree of decrease in intracellular accumulation of the drug[12] and the degree of resistance exhibited by these cells[13].

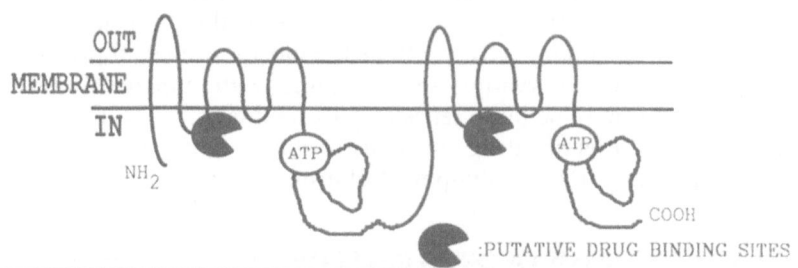

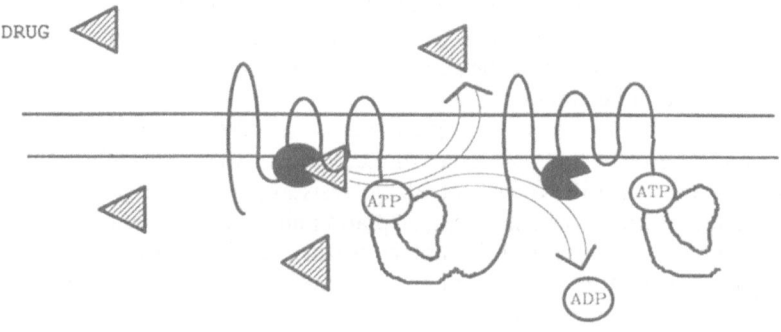

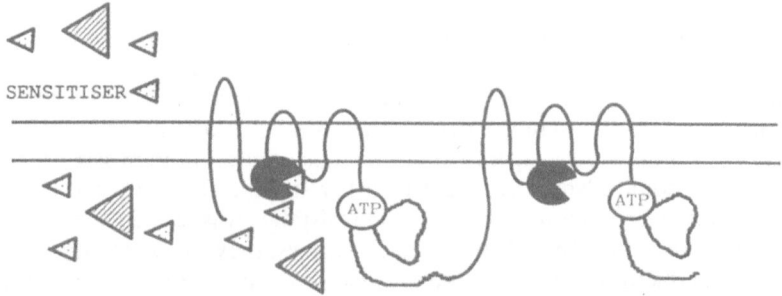

Figure 5.1 Model of P-glycoprotein structure and mechanism of action. (1) The transmembrane domains of P-glycoprotein, the ATP binding sites and potential binding sites for drugs are schematically shown. (2) Drug enters the cell by diffusion, binds to P-glycoprotein; ATP is hydrolysed to ADP and the drug is moved outside the cell. (3) Sensitizer drugs capable of modifying the MDR phenotype may act by competing with cytotoxic drugs for binding to P-glycoprotein

Many subsequent studies have demonstrated that cells with MDR pheno-type have increased expression of the gene encoding the P-glycoprotein, the *mdr1* gene[14-20]. Although *mdr1* is a member of a gene family, there is no evidence for involvement of the other *mdr* genes in the MDR phenotype[21]. An accumulation of evidence suggests that P-glycoprotein acts as an energy-dependent drug efflux pump (see Figure 5.1). Purified P-glycoprotein has been shown to bind photoaffinity-labelled analogues of vinblastine, a reaction that is competitively inhibited by vinblastine as well as anthracyclines[22]. Furthermore, several agents, including the calcium-channel blocker verapamil, can also bind to P-glycoprotein and can compete with the vinblas-tine analogues for binding to P-glycoprotein[23]. Full-length cDNA sequences encoding the mouse[24] and human[25] P-glycoprotein have been isolated and their nucleotide sequence determined. The deduced amino acid sequence of this protein shows structural similarities to well-characterized bacterial membrane transport proteins and, in particular, to the HLY B protein which is involved in actively exporting molecules from the cytoplasm to the external medium[26].

The most direct evidence for the role of P-glycoprotein in the MDR phenotype has come from gene transfer experiments with the *mdr1* gene. Full-length cDNAs for P-glycoprotein have been subcloned into eukaryotic expression vectors and drug-sensitive cells transfected with this gene were shown to have a drug-resistant phenotype[27]. This clearly demonstrates that increased expression of P-glycoprotein can confer the MDR phenotype. However, the frequently observed preferential resistance to the drug used in selection cannot simply be explained by variations in levels of P-glycoprotein expression. Preferential resistance to colchicine has been shown to arise, not only by increased *mdr1* expression, but also to involve a cluster of nucleotide substitutions in the *mdr1* gene, resulting in a single amino acid substitution at position 185 of P-glycoprotein[28]. Transfection of the mutated gene, but not the wild-type, results in preferential resistance to colchicine (see Table 5.1). This has led to the hypothesis that amino acid 185 plays a key role in P-glycoprotein-drug interaction and that its substitution in colchicine-selected cells results in altered affinity of P-glycoprotein for different drugs. This suggests that mutations which increase expression of the *mdr1* gene and/or structural gene mutations in the gene may play a role in MDR.

Post-transcriptional changes in gene expression can lead to differences in activities of proteins. Alternative splicing patterns[29] and polyadenylylation sites[30] have been shown for the *mdr* genes. These observations raise the possibility that modifications of the RNA product of the *mdr* gene may result in varying levels of resistance or differing relative cross-resistance to drugs. However, direct evidence for this hypothesis, such as difference in post-transcriptional modification of *mdr* gene products in resistant cells compared with sensitive cells, has not, as yet, been demonstrated. Alterations in post-translational modifications of the P-glycoprotein, such as phosphoryl-ation, may have a role in determining the degree of resistance[31,32]. Further-more, verapamil and trifluoperazine, which inhibit the active drug efflux and restore drug sensitivity in resistant cells, have been shown to cause an increase in the phosphorylation of the P-glycoprotein[33]. However, it is still not clear

Table 5.1 (a) Properties of multidrug resistant cell lines (adapted from Choi *et al.*, 1988). MDR cell lines were selected by increasing exposure to vinblastine (**KB**-vinblastine) or colchicine (**KB**-colchicine) and have preferential resistance to the drug used in the initial selection. Increased copy number and mRNA expression of the *mdr1* gene has been observed in these MDR cell lines

Cell line	Relative resistance			mdr1 gene copy number	mdr1 mRNA expression	Amino acid 185
	Colchicine	Vinblastine	Adriamycin			
KB	1	1	1	1	0.1	Glycine
KB-vinblastine	171	213	422	100	320	Glycine
KB-colchicine	1750	159	254	30	378	Valine

(b) Sequence around amino acid 185 in P-glycoprotein. The amino acid sequence (top line) and DNA sequence (bottom line) of the **KB** and **KB**-vinblastine cell lines are shown. The **KB**-colchicine cell line has a mutated DNA sequence in this region (alterations are shown in boxes). The numbers on the top line refer to the amino acid sequence of the **P**-glycoprotein and the numbers on the bottom line refer to the nucleotide sequence of the cDNA of *mdr1*. Mutations have been observed at nucleotide numbers 540, 554 and 555. However, only the mutations at 554 and 555 lead to an altered amino acid, substituting valine for glycine in the colchicine-selected line

KB and KB-vinblastine:

							185				
Asp	Val	Ser	Lys	Ile	Asn	Glu	Gly	Ile	Gly	Asp	Lys
GAT	GTC	TC[C]	AAG	ATT	AAT	GAA	[Gly] G[GA]	ATT	GGT	GAC	AAA
		540									

KB-colchicine:

Asp	Val	Ser	Lys	Ile	Asn	Glu	[Val]	Ile	Gly	Asp	Lys
GAT	GTC	TC[T]	AAG	ATT	AAT	GAA	G[TT]	ATT	GGT	GAC	AAA
		540					554 555				

from these studies if phosphorylation is having a direct effect in regulating activity of the P-glycoprotein or if the changes are secondary effects of the pleiotropic activity of these sensitizer drugs.

Although alteration in expression of the P-glycoprotein is, at present, the best characterized mechanism involved in the development of MDR, it is not the only mechanism capable of conferring cross-resistance to structurally unrelated drugs or of increasing resistance to specific drugs[34]. Other changes associated with the plasma membrane have been suggested as being involved in resistance to drugs of the MDR phenotype as well as other drugs. Influx of drug may differ in resistant cells, although this will depend on the mechanism of transport of the particular drug through the membrane and will be limited to the types of change which do not grossly affect normal viability of the cell. Binding of drug by certain molecules present in the plasma membrane, preventing uptake of drug by the cell, has been suggested as leading to reduced cytotoxicity of cisplatin[35]. Intracellular binding of drug by proteins leading to increased localization of drug in vesicles and subsequent exocytosis via the endosome–lysosome system has also been suggested as a possible means of increased resistance to cytotoxic drugs[34,36]. The possible role of the 170 kDa P-glycoprotein in this process has not been fully elucidated.

Cell-to-cell interactions have also been suggested to play a role in response of cells to cytotoxic drugs[37]. Intercellular transfer of small cytoplasmic ions and molecules has long been known to allow metabolic co-operation between cells[38]. This has been shown to allow sensitive cells to survive drug selection[39]. Intercellular transport of drugs via gap junctions has been particularly implicated, since most of the therapeutic drugs used pass through a cytoplasmic pool and are small enough to be able to pass through intercellular gap junctions[40]. This could lead to effective dilution of the drug from the target cells, especially if the adjacent cells have a high capacity for drug detoxification or an active efflux process. Effects of intercellular communication within tumours, as well as communication between tumours and adjacent normal cells, on response of tumours to chemotherapeutic drugs will be an interesting area of future research.

Drug activation and inactivation

There are enzymes present in cells which are able to convert drugs either into more active cytotoxic forms or into inactive non-cytotoxic forms. Changes in any of these metabolic pathways have been suggested as possible mechanisms of increased drug resistance[41,42].

The cytochrome P_1450 enzymes, such as aryl hydrocarbon hydroxylase (AHH), convert many drugs into their active forms by adding oxygen and hydroxyl groups to their structures and making them more hydrophilic and electrophilic. AHH activity has been reported to be reduced in adriamycin-resistant cells[9]. These Adr-resistant cells are also resistant to ellipticine, a cytotoxin that depends on P_1450 for activation into its cytotoxic form, 9-OH-ellipticine. However, the cells remain as sensitive as the wild-type cells if exposed directly to 9-OH-ellipticine. AHH regulation is linked to the risk of carcinogenesis in mice and humans[43,44]. This is an example of how alteration of expression of a gene during carcinogenesis might have a direct effect on how the tumour will respond to chemotherapy.

The drug-conjugating enzymes, including glutathione S-transferase (GST), can bind to and detoxify a variety of cellular toxins[45]. The GST enzymes are a family of enzymes which conjugate electrophilic substrates with the tripeptide glutathione (GSH), thus making a less toxic and more readily excreted metabolite. GST also prevents oxidative damage, induced by free radicals for instance, through its intrinsic organic peroxidase activity. These features have led to the suggestion that increased GSH and GST levels could lead to resistance to a wide range of therapeutic agents. Depletion of GSH levels of cells by buthionine sulphoximine (BSO) has been shown to increase sensitivity of cells to adriamycin, melphalan and cisplatin[46]. Elevated levels of GSH have been detected in cells resistant to melphalan[47], cisplatin and adriamycin[48]. Each isoenzyme of GST exhibits a unique pattern of substrate specificity, so resistance to specific drugs may be mediated via specific isoenzyme forms. The anionic isoenzyme of GST has been shown to be elevated, both at the protein level and at the RNA level, in adriamycin-resistant human breast cancer cell lines[49,50]. Furthermore, increased activity of two different isoenzymes in the basic class of GST has been implicated in resistance to mechlorethamine[51] and chlorambucil[52].

Glutathione peroxidases catalyse the reduction of potentially toxic peroxides to alcohols with the concomitant oxidation of GSH to its disulphide form (GSSG). GSSG is returned to GSH by reduction at the expense of the coenzyme NADPH. This glutathione redox cycle plays an important role in protecting cells from damage due to lipid peroxidation[53]. An adriamycin-resistant clone of MCF-7 human breast tumour cells has been shown to contain increased glutathione peroxidase activity, and fewer toxic hydroxyl radicals are induced by doxorubicin in these cells[54].

Alterations in drug 'targets'

Another means of increasing resistance to a cytotoxic drug is to decrease its effectiveness at the specific biochemical target that leads to toxicity. For instance, if the drug inhibits a specific enzyme, then increasing the levels of this enzyme in the cell, altering the affinity of the enzyme for the drug, or altering the kinetics of the reaction catalysed by the enzyme could all lead to increased resistance to the drug.

Many antineoplastic drugs, such as anthracenes, anthracenediones, aminoacridines and epipodophyllotoxins, are known to produce protein–DNA cross-links and DNA-strand breaks in cultured mammalian cells as well as in isolated nuclei[55,56]. Nuclear proteins involved in double-strand breakage of DNA have been suggested as possible targets for these drugs. Topoisomerases are enzymes that catalyse changes in the secondary and tertiary structure of DNA by breakage and rejoining of the DNA strands. They are essential cellular enzymes required for DNA replication, gene transcription, maintenance of chromatin structure and DNA recombination[57]. Direct evidence that antitumour drugs could promote DNA cleavage by affecting DNA topoiso-

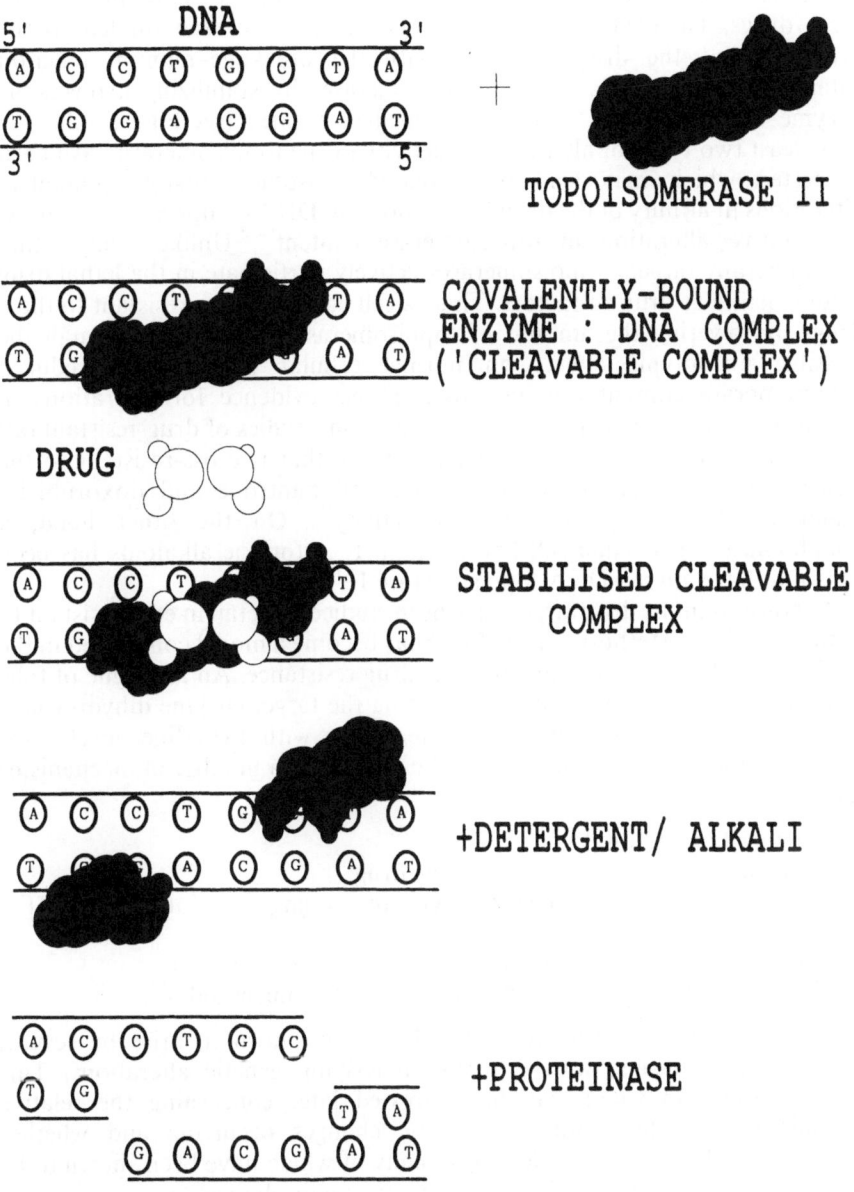

Figure 5.2 Model of action of drugs interacting with topoisomerase II. Topoisomerase II binds covalently to DNA. This step is normally followed by binding of ATP and subsequent strand passage and rejoining. In the presence of drug, the enzyme–DNA complex becomes stabilized. The strand break thus induced can be experimentally observed by detergent or alkali denaturation followed by deproteination

merase and the complex it forms with DNA comes from studies using highly purified topoisomerase II[58,59]. In this purified system, it has been shown that DNA cleavage by topoisomerase II is highly stimulated by the presence of these drugs. Detailed analysis of the DNA cleavage reaction led to the proposal that the drugs interfere with the breakage–reunion reaction catalysed by mammalian DNA topoisomerases by stabilizing a reversible enzyme–DNA complex, termed the 'cleavable complex' (see Figure 5.2).

At least two types of alteration in activity of the topoisomerase have been suggested which may lead to increased resistance: firstly, qualitative alterations in affinity of the drug for the protein–DNA complex; or, secondly, quantitative alteration in topoisomerase content[60]. Unlike many other chemotherapy targets, topoisomerases actively participate in the lethal drug action, acting as drug co-factors. Thus, a cell could become resistant to these drugs by lowering the amount of topoisomerase in the cell, although the possible phenotypic effects on normal cellular processes of reduced topoisomerase content are uncertain. Direct evidence for alterations in topoisomerase is now beginning to emerge from studies of drug-resistant cell lines. An etoposide-resistant hamster cell line that is cross-resistant to the structurally dissimilar agents m-AMSA, mitoxantrone and doxorubicin, manifests altered topoisomerase II activity[60]. On the other hand, a lymphoblastic leukaemic cell line resistant to cytotoxic alkaloids has been shown to have altered DNA topoisomerase I [61].

Alterations in the drug target have been studied in detail in cells resistant to antimetabolites. Methotrexate (MTX) has become a model compound in the study of mechanisms of antimetabolite drug resistance. An analogue of folic acid, its activity is largely due to inhibiting the target enzyme dihydrofolate reductase (DHFR), with consequent interference with thymidine and *de novo* purine synthesis[62]. Resistance to MTX can arise by a number of mechanisms including:

(1) Reduced MTX uptake;
(2) Decreased affinity of DHFR for the drug;
(3) Increased amounts of DHFR enzyme due to amplification of the DHFR gene;
(4) Impaired conversion to polyglutamate species ($MTXglu_n$);
(5) Enhanced salvage of thymidine and/or purine nucleosides[63].

Thus, for a specific drug, resistance has been shown to arise by several different mechanisms, with different underlying genetic alterations. This raises a question which will be addressed later concerning the relative probabilities of these different genetic changes occurring and whether exposure to chemotherapeutic drugs, many of which have been shown to be mutagenic, can influence this probability of genetic change.

5-Fluorouracil (FUra) is another antimetabolite commonly used in chemo-therapy[64]. Two major mechanisms for its cytotoxic activity have been described:

(1) Inhibition of thymidylate synthase (TS) by the FUra metabolite, 5FdUMP, ultimately restricting DNA synthesis, and
(2) Incorporation into RNA following conversion to 5FUTP.

As with MTX, resistance to FUra in cultured cells can be shown to arise through several possible mechanisms. These include:

(1) Inactivation of enzymes involved in metabolizing FUra into the active forms (orotate phosphoribosyl transferase, uridine phosphorylase, uridine kinase);
(2) Structural alterations in TS associated with reduced inhibitor binding affinity;
(3) Elevated levels of TS;
(4) Reduced levels of methylene tetrahydrofolate needed for formation of the FdUMP-TS complex[65].

Repair of drug-induced DNA damage

The majority of chemotherapeutic agents interact directly with DNA and DNA-binding proteins, or inhibit key steps in DNA metabolism. It has, therefore, been suggested that increased resistance to these agents could occur by increased repair of the damage they induce. However, DNA-repair pathways in mammalian cells are poorly understood. Most of our understanding of DNA-repair mechanisms is derived from the analysis of bacterial mutants defective in DNA-repair pathways, which are hypersensitive to DNA-damaging agents[66,67]. A number of mammalian cell lines which display the same characteristics of hypersensitivity towards DNA-damaging agents have now been isolated (including human cell lines from patients with genetic diseases). Many of these cell lines are cross-sensitive to several cytotoxic agents[68], again implying common mechanisms of sensitivity/resistance to structurally unrelated therapeutic agents. Cell lines sensitive to radiation may be of particular use for investigating DNA-repair pathways since, unlike drug-sensitive cells, these clearly cannot be defective in drug transport or metabolism. Isolation of genes able to complement these hypersensitive cell lines is now under way in a number of laboratories[69]. Characterization of these genes will allow a greater understanding of the role of DNA repair, both in carcinogenesis and in resistance to tumour therapy.

The best characterized mammalian DNA-repair protein at present is O^6-alkylguanine-DNA alkyltransferase (O6AT). This enzyme removes covalently bound alkyl adducts from the O^6 position of guanine in DNA, thus repairing a type of DNA damage induced by alkylating agents[70]. The alkyl lesion, which can be a methyl, ethyl, hydroxyethyl or chloroethyl group, becomes covalently bound to a specific sulphydryl group on the protein, which is thereby inactivated. Cell lines deficient in O6AT, termed mer⁻, are much more sensitive than normal cells to a range of alkylating agents and to chloroethylnitrosoureas. Direct evidence for a role of this enzyme in resistance to alkylating agents comes from the transfection of the functional gene into cell lines which are deficient in O6AT: the transfected cells acquire increased resistance to alkylating agents[71].

The antineoplastic activity of cisplatin is almost certainly due to its bifunctional interaction with DNA[72]. Several reports have correlated the number of crosslinks between DNA strands (inter-strand) induced by cisplatin with cytotoxicity in both murine and human tumour cells[73-75]. However, comparisons between sensitive and resistant sublines of tumour cells imply that other lesions are more relevant to cytotoxicity and that the differences in sensitivity are not, in fact, due directly to differences in the kinetics of repair of interstrand crosslinks[76,77]. On the other hand, marked differences in repair capacity towards cisplatin-induced crosslinks within one DNA strand (intrastrand) have been observed between a sensitive testicular cell line and a resistant bladder cell line (although another sensitive testicular cell line did not show this difference)[78]. The increased sensitivity to cisplatin of repair-deficient hamster cells[79] and cells derived from patients suffering from Fanconi's anaemia[80] or xeroderma pigmentosum (XP)[81] support the idea that DNA repair may be involved in cisplatin resistance. The sensitivity of XP cells to cisplatin suggests a role for the excision repair pathway in the removal of cisplatin–DNA adducts. Now that some of the genes involved in excision repair have been cloned[69] and assays are available for measuring excision repair in mammalian cells[82], the role and relative importance of excision repair in resistance/sensitivity to cisplatin can be addressed.

DO THESE MECHANISMS OF DRUG RESISTANCE EXIST IN HUMAN TUMOURS?

In the preceding sections, we have described some of the possible mechanisms that can give rise to drug-resistant variants in cell lines. Many of these variants have the properties of having arisen due to mutations in specific genes[83]. However, resistant variants may also arise by more subtle perturbations of normal genetic mechanisms which affect the level of expression of a given gene. These may include alterations in DNA methylation or DNA-binding proteins affecting gene transcription, factors affecting RNA processing or stability and post-translational protein modifications. Whatever the mechanism,, it is recognized that resistant variants can arise at a detectable, if low, frequency in cell populations. Such drug-resistant variants would have a selective advantage during chemotherapeutic treatment and, with time, could multiply so as to constitute a significant proportion of the tumour. In theory, therefore, the presence of even a single drug-resistant malignant stem cell in a tumour population could result in an incurable cancer. Thus, it is vital to understand the factors that determine the frequency of occurrence of resistant cells *in vivo*. Goldie and Coldman[84] described a mathematical model for progression to resistance in tumours based on theoretical considerations of mutation frequencies. Their model predicts that small tumours are less likely to contain drug-resistant cells and would be more curable than larger ones. It should be noted, however, that rates of mutation are likely to be altered under certain circumstances. Many of the commonly used chemotherapeutic agents are themselves mutagenic[85]. Exposure of cells to these agents may increase mutation frequency at drug resistance loci or even transiently increase drug resistance by interfering with gene transcription. Certain mutations involving 'mutator genes' have been shown to increase rates of gene amplification, and thus generation of drug-resistant mutants[85]. Some virally transformed cell lines[86] and cells from individuals with certain inherited tumour-prone syndromes have been shown to have an increased rate of mutation to drug resistance[87]. Understanding the genesis of drug resistance in tumours and whether alteration in mutation rates plays a role in the frequency of treatment failure may lead to more emphasis on the design of drugs which retain their cytotoxic effects but are not capable of inducing the type of genetic change which leads to drug resistance.

We have discussed a number of mechanisms that can lead to cellular resistance to single agents and combinations of cytotoxic drugs in cultured cells. Do the mechanisms of drug resistance observed in cell lines contribute to treatment failure in human cancer? Exposing cells to drugs in culture is obviously different from treating tumours with therapeutic regimes, even if the same drugs are used. In the whole organism, treatment of the tumour with chemotherapeutic agents is limited by the toxicity to normal cells and organs. The concentration of drug that reaches the tumour cell in clinical practice is generally much lower than the concentration of drug used to select resistant cells *in vitro*. In addition, growth of tumours *in vivo* is dependent on a variety of factors, including the interaction of the cells with hormones and growth factors. In most cases, the cells are capable of progression to a more aggressive or malignant phenotype irrespective of drug exposure. These changes in phenotype can, in some cases, be correlated with alterations in expression and structure of proto-oncogene products[88]. The role of these genes in determining the response of a tumour to chemotherapy is, at this time, unclear, but certain possible correlations between oncogene expression and therapeutic response of tumours are beginning to emerge[89-91].

In order to attempt to answer the question of clinical relevance of resistance mechanisms, combinations of molecular, biochemical and cell biological approaches are being used. Firstly, cytotoxicity assays employing tumour cells which attempt to correlate *in vitro* sensitivity with clinical response of tumours have been developed. Secondly, gene probes and antibodies derived from biochemical and molecular studies of resistant cell lines have been used to analyse responsive and non-responsive tumours for differences in the expression of genes associated with drug resistance. Lastly, direct modification of expression of these genes or their protein products *in vivo* has been proposed. This last approach, as well as demonstrating resistance mechanisms *in vivo*, allows the first tentative steps to be taken towards treatment aimed at overcoming drug resistance in human cancer.

Cell assays of drug resistance of human tumours

The effects of increasing drug concentration on cell viability or metabolism can be measured in short-term assays using cells grown from tumour biopsy material[92]. The major advantages of this type of assay are its short duration and the fact that the majority of all biopsy samples can be evaluated for sensitivity to one or more drugs. The disadvantage is that normal cells may also grow from the biopsy sample, thus confusing the interpretation of tumour sensitivity. Another problem with this type of approach is that the experiments do not necessarily differentiate injured cells that are destined to recover from cells that are reproductively dead. Conversely, the metabolism of cells that will not divide subsequently may not be changed by drugs during the test period.

Clonogenic assays of chemosensitivity deal with the ability of dispersed tumour cells to form colonies in the presence of a drug[93]. They provide a measure of the resistance of cells which have the capacity for self-renewal in the tumour sample rather than simply the total cell population. Clonogenic growth has been achieved with a variety of different tumour types with a 10–70% success rate quoted from different laboratories[92,95]. Colony-forming efficiencies, however, have remained relatively low, predominantly of the order of 0.001–0.1%. This raises the question of the true identity of the minority tumour cell subpopulations which are able to grow in these conditions. Colony-forming cells generally have characteristics representative of the mass of tumour cells, based on histological comparisons, biochemical tumour markers and karyotype. Using suitable polymorphic markers that allow tumour cells to be distinguished from normal cells from the same individual (e.g. mutations in oncogenes or alterations in minisatellite repetitive DNA sequences[94]), it should be possible, in the future, to ensure that it is indeed tumour cells that are being measured for chemosensitivity and not normal cells growing from the biopsy.

One point which emerges from these *in vitro* chemosensitivity assays is that, in almost all studies, a significant correlation has been observed between tumour resistance *in vitro* and the lack of a clinical response in patients treated with the same drug[92,95]. This strongly supports the hypothesis that treatment failure is, in the majority of cases, due to intrinsic phenotypic resistance in the tumour cells, presumably due to specific resistance mechanisms. However, significant correlations between positive chemosensitivity *in vitro* and clinical response of tumours are much less evident. Thus, rather than being used clinically as a predictive tool, the main use of *in vitro* assays on primary human tumour biopsies is, at present, as a research system: to investigate expression of genes associated with resistance to cytotoxic drug activity *in vitro* and as a means of devising ways to overcome cellular drug resistance.

Altered expression of drug resistance-associated gene products in human tumours

The most direct way to address this question with regard to human tumours is to measure the levels of expression of specific genes in tumours from the same patients prior to chemotherapy and after relapse. Demonstration of amplification of the dihydrofolate reductase gene in leukaemic cells from patients after treatment with methotrexate was the first clear example that the same types of resistance mechanisms can operate in human tumours as in experimental systems[96,97]. Similarly, increased binding of a P-glycoprotein monoclonal antibody has been observed in sequential analysis of peripheral blood samples from acute non-lymphoblastic leukaemia patients during chemotherapy[98]. However, for the majority of solid tumours, it is seldom feasible or ethical to obtain sequential samples and alternative means of correlating levels of expression must be sought.

The level of P-glycoprotein expression in tumours and normal tissue has been measured using either probes for *mdr1* RNA levels[99,100] or monoclonal antibodies directed against the protein[101,102]. A recent study of more than 400 human tumours showed high levels of *mdr1* mRNA in many untreated intrinsically resistant tumours; however, there was considerable heterogeneity between patients and some intrinsically resistant tumours, such as melanoma, contained low levels of *mdr1* RNA[103]. Studies of normal tissue showed that the *mdr1* gene is expressed at very high levels in the adrenal gland; at a high level in the kidney and placenta; at intermediate levels in the lung, liver, lower duodenum, colon and rectum; and at low levels in many other tissues. This led to the suggestion that tumours derived from tissues which express *mdr1* at high levels may also express high levels of *mdr1* and consequently be intrinsically resistant to chemotherapy. Indeed, high levels of expression of *mdr1* have been identified in tumours derived from the adrenal gland, colon, liver, pancreas and kidney[99,100,103].

There are a number of problems in explaining intrinsic resistance simply in terms of high *mdr1* expression in the normal tissue from which the tumour arises. Normal tissue adjacent to a tumour is a mixture of a variety of cell types which may not be equivalent to the actual target cell for transformation that gives rise to the tumour. Thus, *mdr1* expression in the target or stem cell which gives rise to the tumour may be considerably different. A large range of expression of *mdr1* is observed both in particular types of tumour and even in normal tissue[103]. This prompts the question: are the differences in expression seen between tissues truly cell type specific or due simply to selection of stem cells in that particular tissue as a result of exposure to toxic agents? Tissues such as colon, lung, liver and rectum are exposed to a wide variety of environmental toxins and carcinogens. High levels of *mdr1* expression in tumours and normal tissue from some patients may be due to selection of resistant stem cells prior to chemotherapy as a consequence of exposure to these toxins. Tissues and tumours that have high levels of *mdr1* expression also often have elevated levels of many other enzymes involved in drug detoxification. Decreased drug accumulation by increased P-glycoprotein-mediated efflux and alterations in drug detoxification by the glutathione redox cycle have been shown to occur together in adriamycin-resistant cells and in human colorectal tumours with *de novo* resistance[42]. This makes it difficult to say which, if any, of these mechanisms might have a greater role in intrinsic drug resistance of tumours. Indeed, it raises the possibility that the respective genes may be regulated in some co-ordinated manner in these cells, similarly to the high expression in erythroid cells of certain enzymes that protect red blood cells and their progenitors from oxidative damage[104,105].

Gene expression can also be compared with response to treatment of tumours of one particular histological type. In breast tumours from patients who have not received chemotherapy, we have observed that about 15% have a high level of *mdr1* expression; 10–100-fold higher than the majority of breast tumours and reaching the level observed in resistant cells isolated in culture (Keith, Stallard and Brown, unpublished). Eventually it will be possible to compare clinical response with level of *mdr1* RNA especially in those patients who undergo chemotherapy. At present, we have compared *mdr1* mRNA expression in the tumour biopsy with chemosensitivity of the tumour to adriamycin as measured by clonogenic assay of cells outgrown from the biopsy. This comparison has shown that the most sensitive cells have low levels of *mdr1*, while those tumours with high levels of *mdr1* are more resistant as measured with this assay. However, not all resistant tumours have high levels of *mdr1* expression. This is perhaps not surprising if different mechanisms can give rise to chemoresistant tumours. These observations support an involvement of *mdr1* in the response of some breast tumours to chemotherapy. However, more conclusive evidence will come from data on the clinical response of these tumours.

As we have already discussed, glutathione and glutathione-dependent enzymes, such as glutathione-S-transferase (GST), are known to play a central role in drug detoxification. However, their role in conferring drug resistance is still circumstantial. Over-expression of the acidic form of GST (GSTpi) has been observed in adriamycin-resistant breast cancer cell lines and in experimental models of preneoplasia[49]. It is interesting to note in this context that an apparent inverse association between GSTpi expression and oestrogen receptor (ER) content in some primary breast cancers has been observed[106]. The basis of this association is unclear, but it suggests that ER-negative breast cancer cells may have a greater GST-mediated protection againt chemotherapeutic drugs than ER-positive tumours. Alterations in several of the glutathione-dependent enzymes have also been observed in two ovarian adenocarcinoma cell lines derived from the same patient before and after the onset of drug resistance to cisplatin, chlorambucil and 5-fluorouracil[107]. However, there is still considerable work to be done to determine whether the differences in GSH-dependent enzymes observed *in vitro* are indeed relevant to clinical observations of drug resistance.

Differences in induction of DNA damage and its repair have also been proposed as mechanisms of tumour resistance to drugs, particularly for resistance to cisplatin[108]. However, until the normal repair processes and the genes coding for the relevant enzymes are understood, evidence for a role of DNA repair in treatment failure will remain circumstantial. Defects in DNA repair have been strongly implicated in human carcinogenesis. A number of human hereditary diseases with apparent deficiencies in the processing of damaged DNA confer predisposition to cancer[67,68]; these include patients with xeroderma pigmentosum, ataxia telangiectasia, Fanconi's anaemia, Bloom's syndrome and Cockayne's syndrome. It has been reported that presumptive ataxia telangiectasia heterozygotes are at increased risk of breast cancer[109]. This raises the possibility that heterozygosity for some of the many DNA-repair deficiencies may be important in cancer susceptibility. Deficiency of DNA ligase has been observed in Bloom's syndrome cells[110,111] and in T-cell acute leukaemia[112], although the genetic basis of these deficiencies and their direct involvement in the diseases has yet to be demonstrated. If defects in DNA repair are indeed involved in human carcinogenesis, then these tumours would be expected to be more sensitive to drugs. Suppression of the DNA-repair deficiency could then subsequently lead to a resistant tumour. This is an important area for future research, since screening of patients and tumours for defects in DNA repair would allow for improved therapeutic strategies.

Most cytotoxic compounds that interact with DNA have been shown to do so in a heterogeneous manner[113]. Alkylating agents, such as the chemotherapeutic chloroethylating agents, react predominantly with guanines in GC-rich regions of the genome[114,115]. Hypomethylated GC-rich regions of the mammalian genome have been observed close to many genes and have been suggested as possible control regions for gene transcription[116]. The effect of methylation or the presence of DNA-binding proteins on preferential reactivity towards alkylating agents has so far not been fully investigated. If there were a differential effect, then large scale changes in levels of methylation or chromatin structure within the nucleus could have an effect on response of a cell to the chemotherapeutic agent. Cisplatin has been shown to bind preferentially to the linker DNA of chromatin[117], suggesting that the accessibility of the DNA does have an effect on binding of drug. Bleomycin has also been shown to interact with DNA in a structure-dependent fashion, being mainly confined to the transcribing regions of chromatin[118]. Similarly, it has been shown that different induced lesions in DNA are differentially repaired depending on their localization[113]. Indeed, one of the proposed targets for the action of chemotherapeutic drugs, topoisomerase II, has been shown to cleave DNA in a sequence-dependent manner[19]. The possible role of this differential damage and repair of the genome is still not fully understood, but it will be extremely interesting to follow up this concept and to see what implications it may hold both for carcinogenesis and drug resistance.

Genetic modulation of drug resistance gene expression

The most direct methods for determining if a given gene is important in a given phenotype are either to block its expression or to over-express it. Over-expression of the *mdr1* gene by transfection into cells in culture has been used to confirm its function[120]. However, this approach only provides circumstantial evidence for the role of the gene *in vivo*. Transgenic mice have been used to examine the role *in vivo* of a number of genes[121], but, so far, drug resistance genes have not been analysed using this approach. Antibiotic resistance genes have been reintroduced into haematopoietic stem cells using retroviral vectors[122]; however, this method has not yet been used to examine resistance to chemotherapeutic agents. Experimentally controlled over-expression of these genes in the normal cells of experimental animals will allow the conceptual gap between cultured cells and human tumours to be bridged. This approach will provide an important direction for future research, yielding considerable information regarding the normal function of these genes and their role in treatment failure.

Another way to study the role of drug resistance genes would be to inactivate them specifically. Site-directed mutagenesis by gene targeting involves the homologous recombination of DNA sequences residing in the chromosome with newly introduced DNA sequences. This could provide a means for specifically inactivating any given gene[123]. Using this approach, the hypoxanthine–guanine phosphoribosyl transferase (HGPRT) gene has been mutated in mouse embryo-derived stem (ES) cells[124]. Selection of HGPRT⁻ ES cells in culture circumvents the relatively low efficiency of gene targeting (about 1/1000 of cells taking up the introduced DNA sequence). ES cells are capable of contributing to the formation of chimeric mice, including contribution to a functional germ line[125]. Thus, the gene-targeted mutation can be inherited by the offspring. This powerful genetical approach will allow the phenotypic consequences of mutations, including drug resistance genes, to be analysed *in vivo*.

Inhibition of expression of specific genes has also been shown to be possible using antisense RNA transcripts[126] or antisense oligonucleotides[127]. Antisense RNA transcripts targeted at the thymidine kinase (TK) gene can inhibit expression of the endogenous TK gene[128]. Likewise antisense oligonucleotides have been shown to inhibit expression of the oncogene *c-myc*[129]. Inactivation of genes implicated in drug resistance using either of these approaches could be a powerful analytical tool to examine the relative contribution any gene makes to drug resistance in a given cell. Indeed, antisense oligonucleotides directed to drug resistance genes or active oncogenes have even been suggested as having therapeutic possibilities[127]. However, there are still vast areas of ignorance concerning the stability, efficiency of uptake, specificity of binding and targeting of the oligonucleotides that have to be resolved before this approach can be considered clinically. A more immediate therapeutic possibility is to use drugs or antibodies as a means of biochemically modulating drug resistance. If a specific drug resistance mechanism is believed to operate in a given tumour, then inhibition of this resistance pathway would directly increase the sensitivity of the cells.

CAN WE MODULATE DRUG RESISTANCE BIOCHEMICALLY TO IMPROVE CLINICAL RESPONSE?

Based on experimental data from several groups, clinical attempts at biochemical modulation of resistance are now being contemplated for a wide range of cytotoxic drugs. However, despite a great deal of interest and activity in the laboratory, relatively few complete clinical trials have actually addressed the issue of modulation of drug resistance. Those which have, and those which are currently being planned, may be considered under the subheadings of the 3 categories of cytotoxic drugs for which mechanisms of resistance have been proposed.

(1) One group of studies has concentrated on the potential for circumventing resistance to drugs mediated via the MDR phenotype. Calcium antagonists (e.g. verapamil) and calmodulin inhibitors (e.g. trifluoperazine) inhibit the active drug efflux and restore drug sensitivity in MDR cells[130–132]. Verapamil can bind to the P-glycoprotein[133,134], suggesting that verapamil may sensitize MDR cells by competing for binding with the drug for the

P-glycoprotein (see Figure 5.1). Verapamil is the most extensively tested of these drugs in randomized and non-randomized studies. The major problem with verapamil is the difficulty in attaining plasma levels equal to those which consistently reverse resistance to the test agents in *in vitro* models[135]. The maximum oral dose achieves plasma levels of $1-2\,\mu$mol, while *in vitro* effects are best seen at concentrations of approximately $6\,\mu$mol. Nevertheless, biological effects have been seen, and studies are continuing. The major metabolite of verapamil, i.e. norverapamil, is present in equimolar concentration following oral administration, and *in vitro* data indicate that it is as efficient at overcoming resistance as the parent compound[136]. It is possible, therefore, that the potential of verapamil has been underestimated. Other studies indicate that agents, such as verapamil, alter hepatic and renal blood flow, and thus interact in the pharmacological distribution of cytotoxic drugs, such as adriamycin[137]. These considerations are important in interpreting the results of clinical trials.

In a continuing randomized study of 172 small-cell lung-cancer patients[138], an apparent increase in myelosuppression was observed in patients who received verapamil (480 mg daily po) in addition to chemotherapy. Although this necessitated dose reductions in 25% of patients in that arm, patients receiving verapamil achieved a slightly higher level of complete response (44% vs. 28%) and a slightly longer median survival for complete responders (14 months vs. 11 months). Firm conclusions from this study will, however, require longer follow-up.

Additional non-randomized studies, using both verapamil (in 12 adriamycin-resistant patients[139]) and verapamil with tamoxifen (in 58 previously untreated patients with small-cell lung cancer[140]) have reported encouraging rates of response. Further studies using this approach are currently being planned in several centres. A large range of hydrophobic non-cytotoxic agents other than verapamil is available for testing as modulators of resistance to natural products. Some of these, including quinidine and bepridil[141,142], show particular promise if only because the levels which may be effective clinically are easily achievable. Some centres aim to concentrate on those tumour types known to be associated with high levels of *mdr* gene expression, e.g. colon cancer and renal cancer. Other investigators will pursue their efforts in tumour types, such as small-cell lung cancer and breast cancer, in which high levels of *mdr* expression are probably seen less frequently, but for which resistance to natural products is a major clinical problem.

(2) Clinical trials on resistance to alkylating agents and cisplatin are scheduled to start within the next year, testing two approaches. Firstly, it is evident that depletion of cellular GSH, using buthionine sulphoximine (BSO), will reverse the resistance to these agents both *in vitro* and *in vivo* in experimental models[143]. The mechanism may be related to reduced inactivation of these cytotoxic agents, and it appears that GSH depletion may be achievable in tumours with doses of BSO lower than those required for normal tissue[144]. Clinical trials with BSO to assess its toxicity are now under way, with the eventual aim of evaluating its potential, in

combination with alkylating agents and cisplatin, to overcome resistance in diseases such as ovarian cancer.

Secondly, as already discussed, resistance to cisplatin has been linked to differences in DNA damage and repair. Thus, agents capable of specifically altering DNA metabolism and repair of the cisplatin–DNA adduct may be useful in circumventing cisplatin resistance. One such agent is aphidocolin, a DNA polymerase α inhibitor. This is effective *in vitro* at reversing cisplatin resistance in ovarian cancer at levels which are non-cytotoxic[108]. Phase I trials with this agent are underway, again with the eventual aim of combination chemotherapy together with cisplatin.

(3) As regards antimetabolites, the major effort in biochemical modulation has concentrated on 5-fluorouracil. As mentioned previously, resistance to this agent may be related to levels of the active metabolite, and several groups have shown that response can be increased by combining 5FU treatment in experimental models with a range of agents, including methotrexate and folinic acid[145,146]. Clinical trials have suggested that such combined treatment may lead to increased activity. The problem is that this type of biochemical modulation seems to be relatively non-selective, and increased normal tissue toxicity has been a common feature of these studies. For example, in a large randomized study in colorectal cancer, the addition of folinic acid to standard doses of 5FU did lead to a significant increase in responses, but the increase in toxicity, particularly myelosuppression and mucositis, was substantial[147]. Further attempts at cirvumventing antimetabolite resistance may depend on the identification of substantially different levels of enzyme activity in malignant and normal cells.

Clearly, all these attempts at biochemical modulation are still at an early stage. It is likely that a major drawback to this approach lies in the probability that multiple mechanisms co-exist. Thus, multiple methods of manipulation may be simultaneously required before a significant impact on cell kill is seen. Nevertheless, the weight of laboratory data is sufficiently compelling to make these studies justifiable, but in planning them two questions arise:

(1) *At what stage during chemotherapy should the modulator be introduced in order to test its efficacy?*
The difficulty with this question is that information on the difference, if any, between 'intrinsic' and 'acquired' resistance is not available. Taking small-cell lung cancer as an example, are drug-resistant cells which will ultimately prove fatal an integral feature of the total tumour cell population when the disease first presents? If they are, it may be logical to introduce the modulating agent with the initial treatment. Alternatively, would it not be better to wait until the disease has relapsed or progressed on treatment, at which time it can be assumed that resistant cells comprise a significant number of the total? At that stage, retreatment with the drugs to which resistance has presumably developed, together with the putative modulator, would constitute a logical type of trial design.

Although theoretically an attractive concept, in practical terms, major problems are likely to arise with this latter trial design. Patients whose disease progresses during chemotherapy are frequently in poor general condition and have short expected survival; meaningful trials in this group of patients are unlikely to be feasible. On the other hand, patients whose disease relapses after a treatment-free period of several months have a reasonable expectation of responding again, at least in the short term, to the same schedule of treatment given initially. Therefore, any trial involving a modulator in this circumstance would need to be randomized. This could lead to difficulties in patient accrual, since repeat chemotherapy is not necessarily appropriate for, or acceptable to, many patients.

An alternative trial design, not yet explored, would involve introducing a modulating agent in a randomized fashion at the end of the planned initial chemotherapy programme. Here the rationale is that standard initial chemotherapy is generally successful in causing tumour reduction, often to a point where residual disease may not be clinically detectable. At this stage, if the microscopic tumour mass contains a significant proportion of resistant cells, then further treatment combined with a modulating agent may be effective in terms of producing a prolonged disease-free interval.

(2) *How can any clinical impact be assessed? To determine a potential improvement in response or survival, is a randomized comparison with a control group necessary?*
This question can be approached by consideration of the type of tumour involved. Studies of modulators in 'inherently resistant' tumours, e.g. colon and renal cancer, need not be large randomized trials and, indeed, this would not be recommended. If, for example, the MDR mechanism is relevant to the ineffectiveness of anthracyclines in treating renal cancer and colon cancer, the addition of a specific modulating agent, e.g. a calcium antagonist, in a non-randomized trial should produce sufficient impact on activity to detect an improvement over expected response. However, for tumours in which resistance is said to be 'acquired', e.g. small-cell lung cancer and breast cancer, the addition of a modulating agent in small non-randomized trials yields relatively little information. For these tumours, large randomized studies involving comparison with standard therapy will be required.

Are approaches to the problem of drug resistance, other than attempts at biochemical modulation as described above, likely to be more fruitful? Drug targeting and the use of high-dose chemotherapy are discussed elsewhere, but, so far, their clinical promise has not been fulfilled. As described already, the mathematical model of Goldie and Coldman[84] has suggested that spontaneous mutations in tumour cells give rise to drug resistance early in tumour development. In an attempt to prevent the growth of resistant cells, they have recommended the use of so-called 'non-cross-resistant' chemotherapy in alternating sequences, early in a treatment programme. The aim is to provide effective therapy for several subsets of tumour cells, but the prerequisite is that the two treatment regimes to be alternated should be roughly equivalent in activity. Unfortunately, this is only rarely the case in clinical practice and positive clinical trials confirming the value of alternating schedules to prevent the emergence of drug resistance, are very few. One study on Hodgkin's disease has suggested a positive benefit for this type of treatment programme[148], but similar studies on solid tumours, such as small-cell lung cancer and breast cancer, have so far proved disappointing. At present the relevance of these models to clinical practice is uncertain, at least for the majority of common solid tumours where drug resistance remains the outstanding challenge.

It is clear that our understanding of possible mechanisms of drug resistance has increased considerably and has led to the invention of treatment regimes intended to circumvent resistance. Isolation and characterization of drug resistance-associated genes and protein products have allowed correlations with altered gene expression and treatment failure in human tumours. However, there are still large areas of ignorance, some of which we have tried to point out. The involvement of P-glycoprotein and other drug resistance-associated genes in acquired resistance of solid tumours is still tenuous. Mechanisms of cisplatin resistance are poorly defined. Changes in the response of tumour cells to drugs during tumour initiation, promotion and progression are unclear. The involvement of DNA-metabolizing enzymes in drug cytotoxicity and resistance needs to be further defined. These are only a few of the most obvious areas requiring further research in this complex area. Perhaps one of the most important challenges will be the need for medical oncologists and research scientists to collaborate to define the important questions to be asked and to design feasible approaches by which they can be answered.

References

1. Young, R. C., Ozols, R. F. and Myers, D. E. (1981). The anthracycline antineoplastic drugs. *N. Engl. J. Med.,* **305**, 139–153
2. Bramwell, V. H. and Pinedo, H. (1980). Bone and soft tissue sarcomas. In Pinedo, H. (ed.) *Cancer Chemotherapy, The EORTC Annual 2,* pp. 393–414. (Amsterdam: Excerpta Medica)
3. Einhorn, L. H. and Williams, S. P. (1979). The role of cisplatin in solid tumour therapy. *N. Engl. J. Med.,* **300**, 289–291
4. Carter, S. K. (1976). Large bowel cancer: the current status of treatment. *J. Natl. Cancer Inst.,* **56**, 3–10
5. Kim, T. H., Hargreaves, H. K., Byrnes, R. K., Lui, V. K., Hawkins, H. K., Woodard, J. and Ragoob, A. L. A. (1981). Pretreatment testicular biopsy in childhood acute lymphocytic leukaemia. *Lancet,* **2**, 657–658
6. Tubiana, M. (1982). Cell kinetics and radiation oncology. *Int. J. Radiat. Oncol. Biol. Phys.,* **8**, 1471–1478
7. Riordan, J. R. and Ling, V. (1985). Genetic and biochemical characterisation of multidrug resistance. *Pharmacol. Ther.,* **28**, 51–75
8. Hill, B. T. (1986). In vitro human tumour model systems for investigating drug resistance. *Cancer Surv.,* **5**, 129–149
9. Moscow, J. A. and Cowan, K. H. (1988). Multidrug resistance. *J. Natl. Cancer Inst.,* **80**, 14–20
10. Biedler, J. L. and Riehm, H. (1970). Cellular resistance to actinomycin D in Chinese

hamster cells in vitro: cross-resistance, radioautoradiographic and cytogenetic studies. *Cancer Res.*, **30**, 1174–1184

11. Juliano, R. L. and Ling. V. (1976). A surface glycoprotein modulating drug permeability in CHO cell mutants. *Biochim. Biophys. Acta*, **455**, 152–162

12. Ling, V. and Thompson, L. H. (1973). Reduced permeability in CHO cells as a mechanism of resistance to colchicine. *J. Cell Physiol.*, **83**, 103–116

13. Kartner, N., Riordan, J. R. and Ling, V. (1983). Cell surface P-glycoprotein is associated with multidrug resistance in mammalian cell lines. *Science*, **221**, 1285–1288

14. Riordan, J. R., Deuchars, K., Kartner, N., *et al.* (1985). Amplification of P-glycoprotein genes in multidrug-resistant mammalian cell lines. *Nature (London)*, **316**, 817–819

15. Fojo, A. T., Whang-Peng, J., Gottesman, M. M., *et al.* (1985). Amplification of DNA sequences in human multidrug-resistant KB carcinoma cells. *Proc. Natl. Acad. Sci. USA*, **82**, 7661 7665

16. Gros, P., Croop, J., Roninson, I., *et al.* (1986). Isolation and characterisation of DNA sequences amplified in multidrug-resistant hamster cells. *Proc. Natl. Acad. Sci. USA*, **83**, 337–341

17. Fairchild, C. R., Ivy, S. P., Kao-Shan, C-S., *et al.* (1987). Isolation of amplified DNA sequences associated with pleiotropic drug resistance from human breast cancer cells. *Cancer Res.*, **47**, 5141–5148

18. Scotto, K. W., Biedler, J. L. and Melera, P. W. (1986). Amplification and expression of genes associated with multidrug resistance in mammalian cells. *Science*, **232**, 751–755

19. Roninson, I. B., Abelson, H. T., Housman, D. E., *et al.* (1984). Amplification of specific DNA sequences correlates with multidrug resistance in Chinese hamster cells. *Nature (London)*, **309**, 626–628

20. Jongsma, A. P. M., Spengler, B. A., Van der Bliek, A. M. and Borst, P. (1987). Chromosomal localisation of three genes coamplified in the multidrug-resistant CHrC5 CHO cell lines. *Cancer Res.*, **47**, 2875–2878

21. Van der Bliek, A. M., Baas, F., Van der Velde-Koerts, *et al.* (1988). Genes amplified and overexpressed in human multidrug-resistant cell lines. *Cancer Res.*, **48**, 5927–5932

22. Safa, A. R., Glover, C. I., Meyers, M. B., *et al.* (1986). Vinblastine photoaffinity labelling of a high molecular weight surface membrane glycoprotein specific for multidrug-resistant cells. *J. Biol. Chem.*, **261**, 6137–6140

23. Cornwell, M. M., Pastan, I. and Gottesman, M. M. (1987). Certain calcium channel blockers bind specifically to multidrug-resistant human KB carcinoma membrane vesicles and inhibit drug binding to P-glycoprotein. *J. Biol. Chem.*, **262**, 2166–2170

24. Gros, P., Croop, J. and Housman, D. (1986). Mammalian multidrug-resistance gene: complex cDNA sequence indicates strong homology to bacterial transport proteins. *Cell*, **47**, 371–374

25. Chen, C-J., Chin, J. E., Ueda, K., *et al.* (1986). Internal duplication and homology to bacterial transport proteins in the *mdr1* (P-glycoprotein) gene from multidrug-resistant human cells. *Cell*, **47**, 381–389

26. Gerlach, J. H., Endicott, J. A., Juranka, P. F., *et al.* (1986). Homology between P-glycoprotein and a bacterial haemolysin transport protein suggests a model for multidrug resistance. *Nature (London)*, **324**, 485–489

27. Ueda, K., Cardarelli, C., Gottesman, M. M. and Pastan, I. (1987). Expression of a full-length cDNA for the human "mdr1" gene confers resistance to colchicine, doxorubicin and vinblastine. *Proc. Natl. Acad. Sci. USA*, **84**, 3004–3008

28. Choi, K., Chen, C., Kriegler, M. and Roninson, I. B. (1988). An altered pattern of cross-resistance in multidrug-resistant human cells results from spontaneous mutations in the mdr1 (P-glycoprotein) gene. *Cell*, **53**, 519–529

29. Van der Bliek, A. M., Baas, F., Ten Houte de Lange, *et al.* (1987). The human mdr3 gene encodes a novel P-glycoprotein homologue and gives rise to alternatively spliced mRNA in liver. *EMBO J.*, **6**, 3325–3331

30. Endicott, J. A., Juranka, P. F., Saranqui, F., *et al.* (1987). Simultaneous expression of two P-glycoprotein genes in drug sensitive CHO cells. *Mol. Cell Biol.*, **7**, 4075–4081

31. Beck, W. T. and Cirtain, M. C. (1982). Continued expression of vinca alkaloid resistance by CCRF-CEM cells after treatment with tunicamycin or pronase. *Cancer Res.*, **42**, 184–189

32. Fine, R. L., Patel, J. and Chabner, B. A. (1988). Phorbol esters induce multi-drug resistance in human breast cancer cells. *Proc. Natl. Acad. Sci. USA*, **85**, 582–586

33. Hamada, H., Hagiwara, K-I., Nakajima, T. and Tsuro, T. (1987). Phosphorylation of the Mr 170,000 to 180,000 glycoprotein specific to multidrug-resistant tumour cells: Effects of verapamil, trifluoperazine and phorbol esters. *Cancer Res.,* **47**, 2860–2865

34. Beck, W. T. (1987). The cell biology of multiple drug resistance. *Biochem. Pharmacol.,* **36**, 2879–2887

35. Rosenberg, B. (1985). Fundamental studies with cisplatin. *Cancer,* **55**, 2302–2310

36. Sehested, M., Skovsgaard, T., Van Deurs, B. and Winter-Neilson, H. (1987). Increase in non-specific adsorption endocytosis in anthracycline- and vinca-alkaloid-resistant Ehrlich ascites tumour cells. *J. Natl. Cancer Inst.,* **78**, 171–177

37. Tofilon, J. P., Buckley, N. and Deen, D. F. (1984). Effect of cell–cell interactions on drug sensitivity and growth of drug sensitive and resistant tumour cells in spheroids. *Science,* **226**, 862–865

38. Pitts, J. D. (1971). Molecular exchange and growth control in tissue culture. In the *Ciba Foundation Symposium of Growth Control in Cell Cultures,* pp. 89–105. (CIBA)

39. Fujimoto, W. Y., Subak-Sharpe, J. H. and Seegmiller, J. E. (1971). Hypoxanthine-quanine phosphoriribosyltransferase deficiency: chemical agents selective for mutant and normal cultured fibroblasts in mixed and heterozygote cultures. *Proc. Natl. Acad. Sci. USA,* **68**, 1516–1519

40. Pitts, J. D. and Finbow, M. E. (1986). The gap junction. *J. Cell. Sci. Suppl.,* **4**, 239–266

41. Wolf, C. R., Lewis, A. D. Carmichael, J., *et al.* (1987). Glutathione-*S*-transferase expression in normal tumour cells resistant to cytotoxic drugs. In Mantle, T. J., Pickett, C. B. and Hayes (eds.) *Glutathione-S-transferases and Carcinogenesis,* pp. 199–212. (London and New York: Taylor and Francis)

42. Kramer, R. A., Zakher, J. and Kim, G. (1988). Role of the glutathione redox cycle in acquired and de novo multidrug resistance. *Science,* **241**, 694–697

43. Kouri, R. E. and Nerbert, D. W. (1977). Genetic regulation of susceptibility to polycyclic-hydrocarbon-induced tumours in mice. In Hiatt, H. H., Watson, J. D. and Winsted, J. A. (eds.) *Origins of Human Cancer,* pp. 811–835. (Cold Spring Harbour, NY: Cold Spring Harbour Laboratory)

44. Kouri, R. E., McKinney, C. E., Sloamiany, D. J., *et al.* (1982). Positive correlation between high aryl hydrocarbon hydroxylase activity and primary lung cancer as analysed in cryo-preserved lymphocytes. *Cancer Res.,* **42**, 1532–1537

45. Jacoby, W. B. (1978). The glutathione-*S*-transferase: a group of multifunctional detoxification proteins. *Adv. Enzymol.,* **46**, 383–414

46. Hamilton, T. C., Winker, M. A., Louie, K. G., *et al.* (1985). Augmentation of adriamycin, melphalan, and cisplatin cytotoxicity in drug resistant and sensitive human ovarian cancer cell lines by buthionine sulphoximine-mediated depletion of glutathione. *Biochem. Pharmacol.,* **4**, 2583–2586

47. Suzukake, K., Vistica, B. P. and Vistica, D. T. (1983). Dechlorination of L-phenylalanine mustard by sensitive and resistant tumour cells and its relationship to intracellular glutathione content. *Biochem. Pharmacol.,* **32**, 165–167

48. Green, J. A., Vistica, D. T., Young, R. C., *et al.* (1984). Potentiation of melphalan cytotoxicity in human ovarian cancer cell lines by glutathione depletion. *Cancer Res.,* **44**, 5427–5431

49. Cowan, K. H., Batist, G., Tulpule, A., *et al.* (1986). Similar biochemical changes associated with multidrug resistance in human breast cancer cells and carcinogen-induced resistance to xenobiotics in rats. *Proc. Natl. Acad. Sci. USA,* **83**, 9328–9332

50. Batist, G., Tulpule, A., Sinha, B. K., *et al.* (1986). Overexpression of a novel anionic glutathione transferase in multidrug resistant human breast cancer cells. *J. Biol. Chem.,* **261**, 15544–15549

51. Buller, A. L., Clapper, M. L. and Tew, K. D. (1987). Glutathione-*S*-transferases in nitrogen mustard-resistant and -sensitive cell lines. *Mol. Pharmacol.,* **31**, 575–578

52. Manoharan, T. H., Puchalski, R. B., Burgess, J. A., *et al.* (1987). Promoter glutathione *S*-transferase Ya cDNA hybrid genes. Expression and conferred resistance to an alkylating molecule in mammalian cells. *J. Biol. Chem.,* **262**, 3739–3745

53. Plaa, G. L. and Witschi, H. (1976). Chemicals, drugs and lipid peroxidation. *Annu. Rev. Pharmacol. Toxicol.,* **16**, 125–141

54. Sinha, B. K., Katki, A. G., Batist, G., *et al.* (1987). Differential formation of hydroxyl

radicals by adriamycin in sensitive and resistant MCF-7 human breast cancer tumour cells; implications for mechanisms of action. *Biochemistry*, **26**, 3776–3781

55. Ross, W., Rowe, T., Glisson, B., *et al.* (1984). Role of topoisomerase II in mediating epipodophyllotoxin-induced DNA cleavage. *Cancer Res.*, **44**, 5857–5860

56. Chen, G. L., Yang, L., Rowe, T. C., *et al.* (1984). Non-intercalative antitumour drugs interfere with the breakage-reunion reaction of mammalian DNA topoisomerase II. *J. Biol. Chem.*, **259**, 13560–13566

57. Wang, J. C. (1985). DNA topoisomerases. *Ann. Rev. Biochem.*, **54**, 665–697

58. Nelson, E., Tewey, K. and Liu, L. (1984). Mechanism of antitumour drugs: poisoning of mammalian DNA topoisomerase II on DNA by an antitumour drug m-AMSA. *Proc. Natl. Acad. Sci. USA*, **81**, 1361–1365

59. Tewey, K. M., Chen, G. L. Nelson, E. M. and Liu, L. F. (1984). Intercalative antitumour drugs interfere with the breakage–reunion reaction of mammalian DNA topoisomerase II. *J. Biol. Chem.*, **259**, 9182–9187

60. Glisson, B., Gupta, R., Hodges, P., *et al.* (1986). Cross-resistance to intercalating agents in an epipodophyllotoxin-resistant CHO cell line: evidence for a common intracellular target. *Cancer Res.*, **46**, 1939–1942

61. Andoh, T., Ishi, K. and Suzuki, Y. (1987). Characterisation of a mammalian mutant with a camptothecin-resistant DNA topoisomerase I. *Proc. Natl. Acad. Sci. USA*, **84**, 5565–5569

62. Schornagel, J. H. and McVie, J. G. (1983). The clinical pharmacology of methotrexate. *Cancer Treat. Rep.*, **10**, 53–75

63. Curt, G. A., Clandeninn, N. J. and Chabner, B. A. (1984). Drug resistance in cancer. *Cancer Treat. Rep.*, **68**, 87–117

64. Heidelberger, C. (1965). Fluoridated pyrimidines. *Prog. Nucleic Acid Res. Mol. Biol.*, **4**, 1–50

65. Ardalam, B, Buscaglia, M. and Schein, P. (1978). Tumour 5-fluorodeoxyuridylate concentration as a determinant of 5-fluorouracil response. *Biochem. Pharmacol.*, **27**, 2009–2013

66. Sancer, A. and Sancar, G. B. (1988). DNA repair enzymes. *Annu. Rev. Biochem.*, **57**, 29–68

67. Lindahl, T. (1982). DNA repair enzymes. *Annu. Rev. Biochem.*, **51**, 61–88

68. Hickson, I. D and Harris, A. L. (1988). Mammalian DNA repair – use of mutants hypersensitive to cytotoxic agents. *Trends Genet.*, **4**, 101–106

69. Thompson, C. H., Salazar, E. P. Brookman, K. W., Collins, C. C., *et al.* (1987). Recent progress with the DNA repair mutants of CHO cells. *J. Cell Sci.*, **6** (Suppl.), 97–110

70. Day, R. S., Babich, M. A., Yarosch, D. B. and Scudiero, D. A. (1987). The role of 06-methylguanine in human cell killing, sister chromatid exchange induction and mutagenesis: a review. *J. Cell Sci.*, **6** (Suppl.), 333–352

71. Margison, C. P. and Brennard, J. (1987). Functional expression of the *E. Coli* alkyltransferase gene in mammalian cells. *J. Cell. Sci.*, **6** (Suppl.). 83–96

72. Roberts, J. J., Knox, R. J. Friedlos, F. and Lydall, D. A. (1986). DNA as the target for the cytotoxic and antitumour action of platinum co-ordination complexes: comparative *in vitro* and *in vivo* studies of cisplatin and carboplatin. In McBrien, D. C. H. and Slater, T. F. (eds.) *Biochemical Mechanisms of Platinum Antitumour Drugs*, pp. 29–64. (Oxford, UK: IRL Press)

73. Zwelling, L. A., Anderson, T. and Kohn, K. W. (1979). DNA-protein and DNA interstrand cross-linking by *cis*- and *trans*- platinum (II) diamminedichloride in L1210 mouse leukaemia cells and relation to cytotoxicity. *Cancer Res.*, **39**, 365–369

74. Pascoe, J. M. and Roberts, J. J. (1974). Interactions between mammalian cell DNA and unorganic platinum compounds. I. DNA interstrand cross-linking and cytotoxic properties of platinum (II) compounds. *Biochem. Pharmacol.*, **23**, 1345–1357

75. Erickson, L. C., Zwelling, L. A. Ducore, J. M. Sharkey, N. A. and Kohn, K. W. (1981). Differential cytotoxicity and DNA crosslinking in normal and transformed human fibroblasts treated with *cis*-diamminedichloroplatinum (II). *Cancer Res.*, **41**, 2791–2794

76. Strandberg, M., Bresnick, E. and Eastman, A. (1982). The significance of DNA cross-linking to *cis*-diamminedichloroplatinum (II) – induced cytotoxicity in sensitive and resistant lines of murine leukaemia L1210. *Chem. Biol. Interact.*, **39**, 169–180

77. Rawlings, C. J. and Roberts, J. J. (1986). Walker rat carcinoma cells are exceptionally sensitive to *cis*-diamminedichloroplatinum (cisplatin) and other bifunctional agents, but

not defective in the removal of platinum-DNA adducts. *Mutation Res.*, **166**, 157–169

78. Bedford, P., Fichtuger-Schepman, A. M. J., Stellard, S. A., *et al.* (1988). Differential repair of platinum-DNA adducts in human bladder and testicular tumour continuous cell lines. *Cancer Res.*, **48**, 3019–3024

79. Meyn, R. E., Jenkins, S. F. and Thompson, L. H. (1982). Defective removal of DNA cross-links in a repair deficient mutant of Chinese hamster cells. *Cancer Res.*, **47**, 388–393

80. Plooy, A. C. M., Van Dijk, M., Berends, F. and Lohman, P. H. M. (1985). Formation and repair of DNA interstrand cross-links in relation to cytotoxicity and unscheduled DNA synthesis in control and mutant human cells treated with *cis*-diamminedichloroplatinum (II). *Cancer Res.*, **45**, 4178–4184

81. Chu, G. and Berg, P. (1987). DNA cross-linked by cisplatin: A new probe for the DNA repair defect in Xeroderma Pigmentosum. *Mol. Biol. Med.*, **4**, 277–290

82. Wood, R. D., Robins, P. and Lindahl, T. (1988). Complementation of the Xeroderma Pigmentosum DNA repair defect in cell-free extracts. *Cell*, **53**, 97–106

83. Lung, V., Chambers, A. F., Harris, J. F. and Hill, R. P. (1985). Quantitative genetic analysis of tumour progression. *Cancer Metastasis Rev.*, **4**, 173–194

84. Goldie, J. H. and Coldman, A. J. (1984). The genetic origin of drug resistance in neoplasms: Implications for systemic therapy. *Cancer Res.*, **44**, 3643–3653

85. Giulotto, E., Knights, C. and Stark, G. R. (1987). Hamster cells with increased rates of DNA amplification, a new phenotype. *Cell*, **48**, 837–845

86. Goldberg, S. and Defendi, V. (1979). Increased mutation rates in doubly viral transformed Chinese hamster cells. *Somat. Cell Genet.*, **5**, 887–895

87. Gupta, R. S. and Goldstein, S. (1980). Diphtheria toxin resistance in human fibroblast cell strains from normal and cancer-prone individuals. *Mutat. Res.*, **73**, 331–338

88. Pickford, I. and Franks, L. M. (1988). Genetic aspects of tumour metastasis. *Cancer Surv.*, **7**, 351–371

89. Johnson, B. E., Ihde, D. C., Makuch, R. W., *et al.* (1987). *myc* family oncogene amplification in tumour cell lines established from small cell lung cancer patients and its relationship to clinical status and course. *J. Clin. Invest.*, **79**, 1629–1634

90. Sklar, M. D. (1988). The *ras* oncogenes increase the intrinsic resistance of NIH 3T3 cells to ionizing radiation. *Science*, **239**, 645–647

91. Riou, G., Monique, G. L. Doussal, V. L., *et al.* (1987). C-*myc* proto-oncogene expression and prognosis in early carcinoma of the uterine cervix. *Lancet*, **2**, 761–763

92. Denby, P. P. and Hill, B. T. (eds.) (1983). *Human Tumour Drug Sensitivity Testing In Vitro.* (London: Acad. Press)

93. Hamburger, A. and Salmon, S. E. (1977). Primary bioassay of human tumour stem cells. *Science*, **197**, 461–463

94. Thien, S. L., Jeffreys, A. J., Gooi, H. C., Cotter, F., *et al.* (1987). Detection of somatic changes in human cancer DNA by DNA fingerprint analysis. *Br. J. Cancer*, **55**, 353–356

95. Hill, B. T. (1986). In vitro human tumour model systems for investigating drug resistance. *Cancer Surv.*, **5**, 129–149

96. Carman, M. D., Schornagel, J. H., Rivest, R. S., *et al.* (1984). Resistance to methotrexate due to gene amplification in a patient with acute leukaemia. *J. Clin. Oncol.*, **2**, 16–20

97. Horns, R. C., Dower, W. J. and Schimke, R. T. (1984). Gene amplification in a leukaemic patient treated with methotrexate. *J. Clin. Oncol.*, **2**, 2–7

98. Ma, D. D. F., Davey, R. A., Harman, D. H., *et al.* (1987). Detection of a multi-drug resistant phenotype in acute non-lymphoblastic leukaemia. *Lancet*, **1**, 135–137

99. Fojo, A. T., Ueda, K., Slamon, D. J., *et al.* (1987). Expression of a multidrug-resistance gene in human tumours and tissues. *Proc. Natl. Acad. Sci. USA*, **84**, 265–269

100. Fojo, A. T., Shen, D-W., Mickley, L. A., Pastan, I. and Gottesman, M. M. (1987). Intrinsic drug resistance in human kidney cancer is associated with expression of a human multi-drug resistance gene. *J. Clin. Oncol.*, **5**, 1922–1927

101. Gerlach, J. H., Bell, D. R., Karakousis, C., *et al.* (1987). P-glycoprotein in human sarcoma: Evidence for multi-drug resistance. *J. Clin. Oncol.*, **5**, 1452–1460

102. Sugawara, I., Kataoka, I., Morishita, Y., *et al.* (1988). Tissue distribution of P-glycoprotein encoded by a multidrug-resistant gene as revealed by a monoclonal antibody, MRK 16. *Cancer Res.*, **48**, 1926–1929

103. Goldstein, L. J., Galski, H., Fojo, A., Wittingham, M. *et al.* (1989). Expression of a multi-drug resistance gene in human cancers. *J. Natl. Cancer Inst.*, **81**, 116–123

104. Chiu, D., Lubin, B. and Shohet, S. B. (1982). Peroxidative reactions in red cell biology. In Pryor, W. A. (ed.) *Free Radicals in Biology,* pp. 115–160. (New York: Academic Press)

105. Harrison, P. R. (1984). Molecular analysis of erythropoiesis. *Exp. Cell Res.,* **155**, 321–344

106. Moscow, J. A., Townsend, A. J., Goldsmith, M. E., *et al.* (1988). Isolation of the human anionic glutathione S-transferase cDNA and the relation of its gene expression to oestrogen receptor content in primary breast cancer. *Proc. Natl. Acad. Sci. USA,* **85**, 6518–6522

107. Lewis, A. D., Hayes, J. D. and Wolf, C. R. (1988). Glutathione and glutathione-dependent enzymes in ovarian adenocarcinoma cell lines derived from a patient before and after the onset of drug resistance: intrinsic differences and cell cycle effects. *Carcinogenesis,* **9**, 1283–1287

108. Masuda, H., Ozols, R. F., Lai, G-M., *et al.* (1988). Increased DNA repair as a mechanism of acquired resistance to *cis*-diamminedichloroplatinum (II) in human ovarian cancer cell lines. *Cancer Res.,* **48**, 5713–5716

109. Swift, M., Reitnauer, P. J., Morrell, D. and Chase, C. L. (1987). Breast and other cancers in families with ataxia-telangiectasia. *N. Engl. J. Med.,* **316**, 1289–1294

110. Chan, J. H. Y., Becker, F. F., German, J. E. E. and Ray, J. H. (1987). Altered DNA ligase I activity in Bloom's syndrome cells. *Nature (London),* **325**, 357–359

111. Willis, J. E. E. and Lindahl, T. (1987). DNA ligase I deficiency in Bloom's syndrome cells. *Nature (London),* **325**, 355–357

112. Rusquet, R. M., Feon, S. A. and David, J. C. (1988). Association of a possible DNA ligase deficiency with T-cell acute leukaemia. *Cancer Res.,* **48**, 4038–4044

113. Bohr, V. A., Phillips, D. H. and Harawatt, P. C. (1987). Heterogeneous DNA damage and repair in the mammalian genome. *Cancer Res.,* **47**, 6426–6436

114. Gibson, N. W., Mattes, W. B. and Hartley, J. A. (1985). Identification of specific DNA lesions induced by three classes of chloroethylating agents. *Pharm. Ther.,* **31**, 153–163

115. Kohn, K. W., Hartley, J. A. and Mattes, W. B. (1987). Mechanisms of DNA sequence selective alkylation of guanine-N7 positions by nitrogen mustards. *Nucleic Acids Res.,* **15**, 10531–10549

116. Bird, A. P. (1986). CpG-rich islands and the function of DNA methylation. *Nature (London),* **321**, 209–213

117. Foka, M. and Paoletti, J. (1986). Interaction of *cis*-diamminedichloroplatinum (II) to chromatin specificity of the drug distribution. *Biochem. Pharmacol.,* **35**, 3282–3295

118. Beckmann, R. P. Agostino, M. J., McHugh, M. M., Sigmund, R. D. and Beerman, T. A. (1987). Assessment of preferential cleavage of an actively transcribed retroviral hybrid gene in murine cells by deoxyribonuclease I, bleomycin, neocarzinostatin or ionising radiation. *Biochemistry,* **26**, 5490–5415

119. Sanders, M. and Hsieh, T. (1983). Double strand DNA cleavage by type II DNA topoisomerase. *J. Biol. Chem.,* **258**, 8421–8428

120. Choi, K., Chen, C-J., Kriegler, M. and Roninson, I. B. (1988). An altered pattern of cross-resistance in multidrug-resistant human cells from spontaneous mutations in the *mdr1* gene. *Cell,* **53**, 519–529

121. Palmiter, R. D. and Brinster, R. L. (1985). Transgenic mice. *Cell,* **41**, 343–345

122. Williams, D. A., Lemischka, I. R., Nathan, D. G. and Mulligan, R. C. (1984). Introduction of new genetic material into pluripotent haematopoietic stem cells of the mouse. *Nature (London),* **310**, 476–480

123. Thomas, K. R. and Capecchi, M. R. (1986). Introduction of homologous DNA sequences into mammalian cells induces mutations in the cognate gene. *Nature (London),* **324**, 34–38

124. Thomas, K. R. and Capecchi, M. R. (1987). Site-directed mutagenesis by gene targeting in mouse embryo-derived stem cells. *Cell,* **51**, 503–512

125. Bradley, A., Evans, M., Kaufman, M. H. and Robertson, E. (1984). Formation of germ-line chimaeras from embryo-derived teratocarcinoma cell lines. *Nature (London),* **309**, 255–256

126. Green, P. J., Pines, O. and Inouye, M. (1986). The role of antisense RNA in gene regulation. *Annu. Rev. Biochem.,* **55**, 569–597

127. Stein, C. A. and Cohen, J. S. (1988). Oligodeoxynucleotides as inhibitors of gene expression: A review. *Cancer Res.,* **48**, 2659–2668

128. Izant, J. G. and Weintraub, H. (1985). Constitutive and conditional suppression of exogenous and endogenous genes by anti-sense RNA. *Science,* **229**, 345–352

129. Wickstrom, E. L., Bacon, T. A., Gonzalez, A., Freeman, D. L., Lyman, G. H. and Wickstrom, E. (1988). Human promyelocytic leukaemia HL60 cell proliferation and c-*myc*

protein expression are inhibited by an antisense pentadecadeoxynucleotide targeted against c-*myc* mRNA. *Proc. Natl. Acad. Sci. USA,* **85**, 1028–1032

130. Tsuruo, T., Iida, H., Tsukagoshi, S. and Sakurai, Y. (1981). Overcoming of vincristine resistance in P388 leukaemia, *in vivo* and *in vitro* through enhanced cytotoxicity of vincristine and vinblastine by verapamil. *Cancer Res.,* **41**, 1967–1972

131. Slater, L. M., Murray, S. L. and Wetrel, M. W. (1982). Verapamil restoration of daunorubicin responsiveness in daumorubicin-resistant Ehrlich ascites carcinoma. *J. Clin. Invest.,* **70**, 1131–1134

132. Garapathi, R. and Grabowski, O. (1983). Enhancement of sensitivity to adriamycin in resistant P388 leukaemia by the calmodulin inhibitor trifluoperazine. *Cancer Res.,* **43**, 3696–3699

133. Cornwell, M. M., Safa, A. R., Felsted, R. L., Gottesman, M. M. and Pastan, I. (1986). Membrane vesicles from multi-drug resistant human cancer cells contain a specific 150 to 170 kDa protein detected by photoaffinity labelling. *Proc. Natl. Acad. Sci. USA,* **83**, 3847–3850

134. Hamada, H., Hagiwara, K.-I., Nakajima, T. and Tsuruo, T. (1987). Phosphorylation of the M170,000 to 180,000 glycoprotein specific to multidrug-resistant tumour cells: effect of verapamil, trifluoperazine and phorbol esters. *Cancer Res.,* **47**, 2860–2865

135. Ozols, R. F., Cunnion, R. E., Klecker, R. W., Hamilton, T. C., Ostchega, Y., Parrillo, J. E. and Young, R. C. (1987). Verapamil and adriamycin in the treatment of drug-resistant ovarian cancer patients. *J. Clin. Oncol.,* **5**, 641–647

136. Merry, S., Kerr, D., Flanigan, P., Milroy, R., Freshney, R. I. and Kaye, S. B. (1987). Inherent adriamycin resistance in a murine tumour line: Circumvention with verapamil and norverapamil. *Br. J. Cancer,* **56**, 185

137. Kerr, D. J., Graham, J., Cummings, J., Morrison, J. G., Thompson, G. G., Brodie, M. J. and Kaye, S. B. (1986). The effect of verapamil on the pharmacokinetics of adriamycin. *Cancer Chemother. Pharmacol.,* **18**, 239–242

138. Milroy, R., Cummings, J., Kaye, S. B. and Banham, S. W. (1987). Phase II clinical and pharmacological study of oral 4-demethoxydaunorubicin in advanced non-pretreated small cell lung cancer. *Cancer Chemother. Pharmacol.,* **20**, 77–77

139. Presant, C. A., Kennedy, P., Wiseman, C., Gala, K., Bouzaglou, A., Wyres, M. and Naessig, V. (1986). Verapamil reversal of clinical doxorubicin resistance in human cancer. *Am. J. Clin. Oncol.,* **9**, 355–357

140. Figueredo, A., Arnold, A., Findlay, M., Goodyear, M., Neville, A., Normandeau, R. and Jones, R. (1988). Pilot study of verapamil and tamoxifen added to chemotherapy of extensive small cell lung cancer. *Proc. ASCO,* **1**, 208

141. Tsuruo, T., Iida, H., Kitatani, Y., Yokata, K., Tsukagoshi, S. and Sakurai, Y. (1984). Effects of quinidine and related compounds of cytotoxicity and cellular accumulation of vincristine and adriamycin in drug-resistant tumour cells. *Cancer Res.,* **44**, 4303

142. Schuurhuis, G. J., Broxterman, H. J., van der Hoeven, J. J., Pinedo, H. M. and Lankelma, J. L. (1987). Potentiation of doxorubicin cytotoxicity by the calcium antagonist bepridil in anthracycline-resistant and -sensitive cell lines. *Cancer Chemother. Pharmacol.,* **20**, 285

143. Tsutsui, K., Komuro, C., Ono, K., Nishidai, J., Shibamato, Y., Takahashi, M. and Abe, M. (1986). Chemosensitisation by BSO in vivo. *Int. J. Rad. Oncol. Biol. Phys.,* **12**, 1183–1186

144. Lee, F. Y., Allaluims-Turner, M. J. and Siemann, D. W. (1987). Depletion of tumour versus normal tissue glutathione by buthionine sulfoximine. *Br. J. Cancer,* **56**, 33–38

145. Cadman, E. C., Heimer, R. and Davis, L. (1979). Enhanced 5-fluorouracil nucleotide formation following methotrexate: Explanation for drug synergism. *Science,* **205**, 1135–1137

146. Kluber, P., Cerna, L. and Meldon, M. A. (1981). Effect of concurrent calcium leucovorin infusion on 5-fluorouracil cytotoxicity against murine L1210 leukaemia. *Cancer Chemother. Pharmacol.,* **6**, 121–125

147. Petrelli, N., Stablein, P., Bruckner, H., Megibow, A., Mayer, R. and Douglas, H. (1988). A prospective randomised trial of 5FU versus 5FU on high dose leucororin in patients with metastatic colorectal cancer. *Proc. ASCO,* **1**, 94

148. Bonnadonna, G., Valagussa, P. and Santoro, A. (1988). Alternating non-cross-resistant combination chemotherapy or MOPP in stage IV Hodgkin's disease. *Ann. Intern. Med.,* **104**, 739–744

6
The detection of minimal disease and implications for cure

B.L. SAMUELS AND J.E. ULTMANN

INTRODUCTION

The limitations of current technology are such that a malignant neoplasm must reach a relatively large size, of the order of hundreds of millions of cells, before it can be detected. This implies that a tumour which is barely detectable nevertheless has considerable malignant potential. The definition of 'minimal disease' thus has important implications for cure of the neoplasm. Minimal disease may mean different things at different times during the life cycle of a tumour, and the implications for cure of the same amount of minimal disease may also change with time.

In animal tumour models, the amount of minimal disease can be precisely defined in terms of the actual number of tumour cells introduced into the experimental animal[1]. In clinical practice, the number of tumour cells is unknown, and minimal disease must, therefore, be operationally defined. Several different parameters might be chosen for this definition, and the amount of tumour constituting minimal disease might well vary according to the parameters chosen.

One operational definition of minimal disease would obviously be 'minimal detectable disease'. In this case, minimal disease would be that amount of tumour that is just detectable. This amount will vary with the technology available for tumour detection. Minimal disease can also be considered in terms of available therapy. This operational view of, for example, testicular cancer, would have been very different before the introduction of cisplatin-based chemotherapy regimens markedly increased the efficacy of chemotherapy in the treatment of this disease[2]. Minimal disease might be defined in terms of patient survival as the greatest amount of tumour compatible with achieving a specified survival parameter. Alternatively, minimal disease might be defined in terms of the life cycle and growth kinetics of the neoplasm as the point at which a specified growth rate is reached or at which the balance of cell proliferation and cell death results in a specified tumour doubling time.

It is important to understand the limitations of the methodology used to detect minimal disease; in certain respects, if tumour can be detected at all, it is, by definition, not minimal. For this reason, 'cure' cannot be distinguished in an individual patient from 'survival with no overt disease'.

THEORETICAL IMPLICATIONS FOR CURE

The human body has between 10^{13} and 10^{14} cells. A tumour will become radiologically detectable at a size of about 100 mg (10^8 cells) and will be just palpable at 1 g (10^9 cells), although many tumours may only become symptomatic and thus come to medical attention at a size of 10^{10} cells[3]. An aggregate tumour mass of 1 kg (10^{12} cells) usually represents a lethal tumour burden. A tumour usually first comes to medical attention at 'minimum size' having already progressed through about three quarters of its life cycle. Thus, any current operational definition of minimal disease would still imply the presence of many tens of millions of tumour cells.

The many factors influencing tumour cell growth and and tumour cell death change during the life cycle of a tumour, so that the net rate of growth is different at various stages of the tumour's natural history. Tumour size is an important determinant. Tumour growth in experimental systems is approximately exponential at small tumour volumes and then follows a sigmoidal Gompertzian function[4] as the tumour volume increases over 1 cm^3. The reasons for the slowing of net tumour growth are not well understood, but it is thought that rapidly growing tumours will begin to outstrip the available blood supply after a certain size, thus tending to reduce the proliferation rate. In addition, the rate of cell loss through cell death and through cells entering a resting, non-dividing stage of the cell cycle increases in tumour nodules over 1 cm^3 in size. The sigmoidal growth curve at larger tumour volumes is a result of the net effects of exponential growth and exponential cell loss. Since chemotherapy and radiation therapy largely affect dividing cells, the higher growth fraction of very small tumours (minimal disease) may mean that the latter may have a more favourable response to therapy than do larger tumours.

Skipper's work in CDF$_1$ mice inoculated with L1210 leukaemia cells showed that chemotherapeutic drugs kill leukaemia cells according to logarithmic, or first order, kinetics, so that a constant fraction rather than a constant number of tumour cells is killed by any specific dose[1]. It is generally accepted that this model applies, at least in part, to the clinical treatment of cancer. Therefore, with a constant fraction, but diminishing absolute number, of cells killed with each successive cycle of therapy, it is again apparent that a small tumour is more likely than a large tumour to be reduced below some theoretical threshold tumour burden within the 3 to 6 cycles of therapy usually tolerable for most regimens. Based on projections from this model, it is apparent that many patients treated for a chemotherapy-sensitive neoplasm do not receive sufficient cycles of therapy for complete tumour cell eradication – although there may, nevertheless, be a significant number of 'cures' in such a group. This has led to the concept of a threshold residual tumour burden which is sufficiently small that the host's own defence mechanisms can deal with it, with the goal of therapy being to reduce tumour burden below that threshold.

84

Goldie and Coldman have developed a mathematical model to predict the development of drug resistance within a tumour[5]. Their work was based on observations made earlier by Luria and Delbruck regarding the capacity of bacteria to develop resistance to infection by bacteriophage[6]. This work showed that some mutant subcultures of parental 'sensitive' bacterial strains were resistant to bacteriophage infection despite the fact that these subcultures had not been exposed to the phage. They concluded that bacterial resistance to bacteriophage infection occurs as a result of random spontaneous mutation rather than as a result of exposure to the phage. As applied by Goldie and Coldman to tumour cells and chemotherapy resistance, the hypothesis assumes that resistance to chemotherapy is a result of spontaneous mutation to a genotype which confers resistance to one or more chemotherapeutic agents. Exposure of the tumour cell to the drug is not required for the mutation to occur and is not part of the mechanism of resistance induction, but, once a cell line with resistance is present, the use of that chemotherapeutic drug will apply selection pressure in favour of the resistant cells. Thus, over time, the proportion of resistant cells in the tumour as a whole will increase. The probability of such a random mutation taking place is related to the spontaneous mutation rate of the tumour (usually between 1 in 10^5 and 1 in 10^6 cell divisions) and also, therefore, to the number of cells available for division and thus at risk for mutation; in other words, it is related to tumour size. Tumour size is a measure of both the number of cells at risk of mutation and, to some extent, a measure of the length of time that has been available for growth of any resistant cells, since, normally, the larger the tumour, the longer it has been present. Thus, the larger the tumour, the more likely it is that a genotype conferring resistance to a given agent would have arisen spontaneously prior to therapy. Therapy using the agent in question is likely to provide selection pressure and potentiate the repopulation of the tumour with resistant cells. The number of resistant cells present in a tumour prior to therapy depends on the point in time prior to therapy at which the mutation to resistance occurred, and, therefore, is to some extent a matter of chance. In most clinical situations, provided that mutation to resistance did not occur very early in the tumour's growth, the proportion of resistant cells when the tumour is first treated is not large and does not affect the initial clinical response. A significant impact on the fractional cell kill would only be expected if the resistant cells constituted more than 50% of the cell population. In the clinical situation, this means that a complete remission (which results from an approximately 2 log cell kill) is achievable even in the presence of a resistant cell population. However, since the resistant cells are not killed by treatment, an increase in the relative proportion of resistant cells and regrowth of a resistant tumour will eventually occur either with or without continued treatment. Thus, unless treatment starts and can be completed before any mutation to resistance has occurred, it is unlikely that any single agent, no matter how potent, could cure a malignant tumour. This prediction is consistent with empirical knowledge regarding the efficacy of chemotherapy treatment and, in fact, single agents are almost never employed in initial therapy. The theoretical exception would be a tumour with an extremely rapid growth rate where the rate of cell division is proportionately much greater than the rate of cell loss. In this situation, relatively few tumour cell divisions would be required before the tumour would be large enough to be diagnosed and treated, and thus there is a lower probability that spontaneous mutation to resistance would occur prior to the start of therapy. The only human tumour predictably curable with single-agent chemotherapy is gestational choriocarcinoma, which does indeed have a rapid doubling time[7]. On the other hand, the simultaneous use of multiple agents allows killing of cells resistant to one drug only by one of the other agents used. Clearly, spontaneous resistance to multiple drugs may arise, but this occurs less frequently assuming that the mechanisms of resistance are independent. This is supported by the demonstrated efficacy of combination chemotherapy in clinical practice. Failure to achieve cure is predicted by the Goldie–Coldman theory with the emergence of cells resistant to multiple agents. In practice, this may occur more often than theoretically predicted, particularly in solid tumours, since many mechanisms of drug resistance are effective against more than one chemotherapeutic agent. Thus, the hypothesis can account for many of the observed results of chemotherapy treatment in the clinic.

We would, therefore, predict from the work of Skipper and his colleagues[1], and later of Goldie and Coldman[5], that tumour bulk would be a significant prognostic factor in the determination of the outcome of chemotherapy. This is borne out in many clinical series in which prognostic models have been developed. In most series, tumour burden has inversely correlated with the degree of success in treatment, whether tumour volume is estimated directly, as during laparotomy for ovarian cancer[8]; by tabulation of the number of sites of disease in large-cell lymphoma[9]; by radiological estimation; or by biochemical quantitation of a tumour product or marker[10]. As such models are further refined and become more accurate, they may allow therapy to be tailored, so that patients with a poor chance of achieving a complete remission with a particular regimen can be identified prospectively and possibly treated with a more aggressive approach.

Since most available antitumour drugs primarily affect cycling cells by interaction with DNA, the proportion of cells in a tumour which are actively cycling at any time represents a potential determinant of the efficacy of therapy. Tumour growth kinetics are such that the proportion of cycling cells (growth fraction) falls as the tumour volume increases[4]. This again has the theoretical implication of decreasing chemotherapeutic efficacy in large, as opposed to small, tumors.

The impact of these hypotheses on clinical planning has been significant. The concept of 'adjuvant chemotherapy' is based on the proposition that, in a clinical situation in which micrometastases exist at the time of excision of the primary tumour, chemotherapy is likely to be more effective immediately postoperatively, in this setting of 'minimal residual tumour burden', than when employed after the metastases have grown to a clinically-detectable volume[11]. This is based on the cell kinetic data as well as on the presumed first-order tumour cell kill kinetics proposed by Skipper. The Goldie–Coldman theory would also suggest that early therapy at low tumour burden is less likely to encounter drug resistance.

This concept can be refined to take into account clinical reality, which enforces a delay in the institution of adjuvant therapy to allow adequate postoperative recuperation and wound healing. Theoretically, a delay in the institution of adjuvant chemotherapy of only a few weeks may allow the emergence of drug-resistant clones of tumour cells. Since the primary object of chemotherapy is to deal with metastases (occult in this situation), there are theoretical advantages to utilizing chemotherapy before surgery in so-called 'neo-adjuvant' or 'proto-adjuvant' fashion, thus avoiding delay in the institution of therapy[12]. Surgery remains the primary modality for achieving local control of tumour; effective chemotherapy will prevent further growth of the primary during the pre-operative period and may even facilitate more complete surgery by shrinking the primary tumour. More importantly, early therapy may prevent drug-resistant cells from developing in the micrometastatic nodules.

In some clinical situations, knowledge of the tumour size will allow determination of appropriate therapy – in some cases suggesting that local therapy alone will be potentially curative, without the risks and morbidity associated with systemic therapy. Tumour size plays a role in most solid-tumour staging schemes but may be of particular importance in tumours, such as those of the head and neck[13] or in extremity sarcomas[14], in which treatment may be determined by primary tumour size even in the absence of evidence of local or distant tumour spread. Thus, a malignant fibrous histiocytoma in the thigh, which has been shown by radiographic studies not to have overt metastases, might be treated by wide excision alone if it were subcutaneous and 2 cm in diameter, but a tumour of the same histologic grade which was 7 cm in size might be treated by excision followed by adjuvant radiation and chemotherapy.

ANIMAL MODELS

Much of the seminal work in tumour biology has been done using animal models, such as the L1210 murine leukaemia model. These tumours have a very high growth fraction, approaching 100%, with up to 60% of cells in S phase (actively synthesizing DNA) at any one time. The growth characteristics of the tumour *in vivo* are very consistent and have been well documented[15]. Skipper *et al.*[1] demonstrated a log linear relationship between the number of tumour cells inoculated and the duration of animal survival after inoculation. A tumour of 10^9 cells constitutes a lethal burden in a mouse. The linear survival plot can be used to determine the size of the initial tumour burden with some degree of accuracy, based on the duration of survival after tumour inoculation[1]. This is obviously useful in the investigation of the concept of minimal disease. However, using this particular model, Skipper *et al.* were able to show that inoculation of even a single clonogenic L1210 cell could lead to the death of the animal, thus confirming an earlier observation made by Furth and Kahn in 1937[16]. The lethal 10^9 cell number is reached in 40 doublings from a single cell. With a 12-hour doubling time for L1210 and a 100% growth fraction, the animals would be expected to die 19 days after inoculation with a single cell. Thus, untreated, in this tumour model, there is no 'minimal disease' in the sense of a non-lethal burden of tumour. Skipper *et al.* also made use of the reproducible relationship of survival time to tumour cell number to generate the data related to the amount of cell kill per unit dose of chemotherapy. The cell kill was determined from the number of days of increased survival resulting from a given dose of the drug. Given a low initial inoculum of tumour and a sufficient number of chemotherapy treatments, it is theoretically possible to reach a point at which less than one tumour cell would be left after therapy, thus truly achieving cure of the tumour. This cure may be defined in terms of the animal's survival for a normal life span or may be defined by the lack of any histological evidence of tumour when the animal is sacrificed at some interval after therapy and an autopsy is performed. The former is an operational definition of cure which more closely approximates the clinical situation.

Recent work with the Brown Norway rat myelocytic leukaemia model in rats has shown that the fraction of cells killed by a given dose of cyclophosphamide decreases as the therapy is administered at increasing time after tumour inoculation[17]. This is consistent with both the Skipper and Goldie–Coldman models, since a greater probability of spontaneous development of drug resistance exists in tumours which have progressed further through their natural history. The importance of this observation resides in the implication that the presence of the same amount of minimal disease has different implications for cure at different times. Thus, a tumour at a size of 10^9 cells, detected for the first time in an asymptomatic person, is more likely to be curable than a residual nodule of tumour, approximately 10^9 cells in size, remaining after resection of a recurrent tumour mass two years after initial surgery.

SIGNIFICANCE OF MINIMAL DISEASE IN HUMANS

Screening and early detection

The data derived from animal models of tumour kinetics, chemotherapeutic drug action, and drug resistance all suggest that the optimal time to treat a tumour is as early as possible during its development. This is clearly true in theory, but the implication that mass screening should therefore be employed to enable tumours to be detected and treated at the earliest opportunity does not necessarily follow. The decision to implement a screening programme for a particular tumour should be based on many parameters, among them the efficacy of available therapy, the cost/benefit ratio of such a screening programme, the limitations of the technology available for screening and the natural history of the tumour screened. Screening, if useful at all, is more likely to have a significant yield when applied to a population that has been predetermined to be at risk for developing the tumour in question. On these theoretical grounds, a screening programme for lung cancer should be directed at heavy smokers over age 50, rather than to the entire adult population or to college athletes under age 20. The ratio of cost-to-yield can clearly be influenced by judicious patient selection, but the ratio of cost-to-benefit may not improve if no effective intervention is possible in many of the identified cases. Thus, patients with Hodgkin's disease who have undergone combined modality chemotherapy and radiation regimens are at relatively high risk of developing acute leukaemia[18]. However, these secondary leukaemias are extremely refractory to treatment, so that the benefits of a screening programme for leukaemia in this population are questionable at best, despite a predicted high yield of positive cases.

In the general population, mass screening could only conceivably be appropriate for the high-incidence tumours, such as lung, breast, colorectal cancer and others for which the entire older adult population could be considered to be at 'high risk'[19]. Various recommendations have been made by such groups as the American Cancer Society[20] for screening for breast cancer[21], colorectal cancer[22], cervical cancer[23], oropharyngeal cancers[24] and skin cancers[25]. The specific recommendations take into account the population involved, the available screening technology and the ease and risk of its application, but not the available therapy, with the implication that therapy will be available if cancer is detected. Thus mammography is suggested with increasing frequency as the patient ages, while breast self-examination is recommended monthly in all adult women. Proctosigmoidoscopy is recommended every 3 to 5 years if initially negative, while stool guaiac testing and digital examination are recommended annually.

A distinction should be made between screening, in which the tests are applied to all members of an asymptomatic population group, and case finding, in which a physician applies the same tests to an asymptomatic individual in whom he detects some indication to warrant application of the tests on an individual basis.

It has been difficult to demonstrate a positive effect for most screening programmes. An important example is lung cancer, now the most common cancer among both men and women in the USA. High-risk groups are readily identifiable, but, even within these groups, screening has little impact[26]. This is because the ultimate test of the efficacy of a screening programme is a reduction of mortality from the tumour in question. Despite a higher proportion of stage I cases and a higher resectability rate in cases identified through screening, no reduction in mortality rates has resulted in the identified cases. Although an increased proportion of early-stage colorectal cancers are reported from screening trials, the evidence for a reduction in overall mortality is equivocal at present, with results of several trials pending[27]. The most widespread and established cancer screening technique is probably the use of the Papanicolaou smear for cytologic detection of cancer of the uterine cervix. No controlled trials of this technique have ever been carried out, but comparison with historical controls does show a decrease in mortality rates which is at least partially due to screening[28]. In the case of breast cancer, a decrease in mortality rates has been demonstrated in several trials, although the long natural history of this cancer means that decades of follow up will be required to determine finally whether mortality from breast cancer is truly reduced or merely delayed[29].

There are many pitfalls in the interpretation of data from screening trials. In particular, there are several forms of statistical bias which must be considered[30]. Lead time bias is the time between administration of the positive screening test and the time at which the tumour ordinarily would have been diagnosed. Even without any intervention, if death occurs at the same point in the natural history of the tumour, the perceived survival time after diagnosis is obviously longer when the tumour is diagnosed earlier in its course. Selection bias occurs because screening is carried out in patients who present themselves for screening and may, therefore, be more health conscious, better educated or have other characteristics which may put them in a better prognostic category than other patients. Over-diagnosis bias is the tendency of screening to detect small and possibly insignificant lesions which, had they not been brought to attention by screening, would not have progressed to the point of being clinically apparent. Related to over-diagnosis bias is length bias, which is a measure of the tendency of screening programmes to detect cases with a more prolonged course (since the patient is, by definition, asymptomatic) and hence potentially with a better prognosis. All of these biases tend to skew the results in the direction of a favourable outcome for patients whose tumour is detected by a screening programme and to lead to the conclusion that survival is prolonged by early detection. Unfortunately, although these biases are known to exist, there is no readily available way to correct for them. Partially for this reason, the only truly valid criterion for success should probably be a reduction in mortality rates for the tumour screened in the population at risk.

The impact of technology on screening programmes is, of course, considerable. As technology advances, the sensitivity of screening techniques will undoubtedly improve. It is less certain, however, that the specificity of testing will improve commensurately. At the same time, if techniques which are both safer (for example, the decline in the radiation exposure necessary to obtain high-quality mammograms) and cheaper to apply can be developed, the cost/benefit balance of many screening programmes could be improved. Without an increase in specificity, however, the cost and danger of the follow-up studies required for a large number of false positive results may continue to offset the benefits to be expected from an increasingly sophisticated screening procedure.

Minimal disease at diagnosis

At the time of tumour diagnosis, procedures are usually undertaken to establish the extent of tumour spread and involvement. This process is codified as tumour 'staging'. Various staging classifications have been developed for different diseases in an attempt to allow more rational treatment choices[13,31]. The data which may contribute to the determination of tumour stage include clinical examination; radiological imaging studies including X-ray, isotope, ultrasound and magnetic resonance imaging; and, in certain tumours, biochemical markers of disease burden, which may be specific tumour markers or non-specific indicators, such as lactate dehydrogenase (LDH). For many tumours, an additional level of staging is provided by surgical intervention, which might take the form of biopsy of a suspicious lesion identified radiologically, determination of depth of tumour invasion in a resected specimen[32] or the knowledge gained by surgical exploration, as, for example, in staging laparotomy for Hodgkin's disease[33].

The importance of the detection of minimal disease here lies in the difference in prognosis and treatment approach associated with the discovery of even minimal tumour spread from the primary lesion. In the case of most solid tumours, this finding means that the tumour is no longer curable by surgical means and therefore probably no longer curable at all. On the other hand, the finding of minimal disease at diagnosis, when there is localized disease only, may have profound implications for cure.

We would expect that, for tumours which respond well to chemotherapy, such as lymphoma, a minimal tumour burden would greatly enhance the probability of cure with chemotherapy, and this is in fact the case[34]. However, local therapy, such as radiation, may also be curative in this situation, and involve less morbidity[35]. The possibility of occult distant disease remains, even in the case of a minimal tumour burden, so that some controversy exists as to the optimal approach to minimal disease. Local therapy may be employed with the expectation that, if occult distant disease were in fact present, it would still be curable with chemotherapy when it eventually became manifest[36]. The Goldie–Coldman theory would predict, however, that cure may be less likely in this situation. Very long-term follow-up of such 'salvage' chemotherapy for patients who had radiation for initially 'localized' Hodgkin's disease indicates that there may indeed be a slightly lower long-term survival rate in this situation[37].

For tumours with a poor response to chemotherapy, such as melanoma[38], non-small-cell lung cancer[39] or squamous carcinoma of the uterine cervix[40], minimal tumour at diagnosis (which, in the case of cervical cancer, may mean non-invasive or *in situ* carcinoma only) means that the possibility of cure with extirpation of the localized disease exists. Chemotherapy cannot be relied upon to eradicate either the known primary disease or any occult micrometastases. If the disease is minimal enough so that no metastases have occurred, then local therapy may be curative. Local therapy may be surgery, as in the case of a lobectomy for localized lung cancer, or radiation, as in localized head and neck cancer, or some other modality, such as cryotherapy or electrocoagulation in the case of *in situ* carcinoma of the cervix. For a minimal primary tumour of the same volume that has already metastasized at the time of diagnosis, cure is very much less likely.

Minimal disease after first intervention

Disease that remains after the first definitive therapeutic intervention is completed has grave implications for curability. In general, the first attempt at cure has the highest probability of success. Minimal disease in this setting is redefined as 'minimal residual disease'. In many situations, the presence of even minimal residual disease also implies some degree of resistance of the tumour to therapy. We would expect, by application of the Goldie–Coldman theory, that, if minimal disease exists after chemotherapy, tumour burden will represent cells which had developed drug resistance prior to the start of chemotherapy. Since chemotherapy is generally used in combination, the implication is that cells with resistance to multiple chemotherapeutic agents are present.

The outcome of therapy is usually defined in terms of tumour response, in which a complete response (sometimes called a complete remission) is defined as complete disappearance of all known disease[41]. Various grades of less than complete response may be defined. The same clinical, radiographic, biochemical and, in some cases, surgical approaches should be used in restaging to determine the outcome of treatment as were employed in the original determination of disease stage. Clearly, there is no possibility of cure if a complete response to therapy has not been achieved. However, a complete clinical response merely implies that disease can no longer be detected by the technology employed to find it. At the time that all radiological evidence of tumour disappears, there may still be up to 10^8 tumour cells present in each tumour site. This theoretical principle is borne out by the clinical observation that patients with acute leukaemia who achieve a complete response after the first cycle of chemotherapy will almost invariably relapse if given no further therapy[42]. Thus, there are still several 'logs of cell kill' required for cure after all evidence of tumour has disappeared. Chemotherapeutic regimens employed with curative intent must, therefore, include therapy which continues after a complete response has been documented. How much additional therapy is required for cure is clearly a difficult matter to resolve. It is unlikely that every last tumour cell could be eradicated by therapy. Thus, there may be a 'threshold' tumour burden below which host-defence mechanisms may be able to cope with the remaining tumour cells, thereby accounting for cures achieved with chemotherapy in such diseases as Hodgkin's disease[43] or testicular carcinoma[44]. Rarely, this may happen on a macroscopic level, as in the few reported cases of spontaneous disappearance of metastatic deposits of renal cell carcinoma after resection of the primary tumour[45].

Thus, for an individual patient, the detection of minimal residual disease after chemotherapy has clear negative implications for curability, but the implications of achievement of a complete response are more difficult to evaluate. For some tumours, such as large-cell lymphoma, it has been demonstrated that the rate of diminution of tumour bulk during initial therapy has prognostic implications for the ultimate outcome[46]. This is probably related to the fraction of cell kill achieved with each cycle of treatment. If a known tumour with 10^9 to 10^{10} cells is no longer detectable after one cycle of therapy (a complete response), then there has probably been at least one to two logs of cell kill, and several further cycles of therapy at the same dose may indeed reduce tumour bulk below the hypothetical curability threshold. On the other hand, if the same tumour is only reduced below the size that is detectable after four cycles of therapy, then, even in the absence of confounding factors, such as cumulative toxicity and the development of drug resistance, at least four times as many cycles of chemotherapy will be required to reach the threshold. In practice, this would be very difficult to administer, since chemotherapy is usually used at the maximum tolerated dose(s) for the maximum tolerated duration.

There are several scenarios in which minimal residual disease might occur that deserve specific consideration, such as the situation in which minimal disease remains after what was intended to be a curative resection. This usually occurs when all of the gross tumour has been removed but later careful histological evaluation shows that the tumour extends right to the edge of the cut specimen. In this situation, it must be assumed that there are at least microscopic deposits of tumour left in the tumour bed, and the operation can no longer be considered to be even potentially curative. In this event, adjuvant therapy with radiation, chemotherapy or both is essential if a cure is to be attempted. The probability of obtaining a cure will, of course, vary according to the sensitivity of the tumour to the adjuvant therapy. One postoperative situation in which minimal residual disease may be identified exists when the tumour is associated with elevated levels of a circulating biochemical or immunological marker. The marker would be expected to decline to undetectable levels after complete resection – if this does not occur, residual disease should be assumed to be present, even if no obvious site of tumour is identified[47]. This finding would be an indication for consideration of systemic therapy. The biological halflife of any tumour marker in the circulation is an important consideration in determining when residual tumour should be evaluated with marker studies, since a marker with a relatively long halflife would be expected to be detectable for some time, even after complete tumour removal[48].

In some situations, the aim of surgery is not to eradicate disease where this is known to be impossible, but to 'debulk' the large volume of known tumour. We would predict that the practice of debulking large tumours in the hope of obtaining an improved cell kinetic situation for chemotherapy is unlikely to be helpful in improving the curability of the disease, although initial response rates to chemotherapy might be improved. Application of the Goldie–Coldman hypothesis suggests that drug-resistant cell lines will be present in the large primary tumour because of its size, and therefore the metastases will probably also contain resistant cells[49]. The ability of chemotherapy to eradicate residual 'minimal' disease in this case is more dependent on the implications of the large original tumour mass for the development of resistant tumour cell lines than on the effect of the small volume of residual disease in increasing the tumour growth fraction. The proportion of resistant cells in the residual tumour would approximate that which would have been found in the large tumour mass before surgery, rather than the proportion to be expected in a newly discovered primary tumour of the same dimensions as the residual tumour.

There are other situations in which the significance of minimal residual disease is clear. After remission induction chemotherapy for patients with acute leukaemia, a bone marrow aspirate which shows any residual leukaemia indicates that further cycles of induction chemotherapy are required, even if the peripheral blood smears do not show any leukaemic blasts[50]. Similarly, patients who have had complete resolution of radiological abnormalities after chemotherapy for carcinoma of the ovary routinely undergo 'second look' laparotomies[51]. In many cases, almost microscopic deposits of tumour may be seen or felt on the peritoneal membrane, or washings of the peritoneal cavity may reveal tumour cells on cytologic evaluation[52]. In this situation, further chemotherapy is usually indicated using either the original or a different regimen.

There are yet other situations in which the significance of minimal residual disease is less clearly defined. This is because of the operational definition of cure which must be used when evaluating therapy for malignancies. For all intents and purposes, when the survival curve of a patient population starts to run parallel to that of an age-matched 'normal population', those patients can be considered 'cured', since the rate at which patients are dying is not different from that which normally would be expected. For example, consider a patient who has been treated for a neoplasm and is clinically in complete remission at the time that he dies of an unrelated cause – but a small amount of residual tumour is found at autopsy. For that patient, the minimal residual disease was of no consequence, and his life was unaffected by whether or not every last tumour cell was eradicated. This may not merely be a case of the tumour not having time to become a problem before death from another cause supervened. In a well-documented series of autopsies performed on patients who were apparently well and had been clinically free of tumour 10 or more years after treatment for Hodgkin's disease, deposits of active Hodgkin's disease were found in a significant proportion of patients[53].

Sometimes minimal residual disease is not occult but is known to be present, yet is deemed to be of little consequence. An example is the finding of residual lymphocytosis after irradiation of bulky lymphadenopathy in a patient with chronic lymphocytic leukaemia[54]. In such situations, the conservative management plan is unchanged by the knowledge that the patient still has tumour cells present. This may occur because the residual tumour is considered inconsequential and unlikely to have an impact on the patient's survival, or because it is felt that current therapy will not increase survival of asymptomatic patients with a particular tumour.

Another possible scenario is that a residual radiographic abnormality is present, but it is not known whether or not this abnormality represents active tumour. An example is the not infrequent occurrence of a residual widening of the mediastinal shadow on radiographs after apparently successful therapy of a patient with Hodgkin's disease who had presented with mediastinal adenopathy. The risk of relapse is not higher in this group than in similar patients without residual abnormalities, nor is disease more likely to recur in the mediastinum if the patient does relapse[55]. Most such patients will go on to show gradual shrinking of the abnormal mediastinal shadow over a period of years. Does this radiological finding represent minimal residual disease which has been reduced by therapy to a size below the threshold at which host defence capability can take over, or does it represent merely residual fibrous stroma which is gradually remodelled over the course of time? A similar phenomenon has recently been documented to occur in patients with non-Hodgkin's lymphoma who are found to have residual abdominal soft tissue masses after therapy[56].

Residual nodules may be identified on radiographs of patients with metastatic germ cell tumours after completion of therapy. The pluripotent nature of germ cell neoplasms is such that during the course of curative therapy, some tumour nodules will undergo differentiation to a more mature form, such as mature teratoma[57]. Rarely, biopsy of such a residual nodule may even show benign cartilage tissue. It may also be that the residual nodule represents active tumour which had not been eradicated by therapy. If the level of a tumour marker, such as α-fetoprotein, was high before therapy, the post-therapy level may give some indication as to the likely nature of the residual nodule – clearly, a residual nodule accompanied by elevated tumour markers has a much graver implication for cure than a nodule of the same size in a patient in whom a previously high marker level has disappeared.

Minimal residual disease at relapse

In most cases, relapse of a malignancy after initial complete remission means that cure can no longer be achieved. Thus, in general, the implications for cure of minimal disease at relapse are no different from the implications of gross disease at relapse. However, some chemotherapy-responsive tumours, such as acute non-lymphocytic leukaemia[58] or carcinoma of the testis[59], may occasionally be cured by aggressive chemotherapy even after a first relapse. In this situation, the implications of minimal disease for cure are similar to the implications of minimal disease at the time of initial diagnosis. The Goldie–Coldman and Skipper hypotheses still apply and suggest that the tumour is less likely to have developed a population of cells resistant to new chemotherapeutic drugs (although random mutation has clearly produced resistance to those already employed) and more likely to be affected significantly by those new drugs if the tumour is small when the second therapy begins. In trials of high-dose chemotherapy with autologous bone marrow rescue for relapsed large-cell lymphoma, the prognosis is better in those patients in whom a second complete remission is induced with conventional-dose chemotherapy prior to the use of the high-dose regimen[60]. It is not clear whether this is because of reduction of tumour bulk to minimal residual disease or, as is more likely, because this merely identifies a group which responds well to chemotherapy.

It should be stated that the implications of minimal disease at relapse for duration and quality of survival after relapse are significant, even in the absence of curative potential, since the ability to achieve effective palliation may well depend on disease bulk and extent.

After a complete response to initial therapy, various means are employed to screen and detect disease recurrence. In general, these techniques are similar to those employed in the initial staging evaluation, but, since such testing is done on an on-going repetitive basis, studies should be selected with careful attention to their potential yield. Regular physical examinations, appropriate blood tests and radiological screening are the most common follow-up methods. In cases where a biochemical or immunological tumour marker was identified prior to initial therapy, renewed detection of this marker is highly suggestive of disease relapse and may occur before any other evidence of disease is present[61].

Iatrogenic minimal disease

The advance of medical technology has given rise to the potential situation in which a minimal tumour load may inadvertently be introduced into a patient as a result of medical manipulation. One such situation might occur in the setting of autologous bone marrow rescue from myelosuppression induced by high-dose chemotherapy. Careful steps are taken to ensure that the bone marrow that is harvested and stored prior to high-dose chemotherapy is free of tumour involvement[62]. The danger here is that occult tumour infiltration of the patient's bone marrow may have occurred prior to harvesting, resulting in reinfusion of stored tumour cells which, like the rescuing bone marrow stem cells, have been spared the effects of the chemotherapy. In this situation, assuming that the chemotherapy has eradicated the tumour in the patient, a minimal tumour burden has been re-introduced into the patient iatrogenically. The implications for cure are not fully understood. Clearly, if the re-introduced disease becomes clinically manifest, for example as a widespread miliary pattern of new tumour nodules, the chances of cure are minimal. On the other hand, many autologous bone marrow rescue programs require only that the bone marrow be histologically free of lymphoma prior to harvesting. It has been shown that 17% of patients with aggressive lymphomas and negative bone marrow biopsies do, in fact, have occult bone marrow infiltration with lymphoma[63]. We can, therefore, infer that, at least in some cases, marrow 'contaminated' with residual lymphoma has been re-infused, but long-term remissions have nevertheless been obtained. Given the fact that marrow involvement with tumour is evaluated by random biopsy, it is likely that this situation may occur more commonly than is documented. In cases where no apparent harm is caused by the re-infusion of lymphoma cells, the re-infused tumour burden may be below the threshold of host defence capability, or the tumour cells may have been selectively damaged by the *in vitro* handling. Techniques used to detect marrow contamination include histologic and immunocytochemical examination of bone marrow biopsies, flow cytometric evaluation of bone marrow using tumour marking antibodies or surface markers in the case of haematologic malignancies, and molecular biological evaluation for specific gene rearrangements known to occur in the tumour cells of interest. Tumour cells which can be detected by antibodies can also be destroyed by antibodies – so-called 'bone marrow purging'[62]. If no suitable antibodies are available, exposure of the bone marrow to very high levels of cytotoxic drugs *in vitro* may cause death of tumour cells without affecting the ability of the hardier marrow stem cells to re-engraft[64].

We might postulate another situation in which inadvertent introduction of minimal tumour occurs when a clinically occult tumour within an organ is transplanted along with that organ from a donor into a recipient. In this situation, the recipient did not have a malignancy prior to the transplant. This may be the closest clinical corollary of the single L1210 cell inoculated into a mouse, since the tumour introduced into the transplant recipient is both clinically occult in the donor and also not visible on direct inspection of the donated organ at the time of transplantation. Unfortunately, the measures taken to prevent host rejection of the transplanted organ may also inhibit the host-defence response to the introduced minimal tumour burden, possibly resulting in the appearance of a clinically apparent tumour in the recipient before the tumour is even apparent in the donor. Interestingly, such a tumour in the recipient may regress if immunosuppression is halted or reduced, drawing attention to the importance of host defence mechanisms in dealing with a minimal tumour burden.

THE IMPORTANCE OF NEW TECHNOLOGIES

The relative lack of benefit of screening programmes may, in part, be related to the large size already attained by the tumour by the time it can be detected using current technology. Similar technologic limitations are important in staging evaluations, in the detection of minimal disease after therapy and in the detection of relapse. The implications of minimal disease for cure may change as improved techniques lead to the detection of corresponding smaller tumours. Several new procedures are promising; all rely on detection of a marker abnormality previously identified as related to the tumour. Premature chromosome condensation is a technique for the visualization of chromosomes at times other than metaphase[65]. If a cytogenetic abnormality was previously noted in the tumour cells, this technique can be used to screen for residual or relapsing cells with the same karyotype. The clonal excess technique relies on flow cytometric detection of κ or λ surface light chains on a lymphoma cell. Since a lymphoproliferative neoplasm is monoclonal, each tumour cell bears the same light chain on its surface. Thus, when there are a number of tumour cells, the usual balance between the number of κ- and the number of λ-bearing cells will be altered by the excess of exclusively κ or λ lymphoma cells circulating[66]. This technique can potentially identify circulating lymphoma cells where none are detected histologically. Lymphoma cells, being B- or T-lymphocytes, have rearrangements of either the immunoglobulin genes[67] or the T-cell receptor genes[68] (or rarely both[69]), which enables a slight excess of cells to be detected by performing a molecular genetic analysis to detect the specific rearrangement in question. In lymphoproliferative and in other tumours, cytogenetic abnormalities may result from specific abnormalities which are important on the molecular level. Frequently, these abnormalities occur in and around the sites of specific oncogenes[70]. If the DNA sequence of the breakpoint or of a known translocation is known, the sequence may be used as a molecular probe to detect even very small numbers of cells bearing this particular abnormality[71]. The recently described polymerase chain reaction allows even greater sensitivity of detection, since any specific DNA sequence can be amplified by enzymatic techniques to a point at which it is detectable by standard molecular biological techniques[72]. This method is capable of detecting one tumour cell in 100 000 normal cells. As these techniques and others yet to be developed come to be introduced into routine clinical use, the current concepts of minimal disease will need to be revised. The implications of detecting minimal disease may well be different in such changed circumstances.

CONCLUSION

It should be axiomatic that, the smaller the amount of tumour present, the more likely that the patient can be cured. Thus, it should follow that minimal disease implies curable disease. However, as we have seen, minimal disease does not always mean the same thing. If minimal disease means barely detectable disease, then, in some cases such as *in situ* carcinoma of the cervix, the disease is curable. In other cases, such as micrometastatic melanoma after excision of the primary, barely detectable disease is not curable. Minimal disease, as detectable in 1989, is certainly not minimal and therein lies the problem. In most situations, the curability of a neoplasm depends on a host of characteristics of that neoplasm, such as prevalence of inherent drug resistance, spontaneous rate of mutation, growth fraction, metastatic potential, patient performance status, status of the patient's immune system, and presence and number of surface tumour markers recognizable by the patient's immune system – to name but a few. In general, minimal disease points to a greater probability of cure than does a larger volume of tumour within a given set of clinical circumstances dictated by these tumour characteristics. However, all the known parameters, of which tumour size is merely one, must be assessed in any individual situation in order to evaluate the likelihood of cure.

References

1. Skipper, H., Schabel, F. and Wilcox, W. (1964). Experimental evaluation of potential anticancer agents XII: On the criteria and kinetics associated with "curability" of experimental leukemia. *Cancer Chemother. Rep.*, **35**, 1–111
2. Einhorn, L. and Donohue, J. (1977). *Cis*-diamminedichloroplatinum, vinblastine, and bleomycin combination chemotherapy in disseminated testicular cancer. *Ann. Int. Med.*, **87**, 293–298
3. DeVita, V. (1983). The relationship between tumor mass and resistance to chemotherapy. *Cancer*, **51**, 1209–1220
4. Laird, A. (1969). Dynamics of growth in tumors and normal organisms. *Natl. Cancer Inst. Monogr.*, **30**, 15–29
5. Goldie, J. and Coldman, A. (1979). A mathematic model for relating the drug sensitivity of tumors to their spontaneous mutation rate. *Cancer Treat. Rep.*, **63**, 1727–1733
6. Luria, S. and Delbruck, M. (1943). Mutations of bacteria from virus sensitivity to virus resistance. *Genetics*, **28**, 491–511
7. Berkowitz, R. and Goldstein, D. (1979). Methotrexate with citrovorum factor rescue for nonmetastatic gestational neoplasms. *Obstet. Gynecol.*, **54**, 725–728
8. Tobias, J. and Griffiths, C. (1976). Management of ovarian carcinoma: Current concepts and future prospects. *N. Engl. J. Med.*, **294**, 818–823
9. Shipp, M., Harrington, D., Klatt, M., Jochelson, M., Pinckus, G., Marshall, J., Rosenthal, D., Skarin, A. and Canellos, G. (1986). Identification of major prognostic subgroups of patients with large-cell lymphoma treated with m-BACOD or M-BACOD. *Ann. Intern. Med.*, **104**, 757–765
10. Javadpour, N. (1980). The role of biologic tumor markers in testicular cancer. *Cancer*, **45**, 1755–1761
11. Martin, D. (1981). The scientific basis for adjuvant chemotherapy. *Cancer Treat. Rev.*, **8**, 169–189
12. Frei, E. (1988). What's in a name – neoadjuvant. *J. Natl. Cancer Inst.*, **80**, 1088–1089
13. Beahrs, O., Henson, D., Hutter, R. and Myers, M. (1988). *Manual for Staging of Cancer*, 3rd Edn. (Philadelphia: Lippincott)

14. Enneking, W. (1986). A system of staging musculoskeletal neoplasms. *Clin. Orthop. Relat. Res.,* **204**, 9–24
15. Yankee, R., DeVita, V. and Perry, S. (1967). The cell cycle of leukemia L1210 cells *in vivo. Cancer Res.,* **27**, 2381–2385
16. Furth, J. and Kahn, M. (1937). The transmission of leukemia of mice with a single cell. *Am. J. Cancer,* **31**, 276–282
17. Martens, A. (1988). *Normal and Leukemic Stem Cells During Minimal Residual Disease: Studies in an Experimental Rat Leukemia Model (BNML). Monograph.* (Rijswijk, Netherlands: Radiobiological Institute TNO)
18. Aisenberg, A. (1983). Acute nonlymphocytic leukemia after treatment for Hodgkin's disease. *Am. J. Med.,* **75**, 449–454
19. Horm, J., Asire, A., Young, J. and Pollack, E. (eds.) (1985). *SEER Program: Cancer Incidence and Mortality in the US, 1973–1981.* (Bethesda: NIH publication no. 85-1837)
20. Hulka, B. (1988). Cancer screening: degrees of proof and practical application. *Cancer,* **62**, 1776–1780
21. Dodd, G. (1988). Screening for the early detection of breast cancer. *Cancer,* **62**, 1781–1783
22. Decosse, J. (1988). Early cancer detection: colorectal cancer. *Cancer,* **62**, 1787–1790
23. Gusberg, S. (1988). Detection and prevention of uterine cancer. *Cancer,* **62**, 1784–1786
24. Silverman, S. (1988). Early diagnosis of oral cancer. *Cancer,* **62**, 1796–1799
25. Kopf, A. (1988). Prevention and early detection of skin cancer/melanoma. *Cancer,* **62**, 1791–1795
26. Newell, G., Boutwell, W., Morris, D., Tilley, B. and Branyon, E. (1982). Epidemiology of cancer. In DeVita, V., Hellman, S. and Rosenberg, S. (eds.) *Principles of Oncology,* pp. 3–32. (Philadelphia: Lippincott)
27. Cummings, K., Michalek, A., Tidings, J., Herrera, L. and Mettlin, C. (1986). Results of a public screening program for colorectal cancer. *NY State J. Med.,* **86**, 68–72
28. Guzick, D. (1978). Efficacy of screening for cervical cancer. *Am. J. Public Health,* **68**, 125–134
29. Shapiro, S. (1977). Evidence on screening for breast cancer from a randomized trial. *Cancer,* **39**, 2772–2782
30. Miller, A. and Ultmann, J. (1989). Application of screening to early detection of malignancies. In Kelley, W. (ed.) *Textbook of Internal Medicine,* pp. 1209–1211. (Philadelphia: Lippincott)
31. Carbone, P., Kaplan, H., Mushoff, K., Smithers, D. and Tubiana, M. (1971). Report of the committee on Hodgkin's disease staging classification. *Cancer Res.,* **31**, 1860–1861
32. Dukes, C. (1932). The classification of cancer of the rectum. *J. Pathol. Bacteriol.,* **35**, 323–332
33. Larson, R. and Ultmann, J. (1982). The strategic role of laparotomy in staging Hodgkin's disease. *Cancer Treat. Rep.,* **66**, 767–774
34. Miller, T. and Jones, S. (1979). Chemotherapy of localised histiocytic lymphoma. *Lancet,* **1**, 358–360
35. Sweet, D., Kinzie, J., Gaeke, M., Golomb, H., Ferguson, D. and Ultmann, J. (1981). Survival of patients with localized diffuse histiocytic lymphoma. *Blood,* **58**, 1218–1223
36. Portlock, C., Rosenberg, S., Glatstein, E. and Kaplan, H. (1978). Impact of salvage treatment on initial relapses in patients with Hodgkin's disease, stages I–III. *Blood,* **51**, 825–833
37. Mauch, P., Goffman, T., Rosenthal, D., Canellos, G., Come, S. and Hellman, S. (1985). Stage III Hodgkin's disease: Improved survival with combined modality therapy as compared with radiation therapy alone. *J. Clin. Oncol.,* **3**, 1166–1173
38. Mastrangelo, M., Rosenberg, S., Baker, A. and Katz, H. (1982). Cutaneous melanoma. In DeVita, V., Hellman, S. and Rosenberg, S. (eds.) *Principles of Oncology,* pp. 1124–1170. (Philadelphia: Lippincott)
39. Mulshine, J., Glatstein, E. and Ruckdeschel, J. (1986). Treatment of non-small cell lung cancer. *J. Clin. Oncol.,* **4**, 1704–1715
40. Malkasian, G., Decker, D. and Jorgenson, E. (1976). Chemotherapy of carcinoma of the cervix. *Gynecol. Oncol.,* **5**, 109–120
41. Grossman, S. and Burch, P. (1988). Quantitation of tumor response to anti-neoplastic therapy. *Semin. Oncol.,* **15**, 441–454

42. Clarkson, B. and Fried, J. (1971). Changing concepts of treatment in acute leukemia. *Med. Clin. N. Am.,* **55**, 561–600
43. DeVita, V., Simon, R., Hubbard, S., Young, R., Berard, C., Moxley, J., Frei, E., Carbone, P. and Canellos, G. (1980). Curability of advanced Hodgkin's disease with chemotherapy. *Ann. Intern. Med.,* **92**, 587–595
44. Greist, A., Roth, B., Einhorn, L. and Williams, S. (1985). Cisplatin combination chemotherapy for disseminated germ cell tumors: long-term followup. *Proc. Am. Soc. Clin. Oncol.,* **4**, C-388
45. Johnson, D., Kaesler, K. and Samuels, M. (1975). Is nephrectomy justified in patients with metastatic renal carcinoma? *J. Urol.,* **114**, 27–29
46. Armitage, J., Weisenburger, D., Hutchins, N., Moravec, D., Dowling, M., Sorenson, S., Mailliard, J., Okerbloom, J., Johnson, P., Howe, D., Bascom, G., Casey, J., Linder, J. and Purtilo, D. (1986). Chemotherapy for diffuse large-cell lymphoma: Rapidly responding patients have more durable remissions. *J. Clin. Oncol.,* **4**, 160–164
47. Paulson, D., Einhorn, L., Peckham, M. and Williams, S. (1982). Cancer of the testis. In DeVita, V., Hellman, S. and Rosenberg, S. (eds.) *Principles of Oncology,* pp. 786–822. (Philadelphia: Lippincott)
48. Bates, S. and Longo, D. (1987). Use of serum tumor markers in cancer diagnosis and management. *Semin. Oncol.,* **14**, 102–138
49. DeVita, V. (1983). The relationship between tumor mass and resistance to chemotherapy. *Cancer,* **51**, 1209–1220
50. Gale, R., Foon, K., Cline, M. and Zighelboim, J. (1981). Intensive chemotherapy for acute myelogenous leukemia. *Ann. Intern. Med.,* **94**, 753–757
51. Berek, J., Hacker, N., Lagasse, L., Nieberg, R. and Elashoff, R. (1983). Survival of patients with ovarian cancer following secondary cytoreductive surgery. *Obstet. Gynecol.,* **61**, 189–193.
52. Copeland, L., Gershenson, D., Wharton, J., Atkinson,, E., Sneige, N., Edwards, C. and Rutledge, F. (1985). Microscopic disease at second-look laparotomy in advanced ovarian cancer. *Cancer,* **55**, 472–478
53. Colby, T., Hoppe, R. and Warnke, R. (1981). Hodgkin's disease at autopsy: 1972–1977. *Cancer,* **47**, 1852–1862
54. Gale, R. and Foon, K. (1985). Chronic lymphocytic leukemia. Recent advances in biology and treatment. *Ann. Intern. Med.,* **103**, 101–120
55. Jochelson, M., Mauch, P., Balikian, J., Rosenthal, D. and Canellos, G. (1985). The significance of the residual mediastinal mass in treated Hodgkin's disease. *J. Clin. Oncol.,* **3**, 637–640
56. Surbone, A., Longo, D., DeVita, V., Ihde, D., Duffey, P., Jaffe, E., Solomon, D., Hubbard, S. and Young, R. (1988). Residual abdominal masses in aggressive non-Hodgkin's lymphoma after combination chemotherapy: Significance and management. *J. Clin. Oncol.,* **6**, 1832–1837
57. Bracken, R., Johnson, D., Frazier, O., Logothetis, C., Trindade, A. and Samuels, M. (1983). The role of surgery following chemotherapy in stage III germ cell neoplasms. *J. Urol.,* **129**, 39–43
58. Grever, M. (1987). Treatment of patients with acute nonlymphocytic leukemia not in remission. *Semin. Oncol.,* **14**, 416–424
59. Hainsworth, J., Williams, S., Einhorn, L., Birch, R. and Greco, A. (1985). Successful treatment of resistant germinal neoplasms with VP-16 and cisplatin: Results of a Southeastern Cancer Study Group trial. *J. Clin. Oncol.,* **3**, 666–671
60. Appelbaum, F., Sullivan, K. and Thomas, E. (1985). Marrow transplantation as treatment for patients with recurrent malignant lymphoma. *Int. J. Cell Cloning,* **3**, 219
61. Anderson, T., Waldman, T. and Javadpour, N. (1979). Testicular germ cell neoplasms: Recent advances in diagnosis and therapy. *Ann. Intern. Med.,* **90**, 373–385
62. Treleaven, J. and Kemshead, J. (1985). Removal of tumor cells from bone marrow: An evaluation of the available techniques. *Hematol. Oncol.,* **3**, 65–75
63. Benjamin, D., Magrath, I., Douglass, E. and Corash, L. (1983). Derivation of lymphoma cell lines from microscopically normal bone marrow in patients with undifferentiated lymphomas: Evidence of occult bone marrow involvement. *Blood,* **61**, 1017–1019
64. Anderson, K. and Nadler, L. (1986). Bone marrow transplantation in the therapy of non-

Hodgkin's lymphomas. In DeVita, V., Hellman, S. and Rosenberg, S. (eds.) *Important Advances in Oncology 1986,* pp. 287–310. (Philadelphia: Lippincott)

65. Hittelman, W., Brousard, L., Dosik, G. and McCredie, K. (1980). Predicting relapse of human leukemia by means of premature chromosome condensation. *N. Engl. J. Med.,* **303,** 479–484

66. Smith, B., Weinberg, D., Robert, N., Towle, M., Luther, E., Pinckus, G. and Ault, A. (1984). Circulating monoclonal B lymphocytes in non-Hodgkin's lymphoma. *N. Engl. J. Med.,* **311,** 1476–1481

67. Arnold, A., Cossman, J., Bakhshi, A., Jaffe, E., Waldman, T. and Korsmeyer, S. (1983). Immunoglobulin gene rearrangements as unique clonal markers in human lymphoid neoplasms. *N. Engl. J. Med.,* **309,** 1593–1599

68. Minden, M. and Mak, T. (1986). The structure of the T cell antigen receptor genes in normal and malignant T cells. *Blood,* **68,** 327–336

69. Kurosawa, Y., von Boehmer, H., Haas, W., Sakano, H., Trauneker, A. and Tonegawa, S. (1981). Identification of D segments of immunoglobulin heavy-chain genes and their rearrangements in T lymphocytes. *Nature (London),* **290,** 565–570

70. Erikson, J., Finan, J., Nowell, P. and Croce, C. (1982). Translocation of immunoglobulin-V_H genes in Burkitt lymphoma. *Proc. Natl. Acad. Sci. USA,* **79,** 5611–5615

71. Tsujimoto, Y., Finger, L., Yunis, J., Nowell, P. and Croce, C. (1984). Cloning of the chromosome breakpoint of neoplastic B-cells with the t(14;18) chromosome translocation. *Science,* **226,** 1097–1099

72. Saiki, R., Gelfand, D., Stoffel, S., Scharf, S., Higuchi, R., Horn, G., Mullis, K. and Erlich, H. (1988). Primer-directed enzymatic amplification of DNA with a thermostable DNA polymerase. *Science,* **239,** 487–491

7
High-dose chemotherapy

R.L. SOUHAMI AND H. EARL

INTRODUCTION

After a decade of exploration of the use of high-dose chemotherapy in the treatment of cancer, we are still unsure of its value in the routine management of any tumour. The aim of the approach is to attempt to overcome drug resistance by increasing drug dosage beyond the usual range employed. The technical advances which have made this approach possible include the development of techniques for the collection and preservation of viable bone marrow and the increasing ability to maintain patients during prolonged periods of myelosuppression by using blood product support and antibiotics. The dose-limiting toxicity of the drugs employed has, therefore, to be myelosuppression, since other toxicities, such as doxorubicin cardiomyopathy, cannot, at present, be circumvented. For this reason, dose escalation is an option for only a restricted range of drugs. At first sight, the aim behind dose intensification seems reasonable since one can imagine tumours which are, as it were, on the brink of cure – where conventional treatment might fail yet an intensive treatment might succeed. The problem is to identify the patients to whom this applies. This will clearly depend on the type of tumour, its response to drugs in conventional doses, the degree to which drug resistance can be overcome by the proportionate dose increase which is feasible, the stage at which the dose intensification is introduced into the treatment programme, and the drugs and drug combinations employed for initial treatment and for intensification. It is this complexity which has meant that a clear evaluation of the approach has been difficult.

Consideration of four types of tumour illustrates some of these general points. In small-cell lung cancer (SCLC) only 2.5% of patients are alive at 5 years[1]. Paradoxically, the tumour is exceptionally sensitive to cytotoxic drugs in comparison with other adult solid tumours. Response rates of over 80% are attained in untreated tumours when combination chemotherapy is used, with complete responses (disappearance of clinical and radiological signs of disease) in up to 50%[2]. The problem is that these responses are usually of relatively short duration and drug resistance quickly emerges. The patients who have a high likelihood of responding and surviving for more than a year are easily identifiable[3]. In treating this tumour, an approach using dose intens-

103

ification seems eminently sensible, especially in those patients who can be identified as likely to benefit. The problem is different in advanced Hodgkin's disease or intermediate and higher grade non-Hodgkin's lymphoma (NHL). In these diseases, response to chemotherapy is usual and often complete. Conventional alternating combination regimens produce complete responses in over 80% of cases in both types of lymphoma[4]. However, unlike SCLC, in advanced Hodgkin's disease, 45–55% of patients appear to be long-term survivors[5] and the same proportion in NHL[4]. The difficulty is, therefore, to identify patients who are at risk from failure with conventional therapy and then to perform clinical studies which allow the role of dose increases to be properly assessed. With other tumours, such as colonic carcinoma, the cancer is primarily resistant to cytotoxic drugs in conventional doses and the aim of dose intensification is to determine whether any worthwhile response can be obtained by this means. The design of studies in this situation will clearly be different, with greater emphasis on dose intensification as the first treatment.

A further advantage of high-dose chemotherapy, apart from increasing the cure rate, might be that it would replace protracted, lower-dose treatments by a single cycle of high-dose drugs. This might be done either as the initial therapy or after remission had been induced when continued treatment might be replaced by the dose intensification. This approach – of getting the treatment over in a shorter time – may be preferable from the patient's point of view.

EVIDENCE FOR A DOSE–RESPONSE EFFECT WITH CYTOTOXIC DRUGS

Is there evidence that by increasing the dose of a cytotoxic drug, an increase in response occurs? In cancer chemotherapy the dose–response relationship has a different meaning from other areas of pharmacology in which the dose–response curves of agonist–receptor interactions define the concentration range over which increasing dose causes an increase in response. With cytotoxic chemotherapy, the effect of a drug on a tumour is much more complex. Some drugs are pro-drugs which are converted to their active form in the liver or in the target cell. Cyclophosphamide is an example of a drug which is first activated to 4-OH cyclophosphamide in the liver. This metabolite is taken up by tumour cells and converted to phosphoramide mustard as one of the main alkylating molecules. Methotrexate is polyglutamated inside the cell which increases its inhibitory effect on its target enzyme, dihydrofolate reductase. The effect of a drug on the tumour may also show marked schedule dependency (see epipodophyllotoxin below). Apart from the complexity of mode of action of cytotoxic agents, the measurement of response also has little in common with that of agonist–receptor interaction. Response usually occurs several days, or weeks, after treatment and only relatively crude methods of measurement are available. For some drugs, it has been possible to describe the relationship between pharmacokinetic parameters, such as area under the curve (AUC), and pharmacodynamic properties, such as haematological toxicity[6]. However, no studies have been carried out, for any drug or tumour, where an attempt has been made to determine if there is a definable relationship between pharmacokinetic measurements and tumour response. The data which exist for dose–response relationships come from clinical trials in which tumour response is assessed in groups of patients treated with different doses of drugs. These studies have seldom been direct comparisons aimed at determining such a relationship. The evidence has to be put together from a variety of different studies with all of the attendant problems of case selection and criteria for assessment of response.

Perhaps the clearest evidence that a dose–response relationship can still pertain above the usual therapeutic ranges comes from studies with alkylating agents. Furthermore, their wide spectrum of tumour reactivity, and the fact that myelosuppression is often the main dose-limiting toxicity, makes this class of agent exceptionally useful for studies of dose escalation.

Cyclophosphamide

Cyclophosphamide is an inactive pro-drug which is converted in the liver to its active principle, 4-OH cyclophosphamide. In the cell, this compound is converted to phosphoramide mustard and nornitrogen mustard which are the active alkylating species[7]. In the process, acrolein is formed which causes single-strand breaks in DNA and depletes intracellular glutathione[8]. This depletion makes the cell more susceptible to further 4-OH cyclophosphamide. In addition, cyclophosphamide appears to be able to induce enzymes in the liver responsible for its own conversion, so that repeated doses of the drug produce successively more alkylating activity in the blood[9]. These considerations mean that 'high-dose' cyclophosphamide will have different properties depending on the schedule according to which it is administered. Administration of the whole dose in a single pulse will produce less alkylating activity than the same total dose given over a more extended time period. The degree of bone marrow suppression is probably less since Smith et al.[10] showed that autologous bone marrow transplantation (ABMT) was not necessary with cyclophosphamide, $7 \, g/m^2$ given as a 12-hour infusion[10], while we have shown that ABMT does contribute to haematological recovery with 50 mg/kg given on each of four successive days[11].

Haemorrhagic cystitis was a dose-limiting toxicity but has been largely overcome by the use of 2-mercaptoethane sulphonate as a sulphydryl donor which protects the urothelium from acrolein liberated by the metabolism of the drug. Carditis has been described as a complication of high-dose treatment but we have not seen a case in over 70 examples of treatment of small-cell lung cancer. Evidence for a dose–response effect has been obtained in treatment of human xenografts[12] and this is supported by studies in small-cell lung cancer where a complete response rate of over 50% has been seen in untreated cases after a single cycle of treatment[13].

Melphalan

This bifunctional alkylating agent is widely used in conventional doses in the treatment of myeloma as well as ovarian and breast cancer. Following intravenous injection at low doses (20 mg/m²), the plasma half-life is short (1 h) and urinary excretion decreases rapidly after 2 h. Similar pharmacokinetics have been found at high doses[14]. These kinetics allow non-cryopreserved bone marrow to be reinfused within 24 h of collection. ABMT of this kind has been shown to accelerate haematological recovery[15]. At doses above 200 mg/m², non-haematological toxicity is dose limiting, particularly oesophagitis, stomatitis and diarrhoea. The effect of 'priming' with cyclophosphamide in reducing these toxicities is somewhat controversial, having been demonstrated in some experimental studies[16] but not in some clinical reports[17].

There is no information with regard to the most effective schedule of administration of the drug. In xenografts, there does appear to be a relationship between dose and growth delay[18] but the most compelling evidence of a dose–response relationship comes from the clinical studies in myeloma and melanoma (see below). Melphalan has been added to high-dose combination regimens in treating a variety of tumours but its contribution to response in these situations cannot be assessed. It seems that it is often assumed that all alkylating agents are equivalent when some of these combinations are constructed. For example, although high-dose melphalan is a common constituent in high-dose regimens for treating lymphomas, there are very little data on response rates to melphalan in conventional doses in these diseases.

Nitrosoureas

Nitrosoureas have been extensively employed in high-dose studies, most experience being with BCNU (*bis*-chloroethylnitrosourea). This drug causes DNA interstrand cross-links and also has carbamoylating activity. The binding of the drug to the O^6 position of guanine is reversed by the enzyme, alkyltransferases (AT), and tumour cell lines low in AT are much more susceptible to cytotoxicity[19]. The drugs are usually lipid soluble, and, for this reason, are widely used in the treatment of brain tumours. Their activity against other tumours is low although preliminary reports of a new analogue, fotemustine, indicate a 30% response rate in melanoma. Absence of single-agent activity has not prevented high-dose BCNU being incorporated into many high-dose protocols.

When given intravenously, the half-life is less than 5 minutes. Myelosuppression is the main toxicity and is characteristically delayed until 4–6 weeks. At higher dose (above 1200 mg/m²), hepatic toxicity and pneumonitis become the major dose-limiting effects[20,21]. In the studies of Phillips et al.[22], 143 patients with refractory cancer were treated with BCNU, 600–2850 mg/m², and ABMT. Ninety-three per cent of patients recovered from severe pancytopenia within 4 weeks and the duration of aplasia did not appear to be related to dose (attesting to the effectiveness of ABMT). Serious extramedullary toxicity occurred at doses of $1200\,mg/m^2$ with a 9.5% incidence of fatal interstitial pneumonitis and 3% fatal hepatic necrosis. It has been frequently noted that the onset of marrow aplasia occurs earlier with higher dose BCNU.

Evidence for a dose–response relationship comes mainly from clinical studies in melanoma and glioma (see below). It should be noted that, while response rates appear to be higher with increased dose, these are almost always partial and short lived. A clinically useful dose–response relationship has not been demonstrated. In spite of a poor record of effectiveness in lymphoma, BCNU is a frequent constituent of high-dose regimens for treatment of these disorders.

Combined alkylating agent therapy

There have been several reports in which combinations of alkylating agents have been given to patients, some of whom have been considered 'refractory' or resistant to a previous treatment containing alkylating agents. The rationale for this approach lies in some clinical and experimental data indicating non-cross-resistance and even synergism between some alkylating agents, such as cyclophosphamide and thiotepa[23,24]. Responses were indeed obtained in some patients whose tumours were previously unresponsive to alkylating agents. These occurred in a wide variety of diseases, including cancers of the breast, colon, ovary, non-small-cell lung cancer and sarcoma. Toxicity was considerable. Eder et al.[25] infused cyclophosphamide and thiotepa (with bolus melphalan in some cases) in 23 patients with advanced cancer, 17 of whom had had previous treatment. Eleven evaluable patients responded for a brief period. Toxicity was manageable although veno-occlusive disease occurred in one patient and there were two deaths. Pharmacokinetic studies revealed marked variability in drug exposures (AUC) in individual patients which correlated with toxicity. Peters et al.[26] used a combination of cyclophosphamide, platinum, BCNU and melphalan in a variety of tumours including five patients with breast cancer (see below). Toxicity was considerable (including veno-occlusive disease) but responses were seen in patients resistant to conventional chemotherapy. Evidently the approach is feasible and may have advantages over simply increasing the dose of a single agent, since the doses of each component were almost equal to the doses used singly.

Etoposide (VP16-213)

This drug is a semisynthetic epipodophyllotoxin whose main toxicities are myelosuppression, mucositis and neuropathy. In conventional dosage, it shows marked schedule dependence, being more effective when given over several days[27]. Its half-life after intravenous administration is 8–14 h and ABMT is usually delayed 1–3 days depending on dose. There is a linear relationship between dose and peak plasma concentrations and AUC[28].

Wolff et al.[29] used etoposide in a variety of refractory malignancies. The extramedullary toxicity limited the maximum dose to $2400\,mg/m^2$. There has been no clear evidence of increased clinical effectiveness associated with a greatly increased dose of etoposide. It is often added to high-dose combination regimens, usually in a conventional dose given over 3–5 days. Examples are the BEAM regimen in non-Hodgkin's lymphoma[30] and, in the studies of Spitzer et al.[31], in small-cell lung cancer.

Mitomycin

This drug is an antibiotic which acts as an alkylating agent. Its main toxicities are myelosuppression, but pneumonitis and haemolytic anaemia with renal failure are often fatal and unpredictable toxic events. Dose increases up to $(40 \, \text{mg}/\text{m}^2/\text{day}) \times 3$ have been made[32]. Early bone marrow suppression occurred and stomatitis, veno-occlusive disease, colitis and pancreatitis were other toxicities. The α (distribution) half-life is 10 minutes and the β (elimination) phase $t_{1/2}$ is 90 minutes. The lack of suggestive evidence of a dose-response effect, and the manifest severe toxicity, limit its usefulness.

THE USE OF MYELOSUPPRESSIVE COMBINATION CHEMOTHERAPY

What are the principles which might guide us in the use of drug combinations which produce bone marrow suppression? The following general points are made as a commentary on what has been done and to indicate the difficulties in assessing results.

It seems reasonable to suppose that, even in higher dosage, combinations of drugs might be more effective than single agents, since this is the case at conventional dose. Nevertheless, when drugs which produce increases in response at very high dose are combined, the dose of each must usually be reduced. 'High dose' then becomes defined on a pharmacodynamic basis in terms of a dose which produces substantial myelosuppression. The fact is, however, that marrow hypoplasia is an unwanted effect; it is tumour response which is needed. The choice of the doses and drugs in the combination is usually partly determined by factors unconnected with the data indicating the range over which a normal dose–response relationship holds. In phase III studies the two main additional factors influencing this choice are:

(1) The combination should contain drugs known to be effective agents against the tumour. This is not always the case for some of the reported drug regimens. With highly sensitive tumours, such as lymphomas, most drugs are active though even here one can question the use of ara-C and BCNU in regimens for Hodgkin's disease[30]. With less sensitive tumours, the use of procarbazine or BCNU for treating e.g. small cell lung cancer has little to support it on the basis of known response rates.

(2) The drugs used in the combination are rational choices *when the previous treatment which the patient has had is considered.* This is the crux of the matter. If a patient with a lymphoma has not responded fully (or has relapsed) after conventional combination therapy containing an

alkylating agent, is it realistic to suppose that he will be cured or enjoy a prolonged remission by using another alkylator in an increased dose? Moreover, is it true that resistance, or incomplete sensitivity, to one class of drugs will not affect response to drugs of a different class? Most phase II studies at conventional doses show, on the contrary, that response rates to a new drug are substantially lower in patients previously treated with drugs of a different type. Is it, therefore, reasonable to save good drugs for a later intensive treatment, thus possibly diminishing the effectiveness of the initial chemotherapy?

The rationale behind the design of 'high-dose' combination regimens is seldom discussed in reports of treatment. Choice of drugs, doses and schedules is varied and occasionally idiosyncratic. When this is added to a lack of uniformity of case selection, the scope for discussion about the validity of, and indications for, high-dose treatment becomes very wide.

SELECTION OF PATIENTS FOR TREATMENT

In order to describe results for individual tumours, we have used a terminology which allows some analysis of the reasons for case selection.

Initial or *induction chemotherapy* means the chemotherapy given to an untreated patient, either as a conventional combination treatment programme or, exceptionally, as a high-dose treatment.

Late intensification means a high-dose treatment given as a planned treatment, to a defined group of patients, at the end of a conventional chemotherapy programme. Such patients are usually those showing complete or partial response to the initial treatment, and/or who are defined as being at high risk of relapse. Examples are responders to chemotherapy in small-cell lung cancer, patients with primary breast cancer with bad prognostic factors who are receiving adjuvant chemotherapy, patients with non-Hodgkin's lymphoma with incomplete response to chemotherapy or judged to be at very high risk of relapse.

Relapse chemotherapy means treatment given to patients who had a remission of their disease but then had a recurrence. Patients with such a relapse might be shown to be *resistant* to conventional chemotherapy or *responding* to it. They may be treated with high-dose chemotherapy after complete or partial response to further conventional chemotherapy.

Clearly the results of high-dose treatments applied in these different circumstances will be widely different, and comparison with what conventional treatment has to offer can only come from randomized studies. There are very few of these and their design and execution presents considerable difficulties which are discussed at the end of the chapter.

With these difficulties in mind, we now give a summary of the evidence for the value of high-dose chemotherapy in treating solid tumours. With such a vast field, this review is inevitably a condensation of available data.

NON-HODGKIN'S LYMPHOMA

High-dose chemotherapy, with or without total body irradiation, and autologous (or sometimes allogeneic) bone marrow transplantation has been used in some patients with high-grade lymphomas since the 1970s[33,34]. The definition of which patients might benefit from this life-threatening intensification of treatment has proved difficult.

Conventional combination chemotherapy for treating intermediate and high-grade non-Hodgkin's lymphoma has been moderately successful. A recent review of 34 studies reporting 1602 patients showed a 62% initial complete response (CR) rate, with 69% of these patients being in continued complete remission at 2 years[4]. Disease-free survival is about 45% at 5 years for intermediate and high-grade poor-prognosis lymphomas which have been treated by conventional combination chemotherapy. However, for patients relapsing after CR, or for those who fail to obtain a CR on first-line therapy, the prognosis is much worse. Salvage regimens for refractory or relapsed intermediate and high-grade poor-risk NHL, among 398 patients reported in 16 studies, produced, on average, complete responses rates of 25%[4]. The numbers of continued complete remissions in this group at 2 years is vanishingly small with 12/398 patients in continuous complete remission (12% of those achieving CR with salvage regimens and only 3% of those treated at relapse).

Although, in early studies, some patients with NHL were treated with high-dose chemotherapy and bone marrow transplantation in first complete remission[35-39], this practice is difficult to justify since 70% of these patients will be alive and free of disease in 2 years without any further treatment and we do not yet know how to identify the 30% who will relapse. However, it seems justifiable to consider some intensification of treatment in patients with NHL who relapse after CR or those who fail to obtain a CR on first-line chemotherapy, since it is in this group that treatment with conventional salvage regimens only produces a 25% CR rate and a 12% 2-year disease-free survival for those who achieve a complete response. It is this group of patients who form the majority of those treated by high-dose chemotherapy and ABMT. In fact, of the 472 patients who have been reported having been treated with high-dose chemotherapy, only 39 patients were treated in first complete remission and only 4 patients with histologically defined poor-prognosis NHL were treated with high-dose chemotherapy as initial treatment[35,40], the rest being treated following relapse or failure to attain a CR.

Table 7.1 details the major reported studies of high-dose chemotherapy with or without total body irradiation with ABMT in patients with poor-risk NHL. This table shows that 81 patients have been treated in CR, 39 in first CR, and 42 in second CR (i.e. chemosensitive relapse entering CR prior to high-dose procedure). 255 patients in first relapse after CR have been treated, usually after some salvage therapy has been given. These patients seem to be clearly divided on a basis of prognosis into 122 patients who have relapse which is refractory (resistant) to conventional salvage chemotherapy and 133 who have chemosensitive relapse. A small group of 25 patients have also been

Table 7.1 High-dose chemotherapy with or without total body irradiation and bone marrow transplantation in poor prognosis non-Hodgkin's lymphoma

Study	Patients	CR	TDR
Phillips et al. (1984)[45] (Toronto)	24	14/24 (58%)	5/24 (21%)
Gorin et al. (1984)[35] (Paris)	12	4/7 (57%)	1/7 (14%)
Verdonck et al. (1985)[36]	14	7/8 (87%)	—
Philip et al. (1986)[38]	28	13/15 (87%)	4/28 (14%)
Armitage et al. (1986)[46]	29	11/29 (40%)	2/29 (7%)
Armitage et al. (1986)[47]	18	9/16 (56%)	9/16 (56%)
Appelbaum et al. (1987)[39]	82	8/69 (11%)	36/82 (44%)
Gribben et al. (1987)[41]	44	16/44 (36%) (CSR 8/12=66%) (RR 3/20=15%)	5/44 (11%)
Philip et al. (1987)[42]	100	PTF 9/34 (26%) RR 10/22 (45%) CSR 19/25 (76%)	No TBI 10/61=16% TBI 11/39=28%
Takvorian et al. (1987)[43]	49	CSR 42/49 (85%)	2/49 (4%)
Gulati et al. (1988)[48]	31	—	5/31 (16%)
Total	431	Chemosensitive disease 101, 76% Chemoresistant disease 207, 30%	With TBI 28% Without TBI 13%

CR = complete response; RR = resistant (chemo) relapse; CSR = chemosensitive relapse; TDR = toxic death rate; TBI = total body irradiation; PTF = primary treatment failure

treated in first partial response, i.e. these are patients who have never been in CR after conventional treatment but who still have chemosensitive disease. There is also a group of 85 patients who have disease which is resistant to first-line chemotherapy, either with initial response followed by progression while on treatment, or because of primary resistance to first-line chemotherapy. Twenty-four patients in the world literature have been treated in relapse, but their response to initial second-line chemotherapy has not been reported.

An overall complete response rate of about 50% is seen after high-dose chemotherapy with or without total body irradiation and ABMT, which means that 70% of patients are in complete remission after the procedure (since 81 patients were in CR before transplantation). In the most recent studies, the patients have been more clearly divided into groups with different status at ABMT and these groups have differing CR rates. The Bloomsbury transplant group[41] reported an overall 36% complete response rate but this was broken down into a 66% CR rate for patients with chemosensitive relapse, a 41% CR rate for patients with a good (but not complete) response to first-line therapy, and a 15% CR rate for patients with chemoresistant relapse. In the report by Philip *et al.*[42] of 100 patients with NHL, there was an overall CR rate of 47%, but only 26% of patients with primary disease resistance had a CR to subsequent high-dose chemotherapy. However, 45% of patients with resistant relapse obtained a CR, and patients with chemosensitive relapse had a CR rate of 76% following high-dose treatment. Because of these clear differences in response rates depending on status of disease at ABMT, and because this is now being mirrored by differing survival figures[42], increasingly, only patients with *chemosensitive* disease are being treated with high-dose chemotherapy. In the recent report from Takvorian *et al.*[43], all patients had chemosensitive relapse. The most recent report from Philip *et al.*[44] described 17 patients in partial remission after first-line induction therapy. This group of patients cannot be compared with the overall results from conventional second-line therapy since they are clearly selected on the basis of the responsiveness of their tumours.

The overall toxic death rate from high-dose procedures was 20%. However, the toxic death rate (TDR) was clearly different depending on whether patients received TBI (TDR=28%) or high-dose chemotherapy alone (TDR=13%). The main causes of death were interstitial pneumonitis, renal failure, haemorrhage, and aspiration pneumonia, with graft-versus-host disease (GVHD) and veno-occlusive disease of the liver in those who received allogeneic transplants. It appears that interstitial pneumonitis is more common when TBI is used in addition to high-dose chemotherapy[39].

It is difficult to ascertain survival data from these studies, but, taking one of the latest and largest studies, Appelbaum *et al.*[39] report a 22% actuarial 5-year disease-free survival. The most common reason for treatment failure was recurrence of disease, with an actuarial probability of 60%. A proportional hazards regression analysis showed (as expected) that disease-free survival was generally shorter in patients transplanted in resistant relapse, and in those who had previously received radiotherapy to the chest. High-dose chemo-radiotherapy and marrow transplantation may offer a better chance for long-term survival than conventional therapy for young patients whose disease has progressed after initial combination chemotherapy. The best results have been obtained in patients in early relapse or second remission who had not received prior chest radiotherapy. Philip *et al.* report[42] on 100 patients who have 19% actuarial 3-year disease-free survival. Survival is clearly related to state of disease at transplantation with refractory disease leading to a 0–14% 3-year disease-free survival, and responding relapse leading to 36% survival expressed in the same terms.

If recent studies are divided into patients with resistant disease and those with chemosensitive disease, the overall survival is 16% at 2 years for those with resistant disease and about 50% at 2 years for patients with chemosensitive disease (either PR to first-line treatment or chemosensitive relapse).

Since patient selection has played such a large part in these studies, the additional benefit of intensive chemotherapy with bone marrow transplantation in poor-risk NHL can only be established by randomized controlled trials. These trials must be designed carefully so that an interpretable result can be obtained. Clearly high-dose chemoradiotherapy and bone marrow transplantation should only be tested in cases where the results of conventional chemotherapy are not good, and where there is a realistic chance that more intensive treatment will produce a significant improvement in long-term survival. These situations are:

(a) Failure to achieve CR with conventional treatment;
(b) First relapse after CR;
(c) Certain very high-grade lymphomas with a low cure rate (e.g. some high-grade T-cell tumours) where high-dose treatment could be introduced as a planned intensification in patients with CR.

National or international collaboration will be needed to generate sufficient numbers in these studies to give a chance of detecting the likely differences in cure rates. In our view, this phase of study is now essential before an imperfectly validated treatment slips into established clinical practice.

HODGKIN'S DISEASE

Hodgkin's disease (HD) responds very well to conventional chemotherapy and radiotherapy. However, some patients with HD have disease resistant to primary treatment or disease which relapses after conventional treatment. There are reports in the literature of 278 patients treated with high-dose chemotherapy and bone marrow transplantation[49-54] (see Table 7.2). Among the 179 patients for whom the status at ABMT was given, 58 (33%) had resistant relapse usually after several different regimens of chemotherapy, whereas 35 patients (20%) had chemosensitive relapse, and 22 patients (12.5%) were given high-dose chemotherapy at relapse without prior standard salvage chemotherapy. Thirty-two patients were treated in their first partial remission and only 28 patients were treated with high-dose chemotherapy because of primary drug resistance.

Overall complete response rates to high-dose chemotherapy and ABMT are about 55%, with a toxic death rate (TDR) of 17%. The follow-up in most studies remains short, but after high-dose chemotherapy some one-third of patients seem to enjoy long-term (3 year) disease-free survival[55].

However, the same questions have to be asked in HD as in poor-prognosis NHL. Which patients are the most suitable to treat? At what point in their illness? Are the response rates and long-term survival good enough to justify the risk of toxic early death ($\sim$ 17%)? Many patients nowadays receive alternating non-cross-resistant chemotherapy at diagnosis, such as LOPP/ABVD*[56] or LOPP/EVAP*[57]. On relapse after treatment with these regimens, second CR rates vary from 4% to 59%[58,59], and it is generally accepted that only a

*LOPP = chlorambucil, vincristine, procarbazine, prednisolone; ABVD = doxorubicin, bleomycin, vinblastine, decarbazine; EVAD = etoposide, vinblastine, doxorubicin, prednisolone

small proportion of patients (probably about 20%) will remain in prolonged CR following second-line chemotherapy. However, some patients with HD survive for many years in various states of relapse, unlike patients with diffuse large-cell lymphomas which, if uncontrolled, are rapidly fatal. Patients who either have primary resistant disease or who have failed two modalities of treatment, should be considered for this approach.

As with NHL, randomized trials are now essential. The clinical situations deserving of study are:

(1) Primary treatment failure;
(2) First relapse;
(3) Patients with partially responding bulky but localized disease (e.g. in the mediastinum) where radiotherapy alone may not be able to control residual disease;
(4) As part of a planned late intensification after induction treatment in patients identified as having a poor prognosis, such as presentation with extensive marrow, pulmonary or hepatic involvement.

Table 7.2 High-dose chemotherapy with or without total body irradiation and bone marrow transplantation in Hodgkin's disease

Study	Patients	CR	TDR	Comments
Philip et al. (1986)[49]	17 11PTF 3RR 3CSR	9/17 (52%)	9/17 (52%)	3 long-term survivors (25–66 m)
Carella et al. (1987)[50]	28 —	15/28 (53%)	2/28 (7%)	
Teillet et al. (1987)[51]	5 5PRI	3/5 (60%)	4/5 (80%)	1 a/w 32 m CR
	5 2PRI 3PTF	5/5 (100%)	0/5	3 patients long-term survivors 6–12 months
Goldstone et al. (1987)[52]	117 4CR 5PRI 32CSR 55RR 12PTF	67/117	—	Failure to achieve CR→poor prognosis. Bulk disease at transplant = poor prognosis
Cabanillas et al. (1988)[53]	62 —	29/62 (47%) (+5 after RT) 55%	—	CR patients. 71% remain in CR. Median FU = 19 m (11–67 m)
Gribben et al. (1989)[54]	44 22RCSU 20PRI 2PTF	21/44 (48%)	2/44 (4.5%)	
Total	278 28PTF 58RR 35CSR 32PRI 22RCSU	154/278 (55%)	17/99 (17%)	

TDR = toxic death rate; PTF = primary treatment failure; RR = resistant relapse; CSR = chemosensitive relapse; PRI = 1st partial response; RCSU = relapse chemosensitivity unknown

As with NHL, the small numbers available in these important subgroups mean that collaborative studies will be essential. One such randomized study has now been started in the UK by the British National Lymphoma Investigation to establish whether high-dose therapy with ABMT is better than conventional second-line chemotherapy after first relapse.

SMALL-CELL LUNG CANCER (SCLC)

Using combination chemotherapy, responses are obtained in 80% of patients with limited disease (disease confined to one lung – LD) and 65% of patients with more extensive disease (ED). These responses are of short duration in most patients. In a study of long-term prognosis, Davis et al.[1] showed that only 2.5% of patients were alive at 5 years. It is these disappointing results that gave rise to an interest in high-dose therapy for SCLC. The results of using high-dose treatment in relapse after previous treatment have been uniformly bad. Although responses can be obtained they are short lived[60]. When high-dose therapy has been used as late intensification, the results are somewhat conflicting. Two studies have used cyclophosphamide alone. Banham et al.[61] used high-dose cyclophosphamide after initial chemotherapy (which included cyclophosphamide) and obtained some short-lived responses. Smith et al.[62] used etoposide, doxorubicin and vincristine as initial treatment in 94 patients, and 36 responding patients then received high-dose cyclophosphamide. Of 15 patients who had measurable disease, 12 experienced a further response but generally of very short duration.

Combination chemotherapy has also been used for late intensification. Spitzer et al.[63] treated patients with either doxorubicin, vincristine and ifosfamide or doxorubicin, vincristine, etoposide and cyclophosphamide. After these drugs in conventional doses, he went on to use higher dose cyclophosphamide and etoposide with vincristine followed by cranial and thoracic radiation. Median survival was only 48 weeks which is rather worse than results from many studies of conventional chemotherapy. Several other negative studies of this type have been published. The only controlled study comes from Humblet et al.[64]. In this trial, patients were treated with conventional combination chemotherapy using methotrexate, vincristine, cyclophosphamide, doxorubicin, cisplatin and etoposide. Patients in complete or partial remission were randomized into groups which received either high-dose treatment using cyclophosphamide, $6 \, g/m^2$, BCNU, $300 \, mg/m^2$ and etoposide, $500 \, mg/m^2$ or the same drugs in conventional dosage. There was no overall survival advantage for the high-dose treatment but there was a suggestion of prolongation of survival in those limited-disease patients who had experienced a complete response to the induction chemotherapy. Of the 101 patients who entered the study, 45 were randomized, so the statistical confidence of the results is low. Nevertheless, this study is the only randomized trial addressing the value of late intensification. The length of time it took to complete (four and a half years) and the small numbers indicate the logistic problems in high-dose therapies. In this study, most of the drugs used in the intensification programme had been given in the initial treatment, which again raises the issue of drug resistance and trial design alluded to earlier.

We have used high-dose cyclophosphamide as the initial treatment in SCLC. In our first study of 25 patients, responses were obtained in 21 and there were 14 complete responses. In our second study, the high-dose treatment was repeated but there was no increase in response rate[65]. Two other studies have been completed, in one of which high-dose cyclophosphamide was given after only two cycles of treatment with doxorubicin, etoposide and vincristine, and, in the other, a high-dose combination therapy was given using cisplatin, etoposide and cyclophosphamide or melphalan[66]. In summary, none of these studies have yielded results suggestive of a higher cure rate compared with conventional chemotherapy applied to patients having comparable prognostic factors. Wolff et al.[67] gave high-dose etoposide for two days without ABMT in untreated patients with extensive disease. Eight of 13 responded but, when subsequently treated with cyclophosphamide, doxorubicin and vincristine, no further responses were seen, once again demonstrating the difficulties which come from the acquisition of collateral resistance. Farha et al.[68] gave two cycles of intensive combination chemotherapy (doxorubicin, cyclophosphamide, vincristine and etoposide), each with ABMT followed by 4 cycles of conventional chemotherapy and thoracic radiation. Responses lasted only 41 weeks – an exceptionally disappointing result.

The problem seems to be the rapid acquisition of drug resistance by what appears to the clinician, perhaps misleadingly, to be a sensitive tumour. Even so, it may yet be possible to devise high-dose strategies for treating this disease. We await evidence of clinically useful lack of cross-resistance between drug regimens. Studies of chemotherapy regimens (in conventional doses) in extensive disease might usefully be directed to a systematic exploration of this question.

GLIOMA

The prognosis of grade III and IV astrocytoma is dismal with less than 10% alive at 2 years. A recent overview of randomized trials[69] has indicated that single-agent CCNU may increase survival by a small amount. Against this background, there has been some interest in the use of high-dose BCNU. Hochberg et al.[70] treated 11 patients with BCNU, up to $1400 \, mg/m^2$, and noted stable disease or improvement in 7. Philips et al.[71] treated 36 patients with doses from $1050–1350 \, mg/m^2$ divided into 3 doses over 3 days. Toxicity was severe. Responses were seen in 12 of 27 patients with recurrent disease, and 3 of 9 patients treated as 'adjuvant' survived 2–5 years. Mbidde et al.[21] have reported 22 patients with grade IV glioma treated with high-dose BCNU ($800–1000 \, mg/m^2$) as the first post-surgical treatment, followed by radiotherapy. They pointed out the difficulty in assessing response, even in these previously untreated patients, and declined to estimate a response rate. They did, however, suggest a slight, but by no means definite, improvement in survival compared with matched controls treated conventionally. Johnson et *al.*[72] were less cautious about their results with 25 patients treated almost identically, and suggested an improvement in survival compared with historical controls although follow-up time was very short at the time of publication.

There is thus a hint that response rate may be increased by high-dose BCNU but it is difficult to be sure. Toxicity is formidable with 16% death rate over all studies. As it stands, the results do not suggest that a randomized trial of high-dose BCNU alone is worthwhile. Etoposide in high dose has been used in a single study[73] where 48-hour infusions up to $1 \, g/m^2$ produced no responses in 24 patients, 12 of whom had been previously treated.

MYELOMA

Although 60% of patients with myeloma respond to melphalan and prednisolone, the response usually only last 2-3 years. Responding patients are more likely to be fit with a smaller tumour mass. McElwain's group at the Royal Marsden Hospital has assessed the use of high-dose melphalan, usually as the initial and sole treatment for the disease – a study design which allows a clear impression of the value of the procedure. They have reported results in 56 patients treated with $140 \, mg/m^2$ (without ABMT)[74]. Forty-one had had no previous treatment and 12 of these (27%) experienced complete remission and 21 (51%) a partial response with a median duration of 19 months. Among the 15 patients who were previously treated, 66% responded but only for a short time.

Subsequently, high-dose methylprednisolone was added to high-dose melphalan with an identical response rate but fewer early deaths[75]. In a continuing study, the authors used high-dose melphalan after preliminary treatment with vincristine, doxorubicin and methylprednisolone. With 36 patients treated, response rate seems similar to the other two studies. The results of a randomized comparison of high-dose melphalan ± methylprednisolone with conventional chemotherapy is now being undertaken by the UK Medical Research Council and the results are awaited with great interest as one of the very few randomized trials of high-dose treatment. Barlogie *et al.*[76] have used total body irradiation and high-dose melphalan in 7 patients with myeloma resistant to VAD* and obtained responses in 6, suggesting an effective combination which may justify a larger study.

NEUROBLASTOMA

Advanced and metastatic neuroblastoma is a lethal disease, only 15% of all cases of stage IV disease surviving 2 years[77]. Modern conventional-dose induction chemotherapy can induce response in 90% of patients with approximately 30% of cases achieving a complete or very good partial response[78]. Like SCLC, responses are readily obtained but poorly maintained. It is for these reasons that there has been interest in high-dose chemotherapy which has nearly always been given as chemotherapy on relapse or as a planned late

*VAD: vincristine, doxorubicin, dexamethasone

intensification. Pritchard et al.[79] treated 12 patients with high-dose melphalan followed by surgery and sometimes radiotherapy. All patients had previously received 6 cycles of triple agent chemotherapy. Two patients were in CR after the melphalan and 4 more went on to CR after surgery. Hartmann et al.[80] treated 15 children with stage III and IV disease. All had been heavily pretreated. Seven were in PR, 4 in very good PR and 4 in CR. Of the PR patients, none responded to high-dose melphalan. Among the others, the effect of melphalan was not measurable clinically, and 4 had other treatments as well, so the effect of high-dose melphalan could not be judged although there were 3 patients who survived more than 3 years. These papers showed that the approach was feasible. In a further study in 10 patients[81], a combination of busulphan and cyclophosphamide was used in previously treated patients (5 with unresponding disease, 4 in first relapse and 1 in second relapse). Two patients had a PR and one CR. The treatment was extremely toxic (7/20 deaths in all types of patients) but showed that responses could occur.

The greatest experience is summarised in two recent reports. Philip et al.[78] treated 56 children with stage IV disease with an induction protocol of cisplatin, tenoposide, cyclophosphamide, doxorubicin and vincristine, followed by surgery when possible, followed by further conventional-dose chemotherapy, followed by intensive therapy with ABMT consisting of infused vincristine, total body irradiation (6×2 Gy) and high-dose melphalan. Twenty-three patients were grafted in PR, 6 in very good PR and 8 in CR. On an actuarial basis, of the 14 in very good PR or CR, 44% (6/14) might be disease free at 2 years, but few of the others. Seven treatment-related deaths occurred, and it should be noted that two-thirds of patients did not achieve CR or very good PR with conventional treatment. Slightly better results were reported by Hartmann et al.[82]. In their study of 62 children, 33 achieved CR or very good PR after chemotherapy and went on to high-dose treatment with BCNU, tenoposide and high-dose melphalan given once or twice. The probability of relapse-free survival at 2 years worked out to be 50% but it must again be stressed that the grafted group were selected on the basis of marked previous chemosensitivity.

A randomized trial of high-dose melphalan as consolidation therapy is being conducted by the European Neuroblastoma Study Group. The results are awaited. The weak results with high-dose melphalan in unrandomized studies suggest that there will be a need for further randomized trials of more effective regimens (if these can be found).

BREAST CANCER

The prognosis for patients with metastatic breast cancer is poor: less than 25% will be disease-free at 2 years, and five-year survival is less than 10%. Some retrospective clinical studies have suggested a dose–response relationship[83], and dose intensity (amount of a drug given over a defined time period) has been shown to be of importance in gaining the best response rates in metastatic breast cancer[84]. In another retrospective analysis, dose intensity has also been shown to be important in adjuvant chemotherapy of patients with stage II breast cancer[85], where dose intensity correlated with 3-year relapse-free survival.

High-dose chemotherapy has been used in the treatment of patients with metastatic breast cancer and the reported studies are summarized in Table 7.3. Small numbers of patients have been treated with single-agent chemotherapy using melphalan, mitomycin C or amsacrine. These trials have, on the whole, been disappointing with a 2% CR rate and 21% PR rate. Response rates to multiagent high-dose chemotherapy are between 27% and 70%. Resistant relapse has, as expected, the lowest response rate (27%).

Patients who were treated with high-dose chemotherapy on first relapse have a CR rate of about 50%, and 70% of patients entering the procedure with chemosensitive relapse went into CR after high-dose chemotherapy. A recent review of high-dose chemotherapy and BMT in advanced breast cancer, assessed 27 trials in 172 patients[93]. The overall response rate was 58%, but response rates were highest in trials involving multiple alkylating agents (76%) or previously untreated patients (81%).

In good performance status patients, conventional chemotherapy regimens can produce responses in 55–70% of patients. Most of the responses achieved by high-dose therapy have been short-lived. Studies have been started which use high-dose treatment as late intensification adjuvant chemotherapy in stage II patients at high risk of relapse with >10 axillary lymph nodes

Table 7.3 High-dose chemotherapy and autologous bone marrow transplantation in breast cancer

Reference	n	High-dose treatment	CR	PR	Response rate(%)	TDR
Single-agent in metastatic disease						
Schnell et al. (1981)[86] Dicke et al. (1981)[87]	24	Mitomycin C	1	5	25	2(8%)
Tannir et al. (1983)[88]	16	Amsacrine	0	6	12	0
Corringham et al. (1983)[89] Lazarus et al. (1983)[17] Herzig et al. (1985)[20]	12	Melphalan	0	6	50	0
Combination chemotherapy in metastatic disease						
Steward et al. (1982)[90]	5	Cyclo TBI	3	0	60	1/5(20%)
Peters et al. (1984)[91]	6	CPBM	3	3	100	2/6(33%)
Peters et al. (1989)[92]	16	RR	—	—	27	—
	22	RCSU CPB	—	—	54	—
	50	CSR	—	—	70	—
Adjuvant chemotherapy						
Peters et al. (1989)[92]	14 (Stage II)	CAF followed by CPB/ABMT	—	—	—	—

TDR = toxic death rate; C = cyclophosphamide; P = cisplatinum; B = BCNU; M = melphalan; A = adriamycin; F = 5-fluorouracil

involved, but follow-up is too short to comment on results at the present time. High-dose chemotherapy does not yet have an established place in the treatment of breast cancer, and the results of current unrandomized studies will be of considerable interest. The value of 'adjuvant' late-intensification high-dose chemotherapy, used after conventional adjuvant treatment, can only be established by prospective randomized clinical trial, comparing the high-dose procedure with no further treatment.

FUTURE DIRECTIONS

The very least we could hope for with high-dose therapy is an increase in response rate. This has been found with many regimens used to treat many tumours even when 'refractory' to conventional therapy. What we need is a clinically important duration of response and increase in cure rate. It is our view that this awaits demonstration in any tumour though the results in myeloma and NHL are perhaps encouraging. Randomized trials are long overdue but only a small proportion of patients is likely to benefit or to be eligible. For most tumours, the increase in proportion of survivors is likely to be 10–20% and the statistical rules mean that large numbers of patients will have to enter a study (say in lymphoma) in order to be able to randomize a subgroup to be treated in, say, first relapse or initial partial response. National and even international collaboration will be needed to design clear protocols. These must be as uncluttered as possible and allow a valid assessment of the high-dose procedure. Just because myelosuppresive chemotherapy *can* be given does not mean it *should* be given. We need to move from the past decade of exploration into a new era of validation.

References

1. Davis, S., Wright, P. W., Schulman, S. F., Scholes, D., Thorning, D. and Hammar, S. (1985). Long-term survival in small-cell carcinoma of the lung: A population experience. *J. Clin. Oncol.*, **3**, 80–91
2. Johnson, D. H., Deleo, M. J., Hande, K. R., Wolfe, S. N., Hainsworth, J. D. and Greco, F. A. (1987). High-dose induction chemotherapy with cyclophosphamide, etoposide, and cisplatin for extensive-stage small-cell lung cancer. *J. Clin. Oncol.*, **5**, 703–709
3. Souhami, R. L., Bradbury, I., Geddes, D. M., Spiro, S. G., Harper, P. G. and Tobias, J. S. (1985). Prognostic significance of laboratory parameters measured at diagnosis in small cell carcinoma of the lung. *Cancer Res.*, **45**, 2878–2882
4. Singer, C. R. J. and Goldstone, A. H. (1986). Clinical studies of ABMT in non-Hodgkin's lymphoma. *Clin. Haematol.*, **15**, 105–150
5. Longo, D. L., Young, R. C. and Wesley, M. (1986). Twenty years of MOPP therapy for Hodgkin's disease. *J. Clin. Oncol.*, **4**, 1295–1306
6. van Groeningen, C. J., Pinedo, H. M., Heddes, J., Kok, R. M., de Jong, A. P. J. M., Wattel, E., Peters, G. J. and Lankelma, J. (1988). Pharmacokinetics of 5-fluorouracil assessed with a sensitive mass spectrometric method in patients in a dose escalation schedule. *Cancer Res.*, **48**, 6956–6961
7. Friedman, O. M., Myles, A. and Colvin, M. (1986). Cyclophosphamide and related phosphoramide mustards. Current status and future prospects. *Adv. Cancer Chemother.*, **1**, 143–204

8. Crook, T. R., Souhami, R. L. and McLean, A. E. M. (1986). Cytotoxicity, DNA cross-linking and single strand breaks induced by activated cyclophosphamide and acrolein in human leukaemia cells. *Cancer Res.,* **40**, 5029-5034

9. Schuler, U., Ehringer, G. and Wagner, T. (1987). Repeated high-dose cyclophosphamide administration in bone marrow transplantation. Exposure to activated metabolites. *Cancer Chemother. Pharmacol.,* **20**, 248-252

10. Smith, I. E., Evans, B. D., Harland, S. J. and Millar, J. (1983). Autologous bone marrow rescue is unnecessary after very high-dose cyclophosphamide. *Lancet,* **1**, 76(L)

11. Twelves, C., Souhami, R., Harper, P. and Goldstone, A. (1989). Haematological recovery following high dose cyclophosphamide with autologous bone marrow transplantation. (submitted)

12. Shorthouse, A. J., Jones, J. M., Steel, G. and Peckham, M. J. (1982). Experimental combination and single agent chemotherapy in human lung tumour xenografts. *Br. J. Cancer,* **46**, 35-45

13. Souhami, R. L., Finn, G., Gregory, W. M., Birkhead, B. G., Buckman, R., Edwards, D., Goldstone, A. H., Harper, P. G., Spiro, S. G., Tobias, J. S. and Geddes, D. (1985). High dose cycloposphamide in small cell carcinoma of the lung. *J. Clin. Oncol.,* **3**, 958-963

14. Tattersall, M. H. N., Jarman, M., Newlands, E. S., Holyhead, L., Milsted, R. A. V. and Weinberg, A. (1978). Pharmocokinetics of melphalan following oral or intravenous administration in patients with malignant disease. *Eur. J. Cancer,* **14**, 507-513

15. McElwain, T. J., Hedley, D. W., Burton, G., Clink, H. M., Gordon, M. Y., Jarman, M., Juttner, C. A., Millar, J. L., Milstedt, R. A. V., Prentice, G., Smith, E. I., Spence, D. and Woods, M. (1979). Marrow autotransplantation accelerates haematological recovery in patients with malignant melanoma treated with high-dose melphalan. *Br. J. Cancer,* **40**, 72-80

16. Millar, J. L., Phelps, T. A., Carter, R. L. and McElwain, T. J. (1978). Cyclophosphamide pretreatment reduces the toxic effect of high dose melphalan on intestinal epithelium in sheep. *Eur. J. Cancer,* **11**, 1283-1285

17. Lazarus, H. M., Herzig, R. H., Graham-Pole, J., Wolff, S. N., Phillips, G. L., Strandjord, S., Hurd, D., Forman, W., Gordon, E. M., Coccia, P., Gross, S. and Herzig, G. P. (1983). Intensive melphalan chemotherapy and cryopreserved autologous bone marrow transplantation for the treatment of refractory cancer. *J. Clin. Oncol.,* **1**, 359-367

18. Selby, P. J., Courtenay, V. D., McElwain, T. J., Peckham, M. J. and Steel, G. G. (1980). Colony growth and clonogenic cell survival in human melanoma xenografts treated with chemotherapy. *Br. J. Cancer,* **42**, 438-448

19. Scudiero, D. A., Meyer, S. A., Clatterbuck, B. E., Mattern, M. R., Ziolkowski, C. H. and Day, R. S. (1984). Sensitivity of human cell strains having different abilities to repair O^6-methylguanine in DNA to inactivation by alkylating agents including chloroethylnitrosoureas. *Cancer Res.,* **44**, 2467-2474

20. Herzig, R. H., Phillips, G. L., Lazarus, H. M. *et al.* (1985). Intensive chemotherapy and autologous bone marrow transplantation for treatment of refractory malignancies. In Diche, K. A., Spitzer, G., Zander, A. R. (eds.) *Autologous Bone Marrow Transplantation*, pp. 197-202. (Houston: University of Texas)

21. Mbidde, E. K., Selby, P. J., Perren, J. J., Dearneley, D. P., Whitton, A., Ashley, S., Workman, P., Bloom, H. J. G. and McElwain, T. J. (1988). High dose BCNU chemotherapy with autologous bone marrow transplantation and full dose radiotherapy for grade IV astrocytoma. *Br. J. Cancer,* **58**, 779-782

22. Phillips, G. L., Fay, J. W., Herzig, G. P., Herzig, R. H., Weiner, R. S., Wolff, S. N., Lazarus, H. M., Karanes, C., Ross, W. E., Kramer, B. S. and the Southeastern Cancer Study Group (1983). Intensive 1,3-*bis*(2-chloroethyl)-1-nitrosourea (BCNU), NSC No. 4366650 and cryopreserved autologous marrow transplantation for refractory cancer. A phase I-II study. *Cancer,* **52**, 1792-1802

23. Teicher, B. A., Holden, S. A., Cuchi, C. A. *et al.* (1988). Combination of N N' N″triethylene-thiophosphoramide and cyclophosphamide in vitro and in vivo. *Cancer Res.,* **48**, 94-100

24. Williams, S. F., Bitran, J. D., Kaminer, L., Westbrook, C., Jacobs, R., Ashenhurst, J., Robin, E., Purl, S., Beschorner, J., Schroeder, C. and Golomb, H. (1987). A phase I-II study of bialkylator chemotherapy, high-dose thiotepa and cyclophosphamide with autologous bone marrow reinfusion in patients with advanced cancer. *J. Clin. Oncol.,* **5**, 260-265

25. Eder, J. P., Antman, K., Elias, A., Shea, T. C., Tercher, B. A., Henner, W. D., Schryber, S. M., Holden, S. A., Finberg, R., Critchlow, J., Flaherty, M., Mick, R., Schrupper, L. E. and Frei, E. (1988). Cyclophosphamide and thiotepa with autologous bone marrow transplantation in patients with solid tumours. *J. Natl. Cancer Inst.*, **80**, 1221–1226

26. Peters, W. P., Eder, J. P., Henner, D. *et al.* (1986). High dose combination alkylating agents with autologous bone marrow support: A phase I trial. *J. Clin. Oncol.*, **4**, 646–654

27. Slevin, M. L., Clerk, P. I., Osborne, R. J., Malik, S., Wood, C. D., Harvey, B. J., Joel, S. P., Malpas, J. S. and Wrigley, P. S. M. (1986). A randomised trial to evaluate the effect of schedule on the activity of etoposide in small cell lung cancer. *Proc. ASCO*, **5**, 175

28. Hande, K. R., Wedlund, P. J., Noone, R. M., Wilkinson, G. R., Greco, F. A. and Wolff, S. N. (1984). Pharmacokinetics of high dose etoposide (VP-16-213) administered to cancer patients. *Cancer Res.*, **44**, 379–382

29. Wolff, S. N., Fer, M. F., McKay, C. M., Hande, K. R., Hainsworth, J. D. and Greco, F. A. (1983). High dose VP-16-213 and autologous bone marrow transplantation for refractory malignancies: A phase I study. *J. Clin. Oncol.*, **1**, 701–705

30. Goldstone, A. H., Souhami, R. L., Linch, D. C. *et al.* (1984). Intensive chemotherapy and autologous bone marrow transplantation for relapsed lymphoma. *Exp. Haematol.*, **12**, (suppl 15), 137

31. Spitzer, G., Farha, P., Valdivieso, M., Dicke, K., Zander, A., Vellekoop, L., Murphy, W. K., Dhingra, H. M., Umsawasdi, T., Chiniten, D. and Carr, D. T. (1986). High dose intensification therapy with autologous bone marrow support for limited small cell bronchogenic carcinoma. *J. Clin. Oncol.*, **4**, 4–13

32. Sarna, G. P., Champlin, J. and Gale, R. P. (1982). Phase I study of high-dose mitomycin with autologous bone marrow support. *Cancer Treat. Rep.*, **66**, 277–282

33. Appelbaum, F. R., Deisseroth, A. B., Graw, R. G., Herzig, G. P., Levine, A. S., Magrath, I. T., Pizzo, P. A., Poplack, D. G. and Ziegler, J. L. (1978). Prolonged complete remission following high dose chemotherapy of Burkitt's lymphoma in relapse. *Cancer*, **41**, 1059–1063

34. Appelbaum, F. R., Herzig, G. P., Ziegler, J. L., Graw, R. G., Levine, A. S. and Deisseroth, A. B. (1978). Successful engraftment of cryopreserved autologous bone marrow in patients with malignant lymphoma. *Blood*, **52**, 85–95

35. Gorin, N. C., Najman, A., Douay, L., Salmon, C. H., David, R., Stachowiak, J., Parlier, Y., Lopez, M., Oppenheimer, M., Lecomte, D., Deloux, J., Petit, J. C., Pene, F., Gerota, I., vand den Akker, J. and Duhamel, G. (1984). Autologous bone marrow transplantation in the treatment of poor prognosis non-Hodgkin's lymphomas. *Eur. J. Cancer Clin. Oncol.*, **20**, 217–225

36. Verdonck, L. F., Dekker, A. W. and van Kemren, M. L. (1985). Intensive cytotoxic therapy followed by autologous bone marrow transplantation for non-Hodgkin's lymphoma of high grade malignancy. *Blood*, **65**, 984–989

37. Philip, T., Biron, P., Maraninchi, D., Goldstone, A. H., Herve, P., Souillet, F., Gastaut, J. L., Plouvier, E., Flesh, Y., Philip, I., Harousseau, J. L., Le Mevel, A., Rebattu, P., Linch, D. C., Freycon, F., Milan, I. J. and Souhami, R. L. (1985). Massive chemotherapy with autologous bone marrow transplantation in 50 cases of bad prognosis non-Hodgkin's lymphoma. *Br. J. Haematol.*, **60**, 599–609

38. Philip, T., Biron, P., Philip, I., Favrot, M., Souillet, G., Frappaz, D., Jaubaert, J., Bordigoni, P., Bernard, J. L., Laporte, J. P., LeMevel, A., Plouvier, E., Marguerite, G., Pinkerton, R., Brizard, C. P., Freycon, F., Forster, H. K., Philippe, N. and Brunat-Mentigny, M. (1986). Massive therapy and autologous bone marrow transplantation in pediatric and young adults Burkitt's lymphoma (30 courses on 28 patients: a 5-year experience). *Eur. J. Cancer Clin. Oncol.*, **22**, 1015–1027

39. Appelbaum, F. R., Sullivan, K. M., Buckner, C. D., Clift, R. A., Deeg, J., Fefer, A., Hill, R., Mortimer, J., Neiman, P. E., Sanders, J. E., Singer, J., Stewart, P., Storb, R. and Thomas, E. D. (1987). Treatment of malignant lymphoma in 100 patients with chemotherapy, total body irradiation, and marrow transplantation. *J. Clin. Oncol.*, **5**, 1340–1347

40. Tannir, N. M., Spitzer, G., Zander, A. R., Jagannath, S., Kanojia, M., Vellekoop, L., McLaughlin, P., Hagemeister, F. J. and Dicke, K. A. (1983). High-dose chemoradiotherapy and bone marrow transplantation in patients with refractory lymphoma. *Eur. J. Cancer Clin. Oncol.*, **19**, 1091–1096

41. Gribben, J. G., Vaughan Hudson, B. and Linch, D. C. (1987). The potential value of very intensive therapy with autologous bone marrow rescue in the treatment of malignant lymphomas. *Hematol. Oncol.,* **5**, 281–293

42. Philip, T., Armitage, J. O., Spitzer, G., Chauvin, F., Jagannath, S., Cahn, J. Y., Colombat, P., Goldstone, A. H., Gorin, N. C., Flesh, M., Laporte, J. P., Maraninchi, D., Pico, J., Bosly, A., Anderson, C., Schots, R., Biron, P., Cabanillas, F. and Dicke, K. (1987). High-dose therapy and autologous bone marrow transplantation after failure of conventional chemotherapy in adults with intermediate-grade or high-grade non-Hodgkin's lymphoma. *N. Engl. J. Med.,* **316**, 1493-1498

43. Takvorian, T., Canellos, G. P., Ritz, J., Freedman, A. S., Anderson, K. C., Mauch, P., Tarbell, N., Coral, F., Daley, H., Yeap, B., Schlossman, S. F. and Nadler, L. M. (1987). Prolonged disease-free survival after autologous bone marrow transplantation in patients with non-Hodgkin's lymphoma with a poor prognosis. *N. Engl. J. Med.,* **316**, 1499–1505

44. Philip, T., Hartmann, O., Biron, P., Cahn, J. Y., Pein, F., Bordigoni, P., Souillet, G., Gartner, M., Lasset, C. and Chauvin, F. (1988). High-dose therapy and autologous bone marrow transplantation in partial remission after first-line induction therapy for diffuse non-Hodgkin's lymphoma. *J. Clin. Oncol.,* **6**, 1118–1124

45. Phillips, G. L., Herzig, R. H., Lazarus, H. M., Fay, J. W., Wolff, S. N., Mill, W. B., Lin, H. S., Thomas, P. R., Glasgow, G. P., Shina, D. C. and Herzig, G. P. (1984). Treatment of resistant malignant lymphoma with cyclophosphamide, total body irradiation and transplantation of cryopreserved autologous marrow. *N. Engl. J. Med.,* **310**, 1557–1561

46. Armitage, J. O., Jagannath, S., Spitzer, G., Bierman, P., Kessinger, A., Kumar, P., Cabanillas, F., Zander, A., Vellekoop, L. and Kicke, K. (1986). High dose therapy and autologous marrow transplantation as salvage treatment for patients with diffuse large cell lymphoma. *Eur. J. Cancer Clin. Oncol.,* **22**, 871–877

47. Armitage, J. O., Gingrich, R. D., Klassen, L. W., Bierman, P. J., Kumar, P. P., Weisenburger, D. D. and Smith, D. M. (1986). Trial of high dose cytorabine, cyclophosphamide, total-body irradiation and autologous bone marrow transplantation for refractory lymphoma. *Cancer Treat. Rep.,* **70**, 871–875

48. Gulati, S. C., Shank, B., Black, P., Yopp, J., Koziner, B., Straus, D., Filippa, D., Kempin, S., Castro-Malaspina, H., Cunningham, I., Berman, E., Coleman, M., Langleben, A., Colvin, M., Fuks, Z., O'Reilly, R. and Clarkson, B. (1988). Autologous bone marrow transplantation for patients with poor-prognosis lymphoma. *J. Clin. Oncol.,* **6**, 1303–1313

49. Philip, T., Dumont, J., Teillet, F., Maraninchi, D., Gorin, N. C., Kuentz, M., Harousseau, J. L., Marty, M., Pinkerton, R. and Herve, P. (1986). High dose chemotherapy and autologous bone marrow transplantation in refractory Hodgkin's disease. *Br. J. Cancer,* **53**, 737–742

50. Carella, A. M., Santini, G., Santoro, A. *et al.* (1985). Massive chemotherapy with non-frozen autologous bone marrow transplantation in 13 cases of refractory Hodgkin's disease. *Eur. J. Cancer Clin. Oncol.,* **21**, 607-613

51. Teillet, F., Pulik, M., Teillet-Thiebaud, F., Blaise, A. M., Kuentz, M., Courtois, F., Andolenko, P., Bleichner, G. and Coste, F. (1987). Autologous bone marrow transplantation (ABMT) in poor prognosis Hodgkin's disese (PPHD). *Bone Marrow Transplant.,* **2** (suppl. 1), 211

52. Goldstone, A. H., Gribben, J. G. and Dones, L. (1987). Fourth report of EBMT experience of autologous bone marrow transplantation in lymphoma. *Bone Marrow Transplant.,* **2** (suppl. 1), 200–203

53. Cabanillas, F., Velasquez, W. S., McLaughlin, P., Jagannath, S., Hagemeister, F. B., Redman, J. R., Swan, F. and Rodriguez, M. A. (1988). Results of recent salvage chemotherapy regimens for lymphoma and Hodgkin's disease. *Semin. Hematol.,* **25** (suppl. 2), 47–50

54. Gribben, J. G., Linch, D. C., Singer, C. R. J., Jarret, M. and Goldstone, A. H. (1989). Successful treatment of refractory Hodgkin's disease by high dose combination chemotherapy and autologous bone marrow transplantation. *Blood,* **73**, 340–345

55. Canellos, G. P., Nadler, L. and Takvorian, T. (1988). Autologous bone marrow transplantation in the treatment of malignant lymphoma and Hodgkin's disease. *Semin. Hematol.,* **25** (suppl. 2), 58–65

56. Bonadonna, G., Santoro, A., Viviani, S. and Valagussa, P. (1988). Treatment strategies for Hodgkin's disease. *Semin. Hematol.,* **25** (suppl. 2), 51–57

57. Hancock, B. W., Vaughan-Hudson, B. and Vaughan-Hudson, G. for British National Lymphoma Investigation (BNLI) (1987). Randomised study of LOPP versus LOPP alternating with EVAP in advanced Hodgkin's disease. Preliminary results. Presented at the *3rd International Conference on Malignant Lymphoma*, June 1987, Abstract No. 25, p. 33

58. Buzard, A. C., Lippman, S. M. and Miller, T. P. (1987). Salvage therapy of advanced Hodgkin's disease. *Am. J. Med.*, **83**, 523–532

59. Selby, P., McElwain, T. J. and Canellos, G. (1987). Chemotherapy for Hodgkin's disease. In Selby, P. (ed.) *Hodgkin's Disease*, pp. 269–300. (Oxford: Blackwell)

60. Spitzer, G., Dicke, K. A., Litam, J., Verma, D. S., Zander, A., Lanzotti, V., Valdivieso, M., McCredie, K. B. and Samuels, M. L. (1980). High dose combination chemotherapy with autologous bone marrow transplantation in adult solid tumours. *Cancer*, **45**, 3075–3085

61. Banham, F., Soukoup, M., Burnett, A. *et al.* (1983). Treatment of small cell carcinoma of lung with a late dosage intensification programme containing cyclophosphamide and mesna. *Cancer Treat. Rep.*, **10**, (suppl), 73–77

62. Smith, I. E., Evans, B. D. and Harland, S. J. (1985). High-dose cyclophosphamide with autologous bone marrow rescue after conventional chemotherapy in the treatment of small cell lung carcinoma. *Cancer Chemother. Pharmacol.*, **14**, 120–124

63. Spitzer, G., Farha, P., Valdivieso, M. *et al.* (1986). High dose intensification therapy with autologous bone marrow support for limited small cell bronchogenic carcinoma. *J. Clin. Oncol.*, **4**, 4–13

64. Humblet, Y., Symann, M., Bosly, A., Delaunois, L., Francis, C., Machiels, J., Beauduin, M., Doyen, C., Weynants, P., Longueville, J. and Prignot, J. (1987). Late intensification chemotherapy with autologous bone marrow transplantation in selected small cell carcinoma of the lung: a randomised study. *J. Clin. Oncol.*, **5**, 1864–1873

65. Souhami, R. L., Finn, G. and Gregory, W. (1985). Very high dose cyclophosphamide as initial treatment for small cell carcinoma of the lung. *J. Clin. Oncol.*, **3**, 958–963

66. Souhami, R. L., Hajichristou, H. T., Miles, D. W., Earl, H. M., Harper, P. G., Ash, C. M., Goldstone, A. H., Spiro, S. G., Geddes, D. M. and Tobias, J. S. (1989). Intensive chemotherapy with autologous bone marrow transplantation for small cell lung cancer. *Cancer Chemother. Pharmacol.*, **24**, 321–325

67. Wolff, S. N., Johnson, D. H., Hande, K. R. *et al.* (1983). High dose etoposide as single agent chemotherapy for small cell carcinoma of the lung. *Cancer Treat. Rep.*, **67**, 957–958

68. Farha, P., Spitzer, G., Valdivieso, M., Dicke, K. A., Zander, A., Dhingra, H. M., Minnhaar, G., Vellekoop, L., Verma, D. S., Umsawasdi, T. and Chiniten, D. (1983). High dose chemotherapy and autologous bone marrow transplantation for the treatment of small cell lung carcinoma. *Cancer*, **52**, 1351–1355

69. Stenning, S. P., Freedman, L. S. and Bleehen, N. M. (1987). An overview of published results from randomized studies of nitrosoureas in primary high grade malignant glioma. *Br. J. Cancer*, **56**, 89–90

70. Hochberg, F., Parker, L., Takvorian, T., Canellos, G. and Zervas, N. (1981). High dose BCNU with autologous bone marrow rescue for recurrent glioblastoma multiforme. *J. Neurosurg.*, **54**, 455–460

71. Philips, G. L., Wolff, S. N., Fay, J. W., Herzig, R. H., Lazarus, H. M., Schold, C. and Herzig, G. P. (1986). Intensive 1,3-bis(2 chlorethyl)-1-nitrosourea (BCNU) monochemotherapy and autologous bone marrow transplantation for malignant glioma. *J. Clin. Oncol.*, **4**, 639–645

72. Johnson, D. B., Thompson, J. M., Corwin, J. A., Mosley, K. R., Smith, M. T., de las Reyes, R. A., Daly, M. B., Petty, A. M., Lamaster, D., Pierson, W. P., Ruxer, R., Leff, R. S. and Messerschmidt, G. L. (1987). Prolongation of survival for high-grade malignant gliomas with adjuvant high dose CNU and autologous bone marrow transplantation. *J. Clin. Oncol.*, **5**, 763–769

73. Finn, G. P., Bozek, T., Slevin, M., Thomas, D. G. and Souhami, R. L. (1985). High dose etoposide (VP16-213) in relapsed malignant glioma. *Cancer Treat. Rep.*, **69**, 603–605

74. Selby, P. J., McElwain, T. J., Nandi, A. C., Perren, T. J., Powles, R. L., Tillyer, C. R., Osborne, R. J., Slevin, M. L. and Malpas, J. S. (1987). Multiple myeloma treated with high dose intravenous melphalan. *Br. J. Haematol.*, **66**, 55–62

75. Selby, P., Zulian, G., Forgeson, G., Nandi, A., Milan, S., Meldrum, M., Viner, C., Osborne, R., Malpas, J. S. and McElwain, T. J. (1988). The development of high dose melphalan and

of autologous bone marrow transplantation in the treatment of multiple myeloma: Royal Marsden and St. Bartholomew's Hospital studies. *Haematol. Oncol.,* **6**, 173–179

76. Barlogie, B., Alexaniou, R., Dicke, K. A., Zagars, G., Spitzer, G., Jagannath, S. and Horwitz, L. (1987). High dose chemoradiotherapy and autologous bone marrow transplantation for resistant multiple myeloma. *Blood,* **70**, 869–872

77. Ninane, J., Pritchard, J. and Malpas, J. S. (1981). Treatment of advanced neuroblastoma: does adriamycin contribute? *Arch. Dis. Child.,* **56**, 544–548

78. Philip, T., Bernard, J. L., Zucker, J. M., Pinkerton, R., Lutz, P., Bordigoni, P., Plouvier, E., Robert, A., Carton, R., Philippe, N., Philip, I., Chauvin, F. and Favrot, M. (1987). High dose chemoradiotherapy with bone marrow transplantation as consolidation treatment in neuroblastoma: an unselected group of stage IV patients over 1 year of age. *J. Clin. Oncol.,* **5**, 266–271

79. Pritchard, J., McElwain, T. J. and Graham-Pole, J. (1982). High dose melphalan with autologous marrow for treatment of advanced neuroblastoma. *Br. J. Cancer,* **45**, 86–94

80. Hartmann, O., Kalifa, C., Benhamou, E., Patte, C., Flamant, F., Jullien, C., Beaujean, F. and Lemerle, J. (1986). Treatment of advanced neuroblastoma with high dose melphalan and autologous bone marrow transplantation. *Cancer Chemother. Pharmacol.,* **16**, 165–169

81. Hartmann, O., Benhamou, E., Beaujean, F., Pico, J. L., Kalifa, C., Patte, C., Flamant, F. and Lemerle, J. (1986). High dose busulfan and cyclophosphamide with autologous bone marrow transplantation support in advanced malignancies in children: A phase II study. *J. Clin. Oncol.,* **4**, 1804–1810

82. Hartmann, O., Benhamou, E., Beaujean, F., Kalifa, C., Lejars, O., Patte, C., Behard, C., Flamant, F., Thyss, A., Deville, A., Vannier, J. P., Pautard-Muchemble, B. and Lemerle, J. (1987). Repeated high dose chemotherapy followed by purged autologous bone marrow transplantation as consolidation therapy in metastatic neuroblastoma. *J. Clin. Oncol.,* **5**, 1205–1211

83. Bonnadonna, G. and Valagussa, P. (1981). Dose response effect of adjuvant chemotherapy in breast cancer. *N. Engl. J. Med.,* **304**, 10–15

84. Hryniuk, W. and Bush, H. (1984). The importance of dose intensity in chemotherapy of metastatic breast cancer. *J. Clin. Oncol.,* **2**, 1281–1288

85. Hryniuk, W. and Levine, M. N. (1986). Analysis of dose intensity for adjuvant chemotherapy trials in stage II breast cancer. *J. Clin. Oncol.,* **4**, 1162–1170

86. Schnell, F. C., Distefano, A. and Spitzer, G. (1981). Phase I study of high dose mitomycin C with autologous bone marrow transplantation in refractory breast cancer. *Proc. AACR* C521.

87. Dicke, K. A., Vellekoop, L., Spitzer, G. *et al.* (1981). Autologous bone marrow transplantation in neoplasia. *Transplant. Proc.,* **13**, 267–269

88. Tannir, N., Spitzer, G., Schell, F., Legha, S., Zander, A. and Blumenschein, G. (1983). Phase II study of high dose amsacrine (AMSA) and autologous bone marrow transplantation in patients with refractory metastatic breast cancer. *Cancer Treat. Rep.,* **67**, 599–600

89. Corringham, R., Gilmore, M., Prentice, H. and Boesen, E. (1983). High dose melphalan with autologous bone marrow transplant treatment of poor prognosis tumours. *Cancer,* **52**, 1783–1787

90. Steward, P. S. (1982). Autologous bone marrow transplantation in metastatic breast cancer. *Breast Cancer Res. Treat.,* **2**, 85–92

91. Peters, W. P., Eder, J. P., Henner, D. *et al.* (1984). High dose combination alkylating agents with autologous bone marrow support: a phase I study. *Proc. ASCO,* **3**, 29

92. Peters, W. P., Jones, R. B., Shpall, E. J. and Shogan, J. (1989). Dose intensification using high dose combination alkylating agents and autologous bone marrow support for the treatment of breast cancer. Submitted. Data reported by kind permission of the authors

93. Antman, K. and Gale, R. P. (1988). Advanced breast cancer: high dose chemotherapy and bone marrow autotransplants. *Ann. Int. Med.,* **108**, 570–574

8
Cytokine therapy

S.A. KELLY, S. MALIK AND F.R. BALKWILL

INTRODUCTION

Cytokines and their inducers have been used in the therapy of cancer for many years, initially as crude preparations, and more recently as purified homogenous proteins. At the turn of the century, William Coley, a New York surgeon, popularized the use of 'Coleys Mixed Toxins', a crude sterile bacterial filtrate which was administered systemically and intratumourally. It is almost certain that this therapy led to the *in vivo* production of several cytokines with antitumour activity. The treatment was highly toxic and was discontinued following the introduction of chemotherapy and radiotherapy. Following his death, however, his daughter reviewed the results and found complete response (CR) in 270 of 1200 patients with advanced, incurable carcinoma and sarcoma[1].

A number of trials using non-specific immunostimulants, e.g. BCG and *C. parvum*, were performed in the 1960s and 1970s. Although some studies suggested response in a variety of neoplasms, particularly renal cell carcinoma and melanoma, overall this therapy failed to demonstrate reproducible benefit[2].

The identification of individual cytokines in tissue fluids and from leukocytes incubated with immunostimulants or viruses proved extremely difficult because of their high specific activity. The antiviral activity of one group of cytokines, the interferons, was first identified in 1957, and many other cell regulatory activities were ascribed to soluble factors from leukocyte, fibroblast and tumour cell cultures. Recombinant DNA technology has subsequently allowed the definitive identification of cytokines and their actions.

Cytokines comprise a heterogeneous group of proteins with a wide variety of overlapping cell regulatory, immune and inflammatory properties. They are of low molecular weight (<80 KDa), often glycosylated, and are produced throughout the body. They usually act in an autocrine or paracrine manner. Occasionally, cytokines may be produced in large amounts and released into the circulation where they may act as hormones. They interact with cell surface receptors, specific for each cytokine or group of cytokines, and are all involved in the regulation of the immune response.

Cytokines may be effective in cancer therapy *via* a number of mechanisms.

127

These include the induction of a host response against the tumour, a direct regulation of tumour cell growth, a direct cytotoxic effect on tumour cells, and interference with the host–tumour relationship.

Table 8.1 summarizes the cytokines discussed in this chapter.

INTERFERONS

Interferons (IFNs) were first described by Isaacs and Lindenmann in 1957[3]. They were initially defined as proteins that exert antiviral activity, not specific to virus type, in at least homologous cells through cellular metabolic processes involving the synthesis of both RNA and protein[4], but it became obvious soon after their discovery that they have many other cell regulatory activities. Interest in IFNs as treatment for cancer began in the late 1960s when Gresser showed that these proteins could inhibit the development and growth of transplantable tumours in mice[5]. Extensive animal studies and anecdotal studies in man subsequently confirmed the antitumour activity.

There are three classes of IFNs – α, β, and γ (see Table 8.1). They share some common functions, e.g. stimulation of natural killer cell (NK) activity, inhibition of cell growth *in vitro*, and enhancement or induction of major histocompatible complex (MHC) class I and β_2 microglobulin expression. IFN-γ differs from the IFN-αs and IFN-β in that it has more immunomodulating activity and increases MHC class II expression on both tumour and accessory cells.

Table 8.1 Cytokines with potential for cancer therapy

	Molecular weight (kDa)	Chromosome	Major source
Interferon-α	17–23	9	Leukocytes
Interferon-β	20	9	Fibroblasts
Interferon-γ	20	12	T, NK cells
Tumour necrosis factor, TNF-α	17 monomer (active as trimer)	6	Monocytes
Lymphotoxin, TNF-β	25	6	T cells
Interleukin-1	17.5	2	Many cells
Interleukin-2, T cell growth factor	17.2	4	T cells
Interleukin-4, B cell-stimulating factor 1	20	5	Many cells
Interleukin-5	18	5	T cells, many cells
Interleukin-6: B cell growth factor, B cell-stimulating factor 2, hybridoma growth factor, hepatocyte-stimulating factor, interferon-β_2	26	7	Many cells
G-CSF	19	17	Many cells
M-CSF	45	5	Many cells
GM-CSF	22	5	Many cells
Multi-CSF (IL-3)	25	5	Many cells
Transforming growth factor-β1, β2, β3	25		Many cells

There are 23 genes coding for IFN-α, of which 15 code for biologically active protein. Most of the IFN-α genes show approximately 90% homology in their nucleotide sequences. They have a clear evolutionary relationship to IFN-β with which they share 25% amino acid identity.

IFN-α and β share a high-affinity cell-surface receptor which is present in low numbers $(2\times10^2-1\times10^4)$[6], and is distinct from that for IFN-γ. Most cells possess IFN-α/β and IFN-γ receptors, although they express more of the latter. The gene for the IFN-γ receptor has now been cloned[7]. Following binding, internalization leads to rapid gene activation. Although all three IFNs induce a common set of genes, some are induced by either IFN-α/β or IFN-γ. For instance, Weil et al.[8] demonstrated that, in addition to those polypeptides induced in common, IFN-γ induces 12 polypeptides that are little, if at all, induced by IFN-α.

Mechanism of antitumour activity

IFNs probably act by a number of different mechanisms dependent on such variables as tumour type, location, and immune and nutritional status of the host[9].

Firstly, they may exert a direct (antiproliferative) effect. IFNs inhibit the growth of both normal and neoplastic cells, slow cell division in all phases of the cell cycle and have varied effects on differentiation. They inhibit the differentiation of some monocyte lines to macrophages, but enhance the differentiation of erythroblasts in the Friend leukaemia line[10]. Human IFNs inhibit the growth of human tumour xenografts growing in the T cell-deficient nude mouse. Secondly, they may act via host immune mechanisms. IFNs may enhance the cytotoxic activity of T cells, NK cells, lymphokine-activated killer (LAK) cells and polymorphs. IFN-γ stimulates macrophage activity. All IFNs enhance class I MHC and β_2 microglobulin expression, but IFN-γ is much more effective in enhancing class II MHC (at least in cell lines), which may facilitate more efficient antigen presentation.

Although the above two mechanisms are well understood, it is uncertain to what extent they are responsible for the antitumour effect of IFN in man. Gresser[10], using a mouse Friend leukaemia cell tumour which is sensitive to IFN in vivo, has demonstrated that regression is not due either to a direct effect or to simulation of the host immune system. It is not clear how IFN is active against this tumour[10]. Other mechanisms of antitumour activity include induction of other cytokines in the tumour or the host, and other alterations in the host/tumour relationship. For example, Sidky and Borden[11] using human xenografts in a nude mouse model have demonstrated, by implanting tumour cells in the cornea and dermis, that tumour-induced angiogenesis was inhibited by IFN. The IFN activity was species specific, with human IFN inhibiting angiogenesis induced by human tumours. This suggests that the signal for angiogenesis was provided by the tumour cells.

Animal studies

All three IFNs have produced tumour regression and increased survival in mice bearing a wide range of tumours. The success of treatment was related to low tumour load and frequent therapy. Human IFNs inhibited the growth of human tumour xenografts growing in nude mice and occasionally complete regression and cure was seen. IFN-α produced a response in a wide variety of subcutaneous (sc) tumours but none showed inhibition of growth by IFN-γ, whether given local, intraperitoneally (ip) or sc, even though sufficient IFN-γ reached the tumour to alter surface antigen expression. IFN-γ is however effective against tumours growing in other sites in nude mice[12].

In animal studies using both xenografts and autochthonous tumours, IFN therapy often produces stable disease; but treatment with IFN alone rarely produces cure.

Cinical studies with IFN-α

Many thousands of patients have been treated with IFNs. Most have received IFN-α of which there are various types. These include single subtypes produced by recombinant DNA technology, e.g. IFN-α_{2a} (Roferon) and IFN-α_{2b} (Intron-A); and Wellferon, a mixture of α subtypes purified from a mass culture of virus-stimulated lymphoblastoid cell lines. There is no evidence to suggest that any single α subtype is superior with respect to activity or incidence of side-effects[9].

A number of neoplasms are responsive to IFN therapy (see Table 8.2). The following section will illustrate some important aspects of IFN treatment in specific tumours.

Hairy cell leukaemia

Therapy with IFN-α has considerably improved the prognosis of patients with hairy cell leukaemia (HCL), with response rates in excess of 90% fre-

Table 8.2 Response rates in phase I and II trials of IFN-α

Disease	Response rate (PR+CR) (%)
Hairy cell leukaemia	80
Chronic myelogenous leukaemia	71
Acute lymphoblastic leukaemia	25
Low-grade lymphoma	65
Chronic lymphocytic leukaemia	11
Cutaneous T cell lymphoma	45
Melanoma	18
Renal cell carcinoma	14
APUD tumours	81
Kaposi's sarcoma	34
Breast cancer	<5

quently reported. The time to response is typically slow. In one study, the median time to partial haematological response was 6 months and to complete haematological response 10 months[13]. The disappearance of leukaemic cells from the circulation enables other indices to return to normal, with a concomitant reduction in the requirement for red cell and platelet transfusions and a decreased incidence of severe infection. However, normalization of the marrow occurs in only about 25% of patients treated. After cessation of therapy, patients may relapse but the majority can achieve a further remission with IFN therapy.

Chronic myeloid leukaemia

The results of treatment of chronic myeloid leukaemia (CML) with IFN-α are at least equivalent to those of conventional therapy in patients in the benign phase of the disease. IFN-α has been demonstrated to increase the leukocyte doubling time, allowing recovery of the normal haematopoietic stem cells[14]. In a study of 51 patients, Talpaz et al.[15] reported a 70% complete haematological remission and 10% partial haematological remission. In contrast to conventional treatment, in 6 of 12 patients who achieved a complete haematological remission, there was complete suppression of the Philadelphia chromosome in the bone marrow.

The place of IFN-α therapy in the accelerated phase of the disease is controversial, but, in a study of 9 patients, Alimena et al.[16] reported 2 partial haematological remissions and 1 complete haematological remission.

Essential thrombocythaemia

There have been a number of reports of the use of IFN-α in this disease[17]. In the study reported by Giles et al.[18], all 18 patients had a rapid fall in platelet counts. In the 14 previously untreated patients, the decrease was greater than 50% and was sustained for 2 to 4 weeks following the completion of induction therapy.

Myeloma

IFN-α is not as effective as chemotherapy in inducing remission of disease. However, Mandelli et al.[19] have reported on the use of IFN-α given as maintenance therapy. Following remission, 101 patients were randomized to receive either no treatment or IFN-α. After a median follow-up of 19 months from the start of maintenance therapy, there were significantly fewer relapses and deaths in the IFN-treated patients[20].

Solid tumours

IFN has little activity in the common solid tumours. However, in patients with carcinoid syndrome, treatment with IFN-α has been demonstrated to produce a high incidence of symptomatic improvement but a much smaller incidence of tumour regression[21]. In renal cell carcinoma and melanoma, studies with various IFN-αs have demonstrated modest but reproducible activity. In renal cell carcinoma, 18 studies using IFN-α have reported responses of 0–31% (overall response 14.2%)[22]. The highest incidence of response was in a subset of patients with pulmonary metastases who had previously undergone nephrectomy.

Local administration

IFNs generally act in a paracrine manner and, in some studies, they have been administered locally. IFN-αs administered intravesically are as effective as conventional therapy in producing remission of superficial bladder tumours[23]. In one small study of ovarian carcinoma[24], intraperitoneal IFN-α₂ was reported to produce 36% (4 of 11) complete pathological remission in patients who had residual tumour at second-look laparotomy. Those with microscopic disease were most likely to respond. However, a recent study using IFN-γ has failed to show similar benefit[25].

Side-effects of IFN-α

The side-effects of IFN-α are varied and are well summarized by Quesada *et al.*[26]. The acute side-effects resemble an influenza-like illness, consisting of fever, chills, tachycardia, myalgias, headache and malaise. In patients receiving continued daily injections, but not patients receiving cyclic or intermittent therapy, the fever usually subsides within 7 to 10 days.

Single doses of up to 150×10^6 units can be given, but patients given daily doses cannot usually tolerate more than 20×10^6 units/day, higher doses producing profound fatigue, and often anorexia and weight loss. Most patients can tolerate daily doses of $3–10 \times 10^6$ units/day on a long-term basis.

Leukopenia is frequent, and the fall in leukocyte counts may be profound, particularly in patients with haematological malignancies. This may lead to septicaemia, but can often be prevented by starting treatment with low-dose IFN and slowly increasing the dose.

Clinical studies with IFN-β

Phase I studies of IFN-β suggest that the side-effects are similar to IFN-α but less severe. In one study using IFN-β ser (a non-glycosylated variant of IFN-β stabilized by the substitution of serine for cysteine at amino acid position 17), a dose of 500×10^6 units/m² could be tolerated[27]. If there was a positive correlation between dose and antiproliferative effect, the less severe side-effects of IFN-β ser might enable higher, more effective doses to be given. However, phase I and II trials show little activity in renal cell carcinoma, melanoma, soft-tissue sarcoma and colon carcinoma[9].

Clinical studies with IFN-γ

Due to its greater immunomodulating properties, it was thought that IFN-γ would exhibit a different spectrum of activity from IFNα/β. There is evidence that it has some activity in chronic lymphocytic leukaemia, where IFN-α has shown little benefit[28]. However, in solid tumours, few responses have been reported. The main side-effects are headache and hypotension, and the reduction in fever seen with continued administration of IFN-α is less frequently seen with IFN-γ.

Dose scheduling

The dose–response relationship in IFN therapy is not clear and may differ in different neoplasms. Standard therapy in HCL is $1-5\times10^6$ units/m^2 thrice weekly ($2.5-12.5\,\mu g/m^2$), but a randomized study[29] comparing Wellferon given in 'standard' (2×10^6 units/m^2) and 'ultralow' (0.2×10^6 units/m^2) dose showed no significant differences between the two dose schedules although there were more objective marrow responses in the standard dose group (59% vs. 36%). In a review of IFN-α in renal cell carcinoma, Krown[30] has demonstrated that moderate dose is more effective in producing remissions than either low- or high-dose treatment. Compared with standard dose, low-dose therapy produces fewer side-effects, the treatment is better tolerated, and the profound drop in white cell count is not seen.

In CML, however, reports suggest that higher doses are most effective. In a study reported by Alimena et al.[16], 20% of patients treated with a dose of 2×10^6 units/m^2 responded compared with 77% of patients given 5×10^6 units/m^2.

IFN antibodies

The incidence and relevance of antibodies to recombinant IFNs is controversial. Naturally occurring IFNs have a high level of species specificity and, as antibodies are not made against 'self antigens', it was thought that recombinant IFNs would not be immunogenic.

Antibodies may be neutralizing (inhibit the antiviral effects of IFN) or non-neutralizing. Speigel et al.[31], using an immunoradiometric assay, found neutralizing antibodies in 2.4% of 537 patients receiving IFN-α_{2b} by systemic therapy, and in <1% in patients receiving intranasal and intralesional therapy. In contrast, Itri et al.[32], using an enzyme immunoassay, found that 25% of patients receiving IFN-α_{2a} had detectable antibodies, the highest incidence being in those with renal cell carcinoma (44%) and AIDS-related Kaposi's sarcoma (34%). The incidence of antibodies was related to length of treatment. Patients who developed neutralizing antibodies were likely to have been treated for longer and to survive for longer than antibody-negative patients. IFN-α_{2a} and IFN-α_{2b} differ only by one amino acid and it is likely that the difference in the incidence of antibodies is mainly due to differences in the sensitivity of the assays used.

Some workers[33] have demonstrated a positive correlation between the appearance of neutralizing antibodies and the loss of response of previously sensitive tumours. It is interesting that, in some patients who develop neutralizing antibodies, a further response can be obtained when the recombinant IFN is substituted by a natural IFN mixture, e.g. Wellferon.

Thus IFNs, particularly IFN-αs, have been shown to have significant activity in a number of malignancies. In hairy cell leukaemia, the place of therapy with IFN-α is well established, but, in other diseases, e.g. chronic myeloid leukaemia, the exact place of IFNs in therapy will only become clear following the results of randomized studies comparing them with conventional therapy. In solid tumours, IFNs have little activity and appear to be of most benefit in neoplasms where there are well-documented cases of spontaneous regression. The mechanism of activity of IFNs in man is unclear although there are many possibilities. Further studies need to be performed to determine the optimal IFN schedule for particular tumours, using IFN alone and in combination with other cytokines, radiotherapy and chemotherapy.

INTERLEUKIN-2

Interleukin-2 (IL-2) is a glycoprotein of molecular weight approximately 15 kDa. It is produced by activated T cells and has a number of functions, the most important being the stimulation of antigen-activated T cell proliferation[34].

The high-affinity IL-2 receptor is composed of 2 non-covalently linked subunits with molecular weights of 55 and 75 kDa. Each alone is able to bind IL-2 with low affinity, but the complex allows binding to IL-2 to occur rapidly and dissociate very slowly. Signal transduction occurs solely *via* the 75 kDa molecule; the 55 kDa molecule appears to act by aiding IL-2 binding[35].

There are a number of mechanisms by which IL-2 may be active against cancer. *In vivo*, IL-2 may induce the secretion of cytokine, such as IFN-γ, tumour necrosis factor (TNF), and lymphotoxin (LT)[36]. IL-2 may also induce the proliferation of antigen-specific T cells. In addition, IL-2 alone without any antigenic stimulation leads to the production of lymphokine-activated killer cells (LAK cells). These are distinct from cytotoxic T lymphocytes (CTLs) in that they do not show antigen specificity or MHC restriction. When assessed in a 4-hour ^{51}Cr release assay, LAK cells are able to lyse a broad range of fresh and cultured NK-resistant and sensitive tumour cells. They have also been demonstrated to lyse some normal cells but to a much lesser degree[37]. LAK activity is exhibited by a number of cell types: mainly NK cells, but T cells, B cells, macrophages, and null cells have also been implicated[38].

In vitro, LAK cells are produced by the incubation of lymphocytes from a variety of sources, e.g. peripheral blood lymphocytes, splenocytes, thoracic duct lymphocytes and tissue infiltrating lymphocytes (TILs), in medium containing IL-2.

Animal studies

The rationale for clinical trials with IL-2 and LAK cells came from *in vitro* and animal work performed mainly by Steven Rosenberg and his colleagues at the National Cancer Institute. They showed that ip IL-2 was effective in reducing the number of established pulmonary and hepatic metastases in mice bearing a variety of immunogenic and non-immunogenic tumours. The combination of LAK and IL-2 was significantly better than IL-2 alone, and the effect correlated with the number of LAK cells infused, the dose of IL-2, and the number of treatments. Repeated doses of IL-2 were necessary to maintain optimal activation of LAK cells. Histological examination of the lungs and liver of mice receiving LAK therapy revealed proliferation of LAK cells[39].

The success of IL-2 therapy was independent of the immune status of the tumour-bearing host. LAK/IL-2 therapy is effective in mice immuno-suppressed by 5 Gy whole body radiation and cyclophosphamide, but infusion of irradiated LAK cells is ineffective[40].

Clinical studies

IL-2 alone

Sondel *et al.*[41] has demonstrated that, following IL-2 infusion, there is a marked lymphocytosis and that freshly isolated lymphocytes show enhanced cytotoxicity against the NK-resistant Daudi cell line. IL-2 alone produced tumour regression, particularly in patients with melanoma and renal cell carcinoma. Although early studies suggested that the response rates were disappointing, the incidence of regression appears to be similar to that found with IL-2/LAK therapy, though the combination therapy produces more CRs. For example, in a study of 85 patients with melanoma, there were no CRs and 9 PRs in 37 patients treated with IL-2 alone and 4CRs and 6PRs in 48 patients given the combination therapy[42].

Table 8.3 Response rates to IL-2/LAK therapy

Author	Number of patients	Complete response	Partial response
Sznol *et al.*[43]	32	1 (3.1%)	5 (18.8%)
Fisher *et al.*[44]	34	1 (3.4%)	4 (11.8%)
Rosenberg *et al.*[45]	106	8 (7.5%)	15 (14.1%)
West *et al.*[46]	102	2 (2%)	19 (18.6%)
Philip *et al.*[47]	15	0	3 (20%)
Bold *et al.*[48]	83	8 (16.9%) CR+PR	
Paciucci *et al.*[49]	25	0	6 (24%)

IL-2/LAK therapy

Treatment with a combination of IL-2 and LAK cells requires a priming course of IL-2, following which the lymphocytes are harvested by leukapheresis. After *in vitro* culture in IL-2, the cells are transferred back into the patient who receives a further course of IL-2.

Table 8.3 summarizes the results of a number of clinical studies using different schedules of IL-2/LAK therapy. Patients treated had advanced disease and a wide range of histological subtypes.

Response rates of between 15% and 30% are typical. Patients with melanoma and renal cell carcinoma are most likely to respond. In some studies, IL-2 has been administered by bolus injection. However, the serum halflife is short (6.9 minutes[50]) and, in an attempt to improve the therapeutic ratio, IL-2 has been delivered by constant infusion. Although some authors[51] have suggested that IL-2 given in this way would be less well tolerated, West et al.[52] found a much reduced incidence of serious side-effects. Infusion has the additional advantage of maintaining a constant exposure of IL-2 which may be necessary for optimal activation of the adoptively transferred cells.

TUMOUR-INFILTRATING LYMPHOCYTES

Tumour-infiltrating lymphocytes (TILs) are isolated by growing single-cell suspensions of tumour in medium containing IL-2. The tumour cells die or are destroyed by the TILs and, eventually, only TILs remain in culture. Freshly isolated TILs appear to be functionally deficient, but, following IL-2 stimulation, they have been demonstrated (in models of micrometastases) to be 50–100 times more cytotoxic than LAK cells[53]. Unfortunately, the yield of TILs is often low and the time taken to produce LAK cells from TILs is much longer than that needed to produce LAK cells from peripheral blood lymphocytes (PBLs). Recent work suggests that activated TILs may be able to home to tumour sites[54].

Rosenberg et al.[55] have recently reported responses in 11 out of 20 patients with metastatic melanoma treated with TILs and IL-2 (1 complete response, 9 partial responses and 1 mixed response). Two of 5 patients responding had failed on the treatment with IL-2 alone. The duration of responses ranged from 2 to >13 months.

Local therapy

Some investigators have reported benefits in patients given local IL-2/LAK therapy. For instance, Steis et al. reported 4 of 5 partial remissions (PR) in patients with peritoneal deposits of ovarian and colorectal tumours who were treated with ip IL-2 and LAK (although at the expense of severe side-effects)[56], and Yoshida et al. reported tumour regression in 6 of 23 patients with recurrent malignant glioma treated intratumourally with IL-2/LAK[57].

Table 8.4 Side-effects of IL-2/LAK therapy

General	Lethargy, fever, chills, infections
Cardiovascular	Hypotension, tachycardia, decreased systemic resistance, arrythmias, myocardial infarction
Respiratory	Respiratory distress, bronchospasm, pleural effusion
Gastrointestinal	Nausea, vomiting, diarrhoea, hepatic impairment
Central nervous	Disorientation, somnolence, coma
Haematological	Anaemia, thrombocytopaenia, neutropaenia, lymphopaenia, lymphocytosis, eosinophilia
Genitourinary	Renal impairment
Endocrine	Hypothyroidism
Cutaneous	Erythema, urticaria

Side-effects of IL-2/LAK therapy

Unfortunately, the side-effects seen in clinical studies are much greater than predicted from animal models. They are summarized in Table 8.4. Almost all are due to IL-2 alone. The most severe dose limiting side-effect is the capillary leak syndrome which consists of increased capillary permeability, vasodilation and hypotension, tachycardia and increased cardiac output. Fluid loss from the vascular space leads to pulmonary oedema, and decreased oxygenation. Patients may require monitoring in an intensive care unit. Although this may be due to IL-2 alone, the syndrome is more severe in patients receiving IL-2 and LAK cells, possibly because LAK cells have been shown to mediate endothelial damage[37].

Thus, IL-2/LAK therapy is potentially an important advance in cancer treatment. Animal studies have shown that IL-2 alone and in combination with LAK cells has significant antitumour activity. There are considerable logistical problems involved in the collection of lymphocytes, and the preparation of LAK cells is time consuming and expensive. The use of more potent effector cells is of great interest as is the combination of LAK therapy and monoclonal antibodies, other cytokines, and chemotherapeutic agents. Other problems that need to be overcome include optimal dosage, alleviation of side-effects, and identification of patients most likely to respond.

INTERLEUKIN-4

Interleukin-4 (IL-4) is a 20 kDa glycoprotein produced by activated T cells originally described for its ability to stimulate the proliferation of human and murine B cells *in vitro*. It is now known to have a much wider spectrum of activity, having effects on T cells, granulocytes, mast cells, erythroid precursors, and megakaryocytes[9].

137

Its most likely potential in cancer therapy is its ability to stimulate the proliferation of cytotoxic T lymphocytes (particularly mitogen stimulated), which are at least as active as those stimulated by IL-2. Thus, IL-4 could be used to generate antigen-specific CTLs which are active against tumours.

Although recent reports have demonstrated that, *in vitro*, IL-4 inhibits IL-2-mediated generation of LAK cells from NK cells[58], Kawakami *et al.* have demonstrated using TILs derived from patients with melanoma that incubation with IL-4 and IL-2 leads to an increased expansion of lymphocyte numbers with enhanced activity against allogenic cells but reduced non-specific killer activity[59].

TUMOUR NECROSIS FACTOR AND LYMPHOTOXIN

The term 'tumour necrosis factor' (TNF) was originally coined to describe a putative serum factor induced by endotoxin challenge in BCG-primed mice, that caused haemorrhagic necrosis of syngeneic murine tumours[60]. Although endotoxin produces complex immunological and metabolic alterations in the host, some of which may contribute to tumour necrosis, this process is largely due to endotoxin-induced synthesis and release of a macrophage-derived cytokine, now referred to as TNF or TNF-α. This protein can constitute 1–5% of the total secretory output of stimulated macrophages, and is a major effector molecule of tumouricidal macrophages[61,62]. The isolation of TNF from a human lymphoblastoid cell line led to the cloning of the cDNA and synthesis of recombinant TNF[63,64]. TNF was also independently purified and sequenced from a macrophage cell line, and was initially called Cachectin, because of its putative role in inducing the profound changes in lipid metabolism in chronically infected cachectic animals[61,65]. Recombinant TNF has similar antitumour effects in murine tumour models to the serum factor originally described by Carswell *et al.*[60]. Subsequent work has shown that TNF can also be produced by normal activated T and B lymphocytes, B-lymphoblastoid cell lines, IL-3-dependent mast cells, and several non-haemopoetic tumour cell lines[66–69]. The stimuli for TNF production are diverse, and include phorbal esters, platelet activating factor, mitogens, viruses, bacterial products, fungi, and complement components[70–75].

A second cytokine called lymphotoxin (LT) was initially described as a mediator in delayed-type hypersensitivity reactions, and was shown to be produced by mitogen and antigen stimulation of T lymphocytes[76,77]. The cDNA for LT was cloned from the B-lymphoblastoid line RPMI 1788[78]. Recombinant LT has essentially identical properties to TNF, although more comparative data are needed. LT is also called TNF-β.

TNF and LT are species non-specific with a high degree of amino acid conservation in all species studied. Human TNF and LT show 31% amino acid identity and 52% DNA sequence homology[79]. The receptor for TNF, not as yet cloned, is thought to be a protein of molecular weight of approximately 60–70 kDa and is present on many cell types, except red cells and platelets[80,81]. LT competes for binding with the TNF receptor, indicating that the two cytokines interact with either the same receptor, or that the respective receptors are in close proximity. The genes for both peptides are located on chromosome 6 in man, in the region of the major histocompatibility (MHC) complex[82]. The following sections will be mainly devoted to TNF, as it has been studied more extensively and is currently being assessed in clinical trials.

TNF is a pleiotropic cytokine, with effects on many different cell populations (Table 8.5). Its central role is probably as a mediator in inflammatory and immune responses, and it may clearly be involved in several physiological and pathological processes, e.g. tissue modelling, cell differentiation, septicaemic shock and autoimmune disease[83-87]. Antibodies to TNF will abrogate the manifestations of septic shock, providing that the antibody is

Table 8.5 Effects of TNF on various cell populations

Fibroblasts
  Growth stimulation at low concentrations
  Cytotoxicity at high concentrations
  Induction of cytokines, e.g. CSFs*, IL-6*, IL-1
  Increased expression of class 1 MHC antigens

Vascular endothelial cells
  Direct cytotoxicity
  Induction of class I MHC antigens
  Induction of cytokines, e.g. CSFs*, IL-1*
  Increased synthesis of platelet-derived growth factor, platelet activating factor*
  Induction of cell-surface adhesion molecules, e.g. ICAM-1
  Coagulation-related changes, e.g. increased tissue factor activity, inhibition and stimulation of plasminogen activator

Bone and cartilage
  Stimulation of bone resorption by osteoclasts*
  Increased cartilage resorption*
  Inhibition of proteoglycan synthesis*

Adipose tissue
  Inhibition of lipoprotein lipase (also in the liver)*
  Suppression of differentiation specific adipose mRNAs

Neutrophil leukocytes
  Increased hydrogen peroxide production
  Increased expression of C3bi receptor
  Enhancement of antibody-dependent cellular cytotoxicity

Eosinophils
  Enhancement of toxicity for intracellular parasites

Macrophages
  Stimulation of tumouricidal activity
  Stimulation of synthesis and release of IL-1, platelet activating factor*, neutrophil activating factor*

T and B lymphocytes
  Growth enhancement of thymocytes *in vivo*
  Co-stimulatory effects with B and T cell mitogens, e.g. IL-2, anti-CD3 antibody
  Enhancement of antibody production *in vivo*

*Actions shared by IL-1

injected before a lethal dose of bacteria and not after[88]. This observation indicates that the release of TNF is an early step in the pathway eventually culminating in the breakdown in homeostasis in septicaemic shock, and TNF-induced release of other molecules, e.g. IL-1, platelet activating factor, and IL-6, is likely to be important in the pathophysiology of septicaemic shock[89-91]. Similarly, substances induced by TNF may regulate its antitumour activity.

The antitumour effect of TNF

Current evidence indicates that the antitumour action of TNF and LT may be due to their direct effects on tumour cells, or indirectly mediated by simulation of host immune cells and alteration of the host–tumour relationship, particularly by effects on tumour vasculature.

Direct effects on tumour cells in vitro

TNF has direct cytostatic or cytocidal effects on 40–50% of tumour cell lines tested *in vitro*. It is relatively non-toxic, and even growth stimulatory for non-transformed cells, except at high concentrations[92,93]. The mechanism of direct cytotoxicity is not known, but may involve activation of phospholipase A2, an endonuclease, ADP ribosylation, generation of cytotoxic lipid inter-mediates, intracellular hydrogen peroxide and free oxygen radicals[94-97]. These mechanisms are not necessarily exclusive. Thus, it has been proposed that activation of membrane phospholipase A2 may lead to mobilization of polyunsaturated fatty acids, such as arachidonic acid. Peroxidation of polyunsaturated fatty acids could generate reactive oxygen radicals, leading to cell damage[98]. The cytotoxic effect requires prolonged exposure to TNF (8–48 h), is pH dependent, does not involve protein synthesis, is enhanced at higher temperatures, and is potentiated by other cytokines, particularly IFN-γ[95,99-102].

Prior incubation of TNF-sensitive cells with low concentrations of TNF can paradoxically protect cells from the cytotoxicity of subsequent exposure to TNF[103]. Furthermore, TNF cytotoxicity is potentiated by inhibitors of RNA and DNA synthesis[104]. These observations suggest that TNF induces the synthesis of proteins that will protect cells against its cytotoxic action. Thus, the induction of IL-6, manganese superoxide dismutase (MnSOD), and TNF itself, in cells exposed to TNF have been linked to TNF resistance[68,105-107]. TNF secretion, rather than induction of TNF messenger RNA only, may be a necessary prerequisite for this effect, possibly because secreted TNF would desensitize cells by down regulating its own surface receptors[108]. The *in vitro* and *in vivo* induction of MnSOD, a mitochondrial enzyme that scavenges free oxygen radicals, strengthens earlier claims suggesting that a major intracellular site of TNF action is the mitochondrion[97]. Whatever the mechanism of the protective effect of prior exposure to TNF, this phenomenon has important implications for clinical trials.

Animal models

The antitumour effect of TNF has been demonstrated in several murine tumour models and in human xenograft models[109-112]. In the Meth-A sarcoma model, although tumour cells are resistant to the cytotoxic effect of TNF *in vitro*, systemic administration of TNF caused haemorrhagic necrosis of subcutaneous (vascular), but not intraperitoneal (avascular) tumour. Histologically, tumour blood vessels were occluded by thrombus, and mice cured of tumour were resistant to subsequent tumour challenge, due to the development of T cell-mediated immunity[111]. The vascular component of TNF action has been elegantly demonstrated by Havell *et al.* by monitoring red-cell influx into subcutaneous implants of the semi-syngeneic SA1 sarcoma in mice[113]. Recombinant murine TNF induced a rapid and prolonged extravasation of red cells into tumours, an effect that was greatly diminished in T cell-deficient mice. It is important to bear in mind, however, that, unlike most human tumours, chemically-induced murine tumours are immunogenic to their hosts.

Our own investigations have centred on the therapy of human tumour xenografts in nude mice, and indicate that intratumoural or locoregional TNF administration is more effective than systemic injection in the treatment of these tumours[114,115]. Treatment of intraperitoneal human ovarian cancer xenografts with intraperitoneal TNF prolongs the survival of mice with two of the three xenografts studied. Early in therapy, free-floating tumour cells undergo necrosis, surrounded by an intense neutrophil and macrophage exudate. These findings suggest that the inflammatory cellular infiltrate induced by TNF in the peritoneal cavity may be part of the antitumour effect, or that TNF is acting directly on the tumour cells. However, even prolonged courses of TNF therapy do not lead to cure of tumour-bearing mice. Indeed, detailed histological examination of the peritoneum reveals that TNF increases the mesothelial and endothelial hyperplasia induced by the tumours, and, more importantly, induces peritoneal adhesion and invasion by viable tumour cells. Thus, TNF has a dual effect in ovarian cancer xenograft models, eradicating ascitic tumour, but also promoting the formation of solid tumour implants on the peritoneal surface. The latter effect is also seen with the xenograft against which TNF has no antitumour activity[116].

Clinical trials

Several phase I trials of treatment with recombinant TNF have been reported in the past three years, employing a variety of administration schedules (Table 8.6)[117-123]. Major tumour responses have not been seen with any TNF administration schedule, although the purpose of phase I trials is primarily to assess toxicity of treatment. The majority of the trials have established that the maximum tolerated dose for recombinant TNF is about $200 \,\mu g/m^{-2}/day^{-1}$ ($500 \,\mu g/m^{-2}/day^{-1}$ with 24 h infusion[121]), with hypotension being the major dose-limiting factor. The serum half-life of recombinant TNF is 15–30 min, although, at higher doses, it tends to be longer[119-122]. Common acute side-

Table 8.6 Phase I clinical trials of recombinant TNF

Schedule	No. of patients	Responses
Bolus injection	20	0
30-min infusion	147	2
60-min infusion	29	0
24-h infusion × 1	50	1
24-h infusion × 5	19	0
Total	265	3(1.1%)

From references 117–123

effects include fever, rigors, chills and headache. In trials where TNF was given as a prolonged infusion, CNS toxicity has been noted[121]. Acute changes in the peripheral blood picture include a transient leukopenia followed by a neutrophil leukocytosis. Prolonged therapy led to anaemia and thrombocytopenia, although this was not clinically significant. Transient and reversible chemical hepatitis has also been seen, and other rare effects include pulmonary toxicity, chest pain and disseminated intravascular coagulation. Metabolic changes following TNF administration include increased oxygen consumption, increased serum triglycerides and free fatty acids, decrease in serum cholesterol and HDL, release of cortisol and ACTH, and increased levels of acute-phase proteins, e.g. C-reactive protein[122,123]. Immunological changes described include increased peripheral blood monocyte superoxide production and decreased natural killer cell activity[124].

The significant antitumour activity of TNF and LT in animal models has yet to be demonstrated in man. In most TNF-sensitive cell lines and animal tumours, a dose–response relationship exists, and it is possible that more intense regimes employing higher doses and prolonged schedules, or selective delivery of TNF to tumour sites would lead to higher response rates. Intratumoural administration of TNF, although of limited clinical use, has been claimed to lead to a 25–40% response rate in a small number of patients[125,126]. Alternative strategies include the use of modified recombinant TNF molecules with increased therapeutic indices[127], and the concomitant administration of drugs that prevent toxicity without diminishing antitumour activity, e.g. antagonists of platelet activating factor[128]. The inductions of endogenous membrane-bound TNF, a recently characterized active 26 kDa protein[129], by appropriate stimuli, may also circumvent the toxicity associated with high levels of TNF in the systemic circulation. Finally, additive or synergistic antitumour activity has been demonstrated by combining TNF therapy with other cytokines, e.g. IFN-γ and IL-2, or cytotoxic drugs[130–131]. Phase I trials assessing these combinations are currently underway.

COLONY STIMULATING FACTORS

All cytokines, for example TNF and the IFNs, have direct or indirect effects on bone marrow-derived cells. This brief section is devoted mainly to the colony-stimulating factors (CSFs), so called because of their ability to support survival, proliferation, and differentiation of haemopoietic colonies in soft agar cultures[132,133]. In addition, CSFs are able to functionally activate mature haemopoietic cells. The four major CSFs are multi-CSF (IL-3), granulocyte-macrophage colony stimulating factor (GM-CSF), granulocyte colony stimulating factor (G-CSF), and macrophage colony stimulating factor (M-CSF). Other cytokines, e.g. IL-1, IL-2, IL-4, IL-5 and IL-6, could also be broadly classified as CSFs[134-138]. IL-1, in particular, has important synergistic activities with other CSFs, as well as direct stimulatory effects on early stem cells. IL-4 and IL-6 have regulatory actions on B-lymphocyte, T-lymphocyte and myeloid populations. IL-5 predominantly affects the development of the eosinophil lineage. Multi-CSF (IL-3), stimulates the growth and development of multipotential stem cells and progenitor cells of the granulocyte/macrophage, erythroid, megakaryocyte, eosinophil, and mast cell lineages[139,140]. The other CSFs show more restricted lineage specificity, although this is determined by the experimental environment. Thus, GM-CSF can, in addition to its effects on granulocyte and macrophage growth and development, affect proliferation of erythroid and eosinophil lineages, albeit at higher concentrations[141]. The actions of G-CSF are restricted to the granulocyte series if pure populations are studied, but, in the presence of accessory cells, resemble the colony-stimulating activities of IL-3 and GM-CSF[142]. M-CSF appears to be more restricted to its effects on the macrophage series but can also affect granulocyte proliferation[143]. The complexity of interactions between the CSFs is further exemplified by the ability of individual cytokines to transmodulate receptors for other CSFs *in vitro*, suggesting an autoregulatory phenomenon that may direct whether differentiation or proliferation occurs[144]. A comprehensive account of the biology of CSFs is beyond the scope of this chapter and has been reviewed in detail elsewhere[145,146].

An issue of interest in whether CSFs are involved in leukaemogenesis. For example, the deletion of the short arm of chromosome 5 (5q-syndrome), with loss of the closely clustered genes for M-CSF, GM-CSF, multi-CSF, IL-4 and IL-5, is a characteristic feature associated with a proportion of acute myeloid leukaemias[147]. Promyelocytic leukaemia is associated with a 17/15 translocation, and, consequently, translocation of the G-CSF gene[148]. It is, therefore, possible that the maturation block that occurs at the level of the promyelocyte may be due to the absence of G-CSF. Although a direct causal link between overexpression of CSF receptors and leukaemia has not been established, another finding of possible relevance to leukaemogenesis is the fact that the protein transcript of the proto-oncogene c-fms, is the receptor for M-CSF[149]. There is evidence for autocrine production of CSFs by a proportion of leukaemic cells from patients with acute myeloid leukaemia, although these findings are controversial[150,151].

143

Recombinant CSFs in cancer therapy

Antitumour activity

To date, there is little evidence that the CSFs are directly cytotoxic or cytostatic for tumour cells in the classical sense. An exception is the inhibition of the growth of small-cell lung cancer lines (SCLC) in clonogenic assays[152]. This is an intriguing finding, as macrophage-related surface antigens are expressed on a proportion of SCLC cells[153].

The ability of CSFs to regulate the functional state of mature haemopoietic cells may contribute to antitumour activity[154]. For example, GM-CSF, IL-3, and M-CSF stimulate macrophages to kill tumour cells by a TNF-dependent mechanism *in vitro*, and peripheral blood monocytes from patients treated with recombinant GM-CSF show enhanced tumouricidal activity[155,156]. We have been unable to demonstrate antitumour activity of intraperitoneal therapy with recombinant murine GM-CSF in ovarian cancer xenograft models. A recent study has demonstrated the cure of a murine B-cell leukaemia with GM-CSF and IL-3 therapy *in vivo* but the mechanisms involved are not known[157]. CSFs may be used to recruit increased numbers of potentially tumouricidal cells for activation by other agents. For example, data from our laboratory indicate that the antitumour activity of the macrophage-activating agent, muramyl tripeptide phosphoethanolamine (MTP-PE), can be enhanced by the concomitant administration of recombinant GM-CSF[158].

The ability of the CSFs to induce differentiation of haemopoietic cells raises the possibility of eradicating leukaemic clones by promoting maturation with consequent loss of malignant potential. Thus, G-CSF, after an initial stage of growth stimulation, induces the terminal differentiation of the murine leukaemia cell line WEHI-3BD+ *in vitro*, leading to the complete suppression of the leukaemic clone[159]. *In vivo* studies with the same leukaemia in mice indicate that indirectly-induced CSFs can also eradicate tumour[160]. G-CSF has been used in patients with the myelodysplastic syndrome, and led to, not only increased numbers of mature neutrophils in the peripheral blood, but also a decrease in bone marrow blast cells[161]. Although induction of differentiation is an attractive approach to the treatment of leukaemias, it must be remembered that CSFs can stimulate growth of leukaemic cells *in vitro*[162,163].

Stimulation of haematopoiesis in vivo

The area of cancer therapy that could be revolutionized by the CSFs is their use to diminish the myelosuppressive effects of current chemotherapeutic and radiotherapy regimes. Early studies in murine and primate models showed that G-CSF or GM-CSF diminished the myelosuppression induced by cytotoxic drugs[164-166]. The simultaneous functional activation of host cells, particularly neutrophils, may confer additional protection against infection[167].

Several phase I/II trials of G-CSF and GM-CSF have been reported in patients receiving chemotherapy[168-170]. An example is the study of Bronchud *et al.*[168], in which patients with small-cell lung cancer received intensive combination chemotherapy, with or without recombinant G-CSF in sequential cycles. The fall in neutrophil count and its duration was significantly diminished by concurrent G-CSF therapy, and this was reflected in the reduction of septicaemic episodes in these patients. Similar results have been reported with GM-CSF in patients undergoing autologous bone marrow transplantation following marrow ablation[171].

To date, no dose-limiting toxicity has been seen with G-CSF, but a clear maximum tolerated dose has been noted for GM-CSF (30–50 μg/kg/day). GM-CSF causes a number of dose-related effects. The commonest side-effects are fatigue, myalgia, fever and bone pain, which can be severe. Other side-effects at higher doses include fluid retention, serositis, diarrhoea, and pleural and pericardial effusions. No clinical trials of multi-CSF have been reported as yet, but, in monkeys, recombinant multi-CSF in combination with GM-CSF has predictably led to increase in all peripheral blood cell populations, including platelets[172]. Mention must also be made of the potential use of recombinant erythropoietin in treating anaemia associated with malignant disease.

INTERLEUKIN-1

Interleukin-1 was originally detected as a thymocyte proliferating factor in the culture supernatants of human adherent lymphocytes[173]. It is now known that at least two distinct proteins, termed IL-1α and IL-1β, have IL-1 activity. Both are available as recombinant proteins. The IL-1α gene codes for a 271 amino acid precursor which is processed into a 159 amino acid 17.5 kDa peptide. The IL-1β gene codes for a 269 amino acid precursor which is secreted as a 153 amino acid 17.5 kDa peptide[174–176]. A membrane-associated form has also been described[177]. Unlike most secreted proteins, the IL-1s do not contain a hydrophobic signal peptide and the mechanism of secretion remains unclear.

The IL-1s are pleiotropic cytokines, which are produced by a range of cell populations, including monocytes, dendritic cells, endothelial cells, epithelial cells, T and B cell lines, and some tumour cell lines. They can be induced by a variety of stimuli, e.g. macrophage production of IL-1 is induced by LPS, immune complexes, UV irradiation, and cytokines, such as IFN-γ and TNF[178,179]. There is considerable overlap with the effects of TNF (see Table 8.5)[180]. A high-affinity receptor for IL-1 has recently been cloned from a murine T cell lymphoma cell line, and, interestingly, shows sequences that suggest that it is part of the immunoglobulin supergene family[181].

The anti-tumour activity of IL-1

Despite the many overlapping actions of the IL-1s and TNF, the antitumour activity of IL-1 has not been as extensively studied as TNF. The stimulatory effects of IL-1 on the immune system, e.g. on T and B cells, macrophages, and

NK cells are potentially important antitumour effector mechanisms. Like TNF, IL-1 has a number of effects on endothelium, for example, it induces procoagulant activity and adhesive cell surface proteins on endothelial cells[182,183]. As IL-1 can be induced by TNF and *vice versa*, it may be an important modulator of the cytotoxic effects of TNF. Thus, IL-1 has been shown to modulate the effects of TNF on macrophage tumouricidal activity, downregulate TNF receptors on tumour cell lines, and inhibit TNF-induced activation of endothelial cells[184-186].

In common with other cytokines, IL-1 can stimulate or inhibit growth of tumour cell lines *in vitro*. In general, the inhibitory effects are cytostatic rather than cytocidal, unless other cytokines are present, e.g. IFN-γ and TNF[187-190]. The mechanisms underlying the growth-inhibitory action of IL-1 are unclear, but are likely to differ from TNF cytotoxicity and cytostasis, for instance IL-1 induced cytostasis is not potentiated by protein-synthesis inhibitors[188].

Recombinant IL-1α has been reported to lead to 70–100% cures of mice with subcutaneous Meth-A sarcoma implants[191]. Antitumour activity was also evident in the B16 melanoma spontaneous metastasis model and metastatic Lewis lung carcinoma. An earlier report of the ineffectiveness of IL-1 in the Meth-A sarcoma model may have been due to the intravenous route of administration employed[111]. Thus, it was shown that intratumoural and intramuscular IL-1 was much more effective than IL-1 given intravenously[191]. Interestingly, the antitumour effect was potentiated by indomethacin[192].

The vascular effects of IL-1 on the murine fibrosarcoma, RIF-1, and a murine pancreatic adenocarcinoma, PANc02, have been described[193]. Red cell influx into both tumours was observed, starting as early as 3 h after injection of recombinant IL-1α. The growth of both tumours was temporarily inhibited.

There is still much to be learnt about the antitumour actions of IL-1, particularly with reference to its contributions to TNF activity *in vivo*. No clinical trials of IL-1 have been conducted as yet.

TRANSFORMING GROWTH FACTOR-β

Transforming growth factor-β (TGF-β) belongs to a family of regulatory peptides whose ancestors go back as far as the fruit fly *Drosophila*[194]. These cytokines are involved in tissue development, remodelling and repair and in the negative control of growth and immune responses. There are at least four closely related mammalian TGF-β molecules, TGF-β1, TGF-β2, TGF-β1.2, and TGF-β3. Other known members of the family include: inhibins, potent and specific inhibitors of follicle stimulating hormone production; Mullerian inhibiting substance (MIS), thought to be responsible for the regression of the Mullerian duct in early male embryos; Vg1 which is thought to be involved in embryonal mesoderm development in *Xenopus*; and the products of the decapentaplegic gene complex which is involved in the development of *Drosophila*.

All members of the family are homo- or heterodimers, which show most homology in their C terminus where there are 7–9 highly conserved cysteine residues. Three structurally distinct cell-surface-binding proteins are thought to be receptors for the TGF-βs and all three are widely distributed on mammalian cells[195]. Little is known about receptors for the other members of the family.

There are at least three reasons why these cytokines have relevance to cancer biology and therapy. First, there is some evidence for defective production or response to TGF-β in human malignancies[196]. The failure of a negative growth signal could be as much a part of the process of malignancy as an increase in a positive growth signal. Most primary tumour cells and tumour cell lines express TGF-β message and protein[197], but there is evidence for altered cellular production or release of TGF-β in mesothelioma, and a breast cancer cell line[198,199]. Moreover, a recent paper has reported that 5 of 6 retinoblastoma cell lines were lacking TGF-β receptors[200]. Second, while it is unlikely that broad-spectrum growth inhibitors, like the TGF-βs, could selectively inhibit cancer without having profound effects on other cells in the body, one particular member of the family, MIS, may specifically inhibit tumours of the female reproductive tract[201]. Third, the immunosuppressive action of these agents may have relevance to the immunosuppression seen in some cancers. A circulating immunosuppressive factor found in glioblastoma patients has been identified as TGF-β2[202]. *In vivo*, TGF-β is a potent inducer of angiogenesis and fibrosis[202], and recent evidence suggests that TGF-β may be a natural mediator of wound healing[204].

CONCLUSION

The availability of recombinant cytokines has made possible the adoption of therapeutic strategies that may complement, or even replace, chemotherapy and radiotherapy for the treatment of malignant disease. However, the only cytokine that has an established role at present in the standard management of cancer is IFN-α for the treatment of selected haematological malignancies, e.g hairy cell leukaemia. In general, the response of most solid tumours to IFNs has been minor. The regression of some chemoresistant tumours, particularly malignant melanoma and renal cell carcinoma, by adoptive transfer of LAK cells or IL-2 expanded tumour infiltrating lymphocytes, therefore, represents an important advance in their management. Much effort is being directed into trials of LAK therapy, particularly towards defining schedules which retain antitumour activity without the extreme toxicities seen in the original trials. It seems unlikely that TNF as a single agent will lead to major responses in cancer and the results of trials of combining this cytokine with other cytokines or cytotoxic drugs are awaited.

The complementary role of cytokines in cancer therapy is underlined by the use of CSFs to diminish chemotherapy-induced myelosuppression. Other cytokines may find such roles, for example TNF and IL-1 have been shown to have radioprotective effects, and TNF treatment can enhance the localization of tumour-specific monoclonal antibodies *in vivo*[205,206].

What considerations should be taken in future to optimize the use of cytokines in cancer therapy? Any generalizations about cytokine therapy are hazardous because of the complexity, multiplicity and interrelatedness of their actions. Most cytokines have pleiotropic cell regulatory activities, which may *contribute* to the pathophysiology of malignant disease. Evidence for this can be found at various levels, e.g. the possible role of IL-1-like peptides in causing the hypercalcaemia of malignancy in squamous cell lung cancers, and enhancement of metastasis by IFN-γ and TNF in experimental animal models[207,208]. Therefore, it is difficult to predict the medium- to long-term effects of administration of pharmacological quantities of cytokines. Therapeutic trials should attempt to keep abreast of laboratory data, taking into account all the inherent limitations in transposing these to the clinical situation. This is exemplified by the scientific data that was meticulously gathered prior to initiation of IL-2/LAK trials, which were subsequently applied with some success in patients. The fundamental basis of cytokine antitumour activity, if known, should enable rational design of dose schedule regimes. Thus, if a cytokine is being used solely as a cytotoxic agent with direct tumouricidal effects, trials may be based on the same sort of considerations as chemotherapeutic regimes, e.g. exploration of dose escalation, dose intensity and selective delivery to tumour sites. On the other hand, if an indirect mechanism is thought to be involved, or the cytostatic activities of a cytokine are to be exploited, the most effective cytokine regimes may use chronic low-dose administration. This indeed was the documented experience in the most effective cures obtained with Coley's toxins nearly a century ago.

References

1. Coley-Nauts, H., Fowler, G. A. and Bogatko, F. H. (1953). A review of the influence of bacterial infection and of bacterial products (Coley's toxins) on malignant tumours in man. *Acta Med. Scand. (Suppl)*, 274–277
2. Oldham, R. K. and Smalley, R. K. (1985). Newer methods of cancer treatment. Biologicals and biological response modifiers. In Devita, V. T. Jr., Hellman, S. and Rosenberg, S. A. (eds.) *Cancer. Principles and Practice of Oncology*, 2nd Edn., pp. 2223–2227
3. Isaacs, H. and Lindenmann, J. (1957). Virus interference 1. The interferon. *Proc. R. Soc. London (Biol.)*, **147**, 257–262
4. Stewart, W. E. II, Blalock, J. E., Burke, D. C., Chany, C., Dunnick, J. K., Falcoff, E., Friedman, R. M., Galasso, G. J., Joklik, W. K., Vileck, J. T., Younger, J. S. and Zoon, K. C. (1980). Interferon nomenclature. *Nature (London)*, **286**, 622–624
5. Gresser, I., Bourali, C., Lévy, J. P., Fontaine-Brouty-Boyé, D. and Thomas, M. T. (1969). Increased survival in mice inoculated with tumour cells and treated with interferon preparations. *Proc. Natl. Acad. Sci. USA*, **63**, 51–57
6. Langer, J. A. and Pestka, S. (1988). Interferon receptors. *Immunol. Today*, **12**, 393–400
7. Aguet, M., Dembic, Z. and Merlin, G. (1988). Molecular cloning and expression of the human interferon-γ receptor. *Cell*, **55**, 273–280
8. Weil, J., Epstein, C. J. and Epstein, L. B. (1983). A unique set of polypeptides is induced by γ interferon in addition to those induced in common with α and β interferon. *Nature (London)*, **301**, 437–439
9. Balkwill, F. R. (1989). Interferons. In *Cytokines in Cancer Therapy*, Chap. 2. (Oxford: University Press)
10. Gresser, I. (1985). How does interferon inhibit tumour growth? *Interferon*, **6**, 93–126
11. Sidky, Y. A. and Borden, E. C. (1987). Inhibition of angiogenesis by interferons: Effects on tumour and lymphocyte induced vascular responses. *Cancer Res.*, **47**, 5155–5161
12. Balkwill, F. R., Stevens, M. H., Griffith, D. B., Thomas, J. A. and Bodmer, J. G. (1987).

Interferon-g regulates HLA-D expression on solid tumours in vivo. *Eur. J. Cancer Clin. Oncol.,* **23**, 101–106

13. Queseda, J. R., Itri, L. and Gutterman, J. U. (1978). Alpha interferon in hairy cell leukaemia (HCL). A five year follow up in 100 patients. *J. Int. Res.,* **6** (suppl. 1), 678

14. Bergsegel, D. E. (1988). Interferon alpha-2b in the management of chronic granulocytic lymphoma. *Cancer Treat. Rev.,* **15**, (suppl. A), 15–20

15. Talpaz, M., Kantarjian, H. M., McCredie, K. B., Keating, M. J., Trujillo, J. and Gutterman, J. (1987). Clinical investigation of human alpha interferon in chronic myelogenous leukaemia. *Blood,* **69**, 1280–1288

16. Alimena, G., Morra, E., Lazzarino, M., Liberati, A. M., Montefusco, E., Inveradi, D., Bernasconi, P., Mancini, M., Donti, E., Grigani, F., Bernasconi, C., Dianzani, F. and Mandelli, F. (1988). Interferon alpha-2b as therapy for Ph'-positive chronic myelogenous leukaemia: A study of 82 patients treated with intermittant or daily administration. *Blood,* **72**, 642–647

17. Velu, T. and Delwiche, F. (1988). Treatment of essential thrombocythaemia by alpha-interferon. *Lancet,* **2**, 628

18. Giles, F. J., Singer, C. R. J., Gray, A. G., Yong, K. L., Brozovic, M., Davies, S. C., Grant, I. R., Hoffbrand, A. V., Macchin, S. J., Metha, A. B., Richards, J. D. M., Thomas, M. J. G., Venutas, S. and Goldstone, A. H. (1988). Alpha-interferon for essential thrombocythaemia. *Lancet,* **2**, 70–72

19. Mandelli, F., Tribalto, M., Avvisati, G., Cantonetti, M., Petrucci, M. T., Boccadoro, M., Pileri, A., Marmont, F., Resgotti, L., Lauta, V. and Dammacco, F. (1988). Recombinant interferon alpha-2b (INTRON A) as post-induction therapy for responding multiple myeloma patients. M84 protocol. *Cancer Treat. Rev.,* **15** (suppl. A), 43–48

20. Mandelli, F. personal communication

21. Öberg, K., Funa, K. and Alm, G. (1983). Effect of leukocyte interferon on clinical symptoms and hormone levels in patients with mid-gut carcinoid tumours and carcinoid syndrome. *N. Engl. J. Med.,* **309**, 129–132

22. Krown, S. E. (1987). Interferon, treatment of renal cell carcinoma. *Cancer,* **59** (suppl.), 647–650

23. Williams, R. D. (1988). Intravesical interferon alpha in the treatment of superficial bladder cancer. *Semin. Oncol.,* **15** (suppl. 5), 10–13

24. Berek, J. S., Hacker, N. F., Lichtenstein, A., Jung, T., Spina, C., Knox, R. M., Brady, J., Greene, T., Ettinger, L. M., Lagasse, L. D., Bonnem, E. M. and Spiegel, R. J. (1985). Intraperitoneal recombinant α-interferon for "salvage" immunotherapy in stage III epithelial ovarian cancer: a gynecologic oncology group study. *Cancer Res.,* **45**, 4447–4453

25. Markman, M., D'Acquisto, R., Hakes, T., Rubin, S., Hoskins, W. and Lewis, J. L. Jr. (1987). Recombinant gamma-interferon (rGI) administered by the intraperitoneal (ip) route as therapy for ovarian cancer. *J. Int. Res.,* **6** (suppl. 1), 681

26. Queseda, J. R., Talpaz, M., Rios, A., Kirzrock, R. and Gutterman, J. U. (1986). Clinical toxicity of interferons in cancer patients: A review. *J. Clin. Oncol.,* **4**, 234–243

27. Reinhart, J., Malspeils, L., Young, D. and Neidhart, J. (1986). Phase I/II trial of human recombinant β-interferon serine in patients with renal cell carcinoma. *Cancer Res.,* **46**, 5364–5367

28. Vadham-Raj, S., Natham, C. F., Sherwin, S. A., Oettgen, H. F. and Krown, S. E. (1986). Phase I trial of recombinant interferon gamma by 1 hour iv infusion. *Cancer Treat. Rep.,* **70**, 609–614

29. Smalley, R. V., Glaspy, J. A., Connors, J. M., Venner, J. M., Bottomley, R. L., Tuttle, R. L. and Whisnant, J. K. (1987), Wellferon (WFN) (interferon alpha-n1) in hairy cell leukaemia (HCL): Effectiveness of several dose schedules. *J. Int. Res.,* **6** (suppl. 1), 679

30. Krown, S. E. (1987). Interferon treatment of renal cell carcinoma. Current status and future prospects. *Cancer,* **59**, 641–657

31. Speigel, R. J., Spicehandler, J. R., Jacobs, S. L. and Olden, E. M. (1986). Low incidence of neutralising factors in patients receiving recombinant alpha-2b interferon (Intron A). *Am. J. Med.,* **80**, 223–228

32. Itri, L. M., Campion, M., Dennin, R. A., Palleroni, A. V., Gutterman, J. U., Groopman, J. E. and Trown, P. W. (1987). Incidence and clinical significance of neutralising antibodies in patients receiving recombinant interferon alpha-2a by intramuscular injection. *Cancer,* **59** (suppl.), 668–674

33. Steis, R. G., Smith, J. W., Urba, W. J., Clark, J. W., Itri, L. M., Evans, L. M., Schoenberger, C. and Longo, D. L. (1988). Resistance to recombinant interferon alpha-2a in hairy-cell leukaemia associated with neutralising anti-interferon antibodies. *N. Engl. J. Med.*, **318**, 1409–1413

34. Smith, K. A. (1988). Interleukin-2: Inception, impact, and implications. *Science*, **240**, 1169–1176

35. Smith, K. A. (1988). The bimolecular structure of the interleukin 2 receptor. *Immunol. Today*, **9**, 36–37

36. Gemlo, B. T., Palladino, M. A., Jaffe, H. S., Espevik, T. P. and Rayner, A. A. (1988). Circulating cytokines in patients with metastatic cancer treated with recombinant interleukin-2 and lymphokine activated killer cells. *Cancer Res.*, **48**, 5864–5867

37. Ettinghausen, S. E., Puri, R. K. and Rosenberg, S. A. (1988). Increased vascular permeability in organs mediated by the systemic administration of lymphokine-activated killer cells and recombinant interleukin-2 in mice. *J. Natl. Cancer Inst.*, **80**, 177–188

38. Grimm, E. A. (1986). Human lymphokine-activated killer cells (LAK cells) as a potential immunotherapeutic modality. *B.B.A.*, **865**, 267–279

39. Rosenberg, S. A. (1986). Adoptive immunotherapy of cancer using lymphokine activated killer cells and recombinant interleukin-2. In DeVita, V. T., Hellman, S. and Rosenberg, S. A. (eds.) *Important Advances in Oncology 1986*, pp. 55–91. (Philadelphia: J. B. Lippincott)

40. Mule, J. J., Shu, S., Schwarz, S. L. *et al.* (1984). Adoptive immunotherapy of established pulmonary metastases with LAK cells and recombinant interleukin-2. *Science*, **225**, 1487

41. Sondel, P. M., Kohler, P. C., Hank, J. A., Moore, K. H., Rosenthal, N. S., Sosman, J. A., Bechhofer, R. and Storer, B. (1988). Clinical and immunological effects of recombinant interleukin 2 given by repetitive weekly cycles to patients with cancer. *Cancer Res.*, **48**, 2561–2567

42. Rosenberg, S. A. (1988). Clinical immunotherapy studies in the Surgery Branch of the U.S. National Cancer Institute: Brief review (1989). *Ca. Treat. Rev.*, **16** (Suppl. A), 115–22

43. Sznol, M., Dutcher, J. P., Atkins, M. B., Rayner, A. R. A., Margolin, K. A., Gaynor, E. R., Weiss, G. R., Aronson, F., Parkinson, D. R. and Hawkins, M. J. (1989). Review of interleukin-2 alone and interleukin-2/LAK clinical trials in malignant melanoma. *Ca. Treat. Rev.*, **16** (Suppl. A), 29–38

44. Fisher, R. J., Coltman, C. A., Doroshow, J. H., Rayner, A. A., Hawkins, M. J., Mier, J. W. and Wiernik, P. (1987). Phase II clinical trial of interleukin II plus lymphokine activated killer cells (IL-2/LAK) in metastatic renal cancer. *Proc. Am. Soc. Clin. Oncol.*, **6**, 244

45. Rosenberg, S. A., Lotze, M. T., Muul, L. M., Chang, A. E., Avis, F. P., Leitman, S., Lineham, W. M., Robertson, C. N., Lee, R. E., Rubin, J. T., Seipp, C., Simpson, C. G. and White, D. E. (1987). A progress report on the treatment of 157 patients with advanced cancer using lymphokine-activated killer cells and interleukin-2 or high dose interleukin-2 alone. *N. Engl. J. Med.*, **316**, 889–897

46. West, W. H. (1988). Continuous infusion recombinant interleukin-2 (rIL-2) and adoptive cellular therapy of renal cell carcinoma and other malignancies. *Ca. Treat. Rev.*, **16** (Suppl. A), 83–91

47. Philip, T., Mercatello, A., Negrier, S., Rebattu, P., Kammerlin, P., Gaspard, M., Tognier, E., Combaret, V., Bijmann, J. T., Franks, C. R., Chauvin, F., Moskovtchenko, J. F., Favrot, M. and Clavel, M. (1988). IL-2 with or without LAK cells in metastatic renal cell carcinoma. *Ca. Treat. Rev.*, **16** (Suppl. A), 91–104

48. Boldt, D. H., Mills, B. J., Gemlo, B. T., Holden, H., Mier, J., Paietta, E., McMannis, J. D., Escobedo, L. V., Sniecinski, I., Rayner, A. A., Hawkins, M. J., Atkins, M. B., Ciobanu, N. and Ellis, T. M. (1988). Laboratory correlates of adoptive immunotherapy with recombinant interleukin-2 and recombinant lymphokine activated killer cells in humans. *Cancer Res.*, **48**, 4409–4416

49. Paciucci, P. A., Holland, J. F., Ryder, J. S., Konefal, R. G., Odichamar, R., Gordon, R. (1982). Immunotherapy with interleukin-2 by constant infusion with and without adoptive cell transfer and weekly doxorubicin. *Ca. Treat. Rev.*, **16** (Suppl. A), 67–82

50. Lotze, M. T., Matory, Y. L., Ettinghausen, S. E., Rayner, A. A., Sharrow, S. O., Seipp, C. A. Y., Custer, M. C. and Rosenberg, S. A. (1985). In vivo administration of purified human interleukin-2. II. Half life, immunologic effects, and expansion of peripheral lymphoid cells in vivo with recombinant IL-2. *J. Immunol.*, **135**, 2865–2875

51. Thompson, J. A., Lee, D. J., Lindgren, C. G., Benz, L. A., Collins, C., Levitt, D. and Fefer,

A. (1988). Influence of dose and duration of infusion of interleukin-2 on toxicity and immunomodulation. *J. Clin. Oncol.,* **6**, 669–678

52. West, W. H., Tauer, K. W., Yanelli, J. R., Marshall, G. D., Orr, D. W., Thurman, G. B. and Oldham, R. K. (1987). Constant infusion recombinant interleukin-2 in adoptive immunotherapy of advanced cancer. *N. Engl. J. Med.,* **316**, 898–905

53. Spies, P. J., Yang, J. C. and Rosenberg, S. A. (1987). *In vivo* anti-tumour activity of tumour infiltrating lymphocytes expanded in interleukin-2. *J. Natl. Cancer Insti.,* **79**, 1067–1075

54. Fisher, B., Packard, B. S., Read, E. J., Carrasquillo, J. A., Carter, C. S., Toplian, S. L., Yang, J. C., Yolles, P. Y., Larsan, S. M., Rosenberg, S. A. (1989). Tumor localization of adoptively transferred indium-111 labeled tumor inflitrating lymphocytes in patients with metastatic melanoma. *J. Clin. Oncol.,* **7**, 250–261

55. Rosenberg, S. A., Packard, B. S., Aebersold, P. M., Soloman, D. S., Topalian, S. L., Toy, S. T., Simon, P., Lotze, M. T., Yang, J. C., Seipp, A., Simpson, C., Carter, C., Bock, S., Schwartzentruber, D., Wei, J. P. and White, D. E. (1988). Use of tumour-infiltrating lymphocytes and interleukin-2 in the immunotherapy of patients with metastatic melanoma. *N. Engl. J. Med.,* **319**, 1676–1680

56. Steis, R., Bookamn, M., Clark, J., Urba, W., McKnight, J., Smith, J., Schoennerger, C., Ozols, R., Young, R., Maluish, A., Beckner, S. and Longo, D. (1987). Intraperitoneal lymphokine activated killer (LAK) cells and interleukin-2 (IL-2) therapy for peritoneal carcinomatosis: Toxicity, efficacy, and laboratory results. *Proc. Am. Soc. Clin. Oncol.,* **6**, 250

57. Yoshida, S., Tanaka, R., Takai, N. and Ono, K. (1988). Local administration of autologous lymphokine-activated killer cells and recombinant interleukin 2 to patients with malignant brain tumours. *Cancer Res.,* **48**, 5011–5016

58. Nagler, A., Lanier, L. L. and Phillips, J. H. (1988). The effects of IL-4 on human natural killer cells. A potent regulator of IL-2 activation and proliferation. *J. Immunol.,* **141**, 2349–2351

59. Kawakami, Y., Rosenberg, S. A. and Lotze, M. T. (1988). Interleukin 4 promotes the growth of tumour-infiltrating lymphocytes cytotoxic for human autologous melanoma. *J. Exp. Med.,* **168**, 2183–2191

60. Carswell, E. A., Old, L. J., Kassel, R. J., Green, S., Fiore, N. and Williamson, B. (1975). An endotoxin-induced serum factor that causes necrosis of tumours. *Proc. Natl. Acad. Sci. USA,* **72**, 3666–3670

61. Beutler, B., Mahoney, J., Le Trang, N. P. and Cerami, A. (1985). Purification of cachectin, a lipoprotein lipase-suppressing hormone secreted by endotoxin induced Raw 264. 7 cells. *J. Exp. Med.,* **161**, 984–985

62. Urban, J. L., Shepard, H. M., Rothestin, J. L., Sugarman, B. J. and Schreiber, J. (1986). Tumor necrosis factor: a potent effector molecule for tumour cell killing by activated macrophages. *Proc. Natl. Acad. Sci. USA,* **83**, 5233–5237

63. Williamson Barbara, D., Carswell, E. A., Rubin Beresh, Y. and Prendergast Jay, S. (1983). Human tumour necrosis factor produced by human B-cell lines: Synergistic cytotoxic interaction with human interferons. *Proc. Natl. Acad. Sci. USA,* **80**, 5397–5401

64. Pennica, D., Nedwin, G. E., Hayflick, J. S., Seeburg, P. H., Derynck, R., Palladino, M. A., Kohur, W. J., Aggarwal, B. B. and Goeddel, D. V. (1984). Human tumour necrosis factor: precursor structure, expression and homology to lymphotoxin. *Nature (London),* **312**, 724–729

65. Beutler, G., Greenwald, D., Hulmes, J. D., Chang, M., Pan, Y., Mathison, J., Ulevitch, R. and Cerami, A. (1985). Identity of tumour necrosis factor and the macrophage-secreted factor Cachetin. *Nature (London),* **316**, 552–554

66. Sung, S. J., Jung, L. K. L., Walters, J. A., Chen, W., Wang, C. Y. and Fu, S. M. (1988). Production of tumour necrosis factor/cachectin by human B cell lines and tonsillar B cells. *J. Exp. Med.,* **168**, 1539–1551

67. Sung, S. J., Bjorndahk, J. M., Wang, C. Y., Kao, Ht and Fu, Sm (1988). Production of tumour necrosis factor/cachectin by human T cell lines and peripheral blood T lymphocytes stimulated by phorbol myristate acetate and anti-CD3 antibody. *J. Exp. Med.,* **167**, 937–953

68. Spriggs, D., Imamura, K., Rodriguez, C., Horiguchi, J. and Kufe, D. W. (1987). Induction of tumour necrosis factor expression and resistance in a human breast tumour cell line. *Proc. Natl. Acad. Sci. USA,* **84**, 6563–6566

69. Richards, A. L., Okuno, T., Takagaki, Y. and Djeu, J. Y. (1988). Natural cytotoxic cell-specific cytotoxic factor produced by IL-3-dependent basophilic/mast cells. *J. Immunol.*, **141**, 3061–3066

70. Izumi, S., Hirai, O., Haysashi, K-I., Konishi, Y., Okuhara, M., Kohsaka, M., Aoki, H. and Yamamura, Y. (1987). Induction of a tumour necrosis factor like activity by nocardia rubra cell wall skeleton. *Cancer Res.*, **47**, 1785–1792

71. Aderka, D., Holtmann, H., Toker, L., Hahn, T. and Wallach, D. (1986). Tumour necrosis factor induction by Sendai virus. *J. Immunol.*, **136**, 2938–2942

72. Gifford, G. E. and Flick, D. A. (1987). Natural production and release of tumour necrosis factor. In *Tumour Necrosis Factor and Related Cytotoxins. Ciba Found. Symp.*, **131**, pp. 3–20

73. Okusawa, S., Yancey, K. B., Van Der Meer, J. W. M., Endres, S., Lonnemann, G., Hefter, K., Frank, M. M., Burke, J. F., Dinarello, C. A. and Gelfand, J. A. (1988). C5a stimulates secretion of tumour necrosis factor from human mononuclear cells in vitro. *J. Exp. Med.*, **168**, 443–448

74. Cuturi, M. C., Murphy, M., Costa-Giomi, M. R., Weinmann, R., Perussia, B. and Trinchieri, G. (1987). Independent regulation of tumour necrosis factor and lymphotoxin production by human peripheral blood lymphocytes. *J. Exp. Med.*, **165**, 1581–1594

75. Valone, F. H., Philip, R. and Debs, R. J. (1988). Enhanced human monocyte cytotoxicity by platelet-activating factor. *Immunology*, **64**, 715–718

76. Ruddle, N. H. and Waksman, B. H. (1968). Cytotoxicity mediated by soluble antigen and lymphocytes in delayed hypersensitivity. III. Analysis of mechanism. *J. Exp. Med.*, **128**, 1267–1279

77. Ruddle, N. H. (1985). Lymphotoxin redux. *Immunol. Today*, **6**, 156–159

78. Gray, P. W., Aggarwal, B. B., Benton, C. V., Bringman, T. S., Henzel, W. J., Jarett, J. A., Leung, D. W., Moffat, B. N. G. P., Suederskey, L. P., Palladino, M. A. and Nedwin, G. E. (1984). Cloning and expression of cDNA for human lymphotoxin, a lymphokine with tumour necrosis activity. *Nature (London)*, **312**, 721–724

79. Aggarwal, B. B., Aiyer, R. A., Pennica, D., Gray, P. W. and Goeddel, D. V. (1987). Human tumour necrosis factors: structure and receptor interactions. In *Tumour Necrosis Factor and Related Cytokines. Ciba Foundation Symp.*, **131**, pp. 39–51

80. Kull, F. C. Jnr., Jacobs, S. and Cuatrecasas, P. (1985). Cellular receptor for 125I1-labelled tumour necrosis factor: specific binding, affinity labelling, and relationship to sensitivity. *Proc. Natl. Acad. Sci. USA*, **82**, 5756–5760

81. Munker, R., Dipessio, J. and Koeffler, H. P. (1987). Tumour necrosis factor receptors of haemopoietic cells. *Blood*, **70**, 1730–1734

82. Spies, T., Morton, C. C., Nedospasov, S. A., Fiers, W., Pious, D. and Strominger, J. L. (1986). Genes for the tumour necrosis factors alpha and beta are linked to the human major histocompatibility complex. *Proc. Natl. Acad. Sci. USA*, **83**, 8699–8702

83. Bertolini, D. R., Nedwin, G. E., Bringman, R. S., Smith, D. D. and Mundy, G. R. (1987). Stimulation of bone resorption and inhibition of bone formation in vitro by human tumour necrosis factors. *Nature (London)*, **319**, 516–518

84. Filipak, M., Sparks, R. L., Tzen, C. and Scott, R. E. (1988). Tumor necrosis factor inhibits the terminal event in mesenchymal stem cell differentiation. *J. Cell Physiol.*, **137**, 367–373

85. Tracey, K. J., Beutler, B., Lowry, S., Merryweather, J., Wolpe, S., Milsark, I. W., Hariri, R. J., Fahey, T. J., Zentella, A., Albert, J. D., Shires, T. and Cerami, A. (1986). Shock and tissue injury inducted by recombinant human cachectin. *Science*, **234**, 471–474

86. Waage, A., Halstensen, A. and Espevik, T. (1987). Association between tumour necrosis factor in serum and fatal outcome in patients with meningococcal disease. *Lancet*, **1**, 355–357

87. Pujol-Borrell, R., Todd, I., Doshi, M., Bottazzo, G. F., Sutton, R., Gray, D., Adolf, G. R. and Feldmann, M. (1987). HLA class II induction in human islet cells by interferon-gamma plus tumour necrosis factor lymphotoxin. *Nature (London)*, **326**, 304–305

88. Tracey, K. J., Fong, Y., Hesse, D. G., Manogue, K. R., Lee, A. T., Kuo, G. C., Lowry, S. F. and Cerami, A. (1987). Anti-cachectin/tnf monoclonal antibodies prevent septic shock during lethal bachteraemia. *Nature (London)*, **330**, 662–665

89. Dinarello, C. A., Canno, J. G., Wolff, S. M., Bernheim, H. A. A., Beutler, B., Cerami, A., Figari, I. S., Palladino, M. A. Jnr and O'Connor, J. V. (1986). Tumour necrosis factor (cachectin) is an endogenous pyrogen and induces production of interleukin 1. *J. Exp.*

Med., **163**, 1433–1450

90. Kohase, M., Henriksen-Destefano, D., May, Lt, Vilcek, J. and Sehgal, P. B. (1986). Induction of B2-interferon by tumour necrosis factor: a homeostatic mechanism in the control of cell proliferation. *Cell,* **45**, 659–666

91. Camussi, G., Bussolino, F., Salvidio, G. and Baglioni, C. (1987). Tumour necrosis factor/cachectin stimulates peritoneal macrophages, polymorphonuclear neutrophils vascular endothelial cells to release platelet activating factor. *J. Exp. Med.,* **166**, 1390–1404

92. Sugarman, B. J., Aggarwal, B. B., Hass, P. E., Figari, I. S., Palladino, M. A. Jnr and Shepard, H. M. (1985). Recombinant human tumour necrosis factor alpha: effects of proliferation on normal and transformed cells in vitro. *Science,* **230**, 943–945

93. Fransen, L., Ruysschaert, M-R., Van Der Heyden, J. and Fiers, W. (1986). Recombinant tumour necrosis factor: species specificity for a variety of human and murine transformed cell lines. *Cell Immunol.,* **100**, 260–267

94. Suffys, P., Beyaert, R., Van Roy, F. and Fiers, W. (1987). Reduced tumour necrosis factor-induced cytotoxicity by inhibitors of the arachidonic acid metabolism. *Biochem. Biophys. Res. Commun.,* **149**, 735–743

95. Dealtry, G. B., Naylor, M. S., Fiers, W. and Balkwill, F. R. (1987). The effect of recombinant human tumour necrosis factor on growth and macromolecular synthesis of human epithelial cells. *Exp. Cell Res.,* **170**, 428–438

96. Agarwal, S., Drysdale, B. E. and Shin, H. S. (1988). Tumour necrosis factor-mediated cytotoxicity involves ADP-ribosylation. *J. Immunol,* **140**, 4187–4192

97. Matthews, N. (1983). Anti-tumour cytotoxin produced by human monocytes: studies on its mode of action. *Br. J. Cancer,* **48**, 405–410

98. Fiers, W., Bronchkaert, P. and Devos, R. (1986). Lymphokines and monokines in anticancer therapy. *Cold Spring Harbor Symp. Quant. Biol.,* **51**, 587–595

99. Laster, S. N., Wood, J. G. and Gooding, L. R. (1988). Tumour necrosis factor can induce both apoptic and necrotic forms of cell lysis. *J. Immunol,* **141**, 2629–2634

100. Baldwin, R. L., Chang, M. P., Bramhall, J., Graves, S., Bonavida, B. and Wisnieski, B. J. (1988). Capacity of tumour necrosis factor to bind and penetrate membranes is pH-dependent *J. Immunol.,* **141**, 2352–2357

101. Watanabe, N., Niitsu, Y., Umeno, H., Sone, H., Neda, H., Yamamuchi, N., Maeda, M. and Urushizaki, I. (1988). Synergistic cytotoxic and antitumour effects of recombinant human tumour necrosis factor and hyperthermia. *Cancer Res.,* **48**, 654–657

102. Fransen, L., Van Der Heyden, J., Ruysschaert, R. and Fiers, W. (1986). Recombinant tumour necrosis factor: its effect and its synergism with interferon gamma on a variety of normal and transformed human cell lines. *Eur. J. Cancer Clin. Oncol.,* **22**, 419–426

103. Hahn, T., Toker, L., Budilovshy, S., Aderka, D., Eshhar, Z. and Wallach, D. (1985). Use of monoclonal antibodies to a human cytotoxin for its isolation and for examining the self-induction of resistance to this protein. *Proc. Natl. Acad. Sci. USA,* **82**, 3814–3818

104. Fiers, W., Brouckaert, P., Goldberg, A., Kettelhut, I., Suffys, P., Tavernier, J., Haesebroeck, B. and Van Roy, F. (1987). Structure–function relationship of TNF and its mechanism of action. In *Tumour Necrosis Factor and Related Cytokines. Ciba Foundation Symp.,* **131**, pp. 109–123

105. Defilippi, P., Poupart, P., Tavernier, J., Fiers, W. and Content, J. (1987). Induction and regulation of mRNA encoding 26-kDa A protein in human cell lines. *Proc. Natl. Acad. Sci. USA,* **84**, 4557–4561

106. Wong, G. H. W. and Goeddel, D. V. (1988). Induction of manganous superoxide dismutase by tumour necrosis factor: possible protective mechanism. *Science,* **242**, 941–943

107. Niitsu, Y., Watanabe, N., Neda, H., Yamauchi, N., Maeda, M., Sone, H. and Kuriyama, H. (1988). Induction of synthesis of tumour necrosis factor in human and murine cell lines by exogenous recombinant human tumour necrosis factor. *Cancer Res.,* **48**, 5417–5421

108. Kronke, M., Hensel, G., Schluter, C., Scheurich, P., Schutze, S. and Pfizenmaier, K. (1988). Tumour necrosis factor and lymphotoxin gene expression in human tumour cell lines. *Cancer Res.,* **48**, 5417–5421

109. Haranaka, K., Satomi, N. and Sakurai, A. (1984). Antitumour activity of murine tumour necrosis factor (TNF) against transplanted murine tumours and heterotransplanted human tumours in nude mice. *Int. J. Cancer,* 263–267

110. Manda, T., Shimomura, K., Mukumoto, S., Kobaysashi, K., Mizota, T., Hirai, O.,

Matsumoto, S., Oku, T., Nishigaki, F., Mori, J., Kikuchi, H. (1987). Recombinant human tumour necrosis factor alpha: evidence of an indirect mode of antitumour activity. *Cancer Res.*, **47**, 3707–3711

111. Palladino, M. A. J. R., Refaat Shalaby, M., Kramer, S. M., Ferraiolo, B. L., Baughman, R. A., Deleo, A. B., Crase, D., Marafino, B., Aggarwal, B. B. and Figari, I. S. (1987). Characterization of the antitumour activities of human tumour necrosis factor alpha and the comparison with other cytokines: induction of tumour-specific immunity. *J. Immunol.*, **138**, 4023–4032

112. Balkwill, F. R., Ward, B. G. and Fiers, W. (1987). Effects of tumour necrosis factor on human tumour xenografts in nude mice. In *Tumour Necrosis Factor and Related Cytokines. Ciba Foundation Symp.*, **131**, pp. 154–169

113. Havell, E. A., Fiers, W. and North, R. J. (1988). The antitumour function of tumour necrosis factor (TNF) 1. Therapeutic action of TNF against an established murine sarcoma is indirect, immunologically dependent, and limited by severe toxicity. *J. Exp. Med.*, **167**, 1067–1085

114. Balkwill, F. R., Lee, A., Aldam, G., Moodie, E., Thomas, A., Tavernier, J. and Fiers, W. (1986). Human tumour xenografts treated with recombinant human tumour necrosis factor alone or in combination with interferons. *Cancer Res.*, **46**, 3990–3993

115. Balkwill, F. R., Ward, B. G., Moodie, E. and Fiers, W. (1987). Therapeutic potential of tumour necrosis factor alpha and gamma interferon in experimental human ovarian cancer. *Cancer Res.*, **47**, 4755–4758

116. Malik, S. T. A., Griffin, D. B., Fiers, W. and Balkwill, F. R. (1989). Tumour necrosis factor prolongs survival of mice with human tumour xenografts but promotes tumour invasion. *Int. J. Cancer* (in press)

117. Feinberg, B., Kurzrock, R., Talpaz, M., Blick, M., Saks, S. and Gutterman, J. U. (1988). A phase I trial of intravenously-administered recombinant tumour necrosis factor-alpha in cancer patients. *J. Clin. Oncol.*, **6**, 1328–1334

118. Blick, M., Sherwin, S. A., Rosenblaum, M. and Gutterman, J. (1987). Phase I study of recombinant tumour necrosis factor in cancer patients. *Cancer Res.*, **47**, 2986–2989

119. Creaven, P. J., Plager, J. E., Dupere, S., Huben, R. P., Takita, H., Mittelman, A. and Proefrock, A. (1987). Phase I clinical trial of recombinant human tumour necrosis factor. *Cancer Chemother. Pharmacol.*, **20**, 223–229

120. Kimura, K., Taguchi, T., Urushizaki, I., Ohno, R., Abe, O., Furue, H., Hattori, T., Ichihashi, H., Inoguchi, K., Majima, H., Niitani, H., Ota, K., Saito, T. and Suga, S. (1987). Phase I study of recombinant human tumour necrosis factor. *Cancer Chemother. Pharmacol.*, **20**, 223–229

121. Spriggs, D. R., Sherman, M. L., Michie, H., Arthur, K. A. A., Imamura, K., Wilmore, D., Frei, E. and Kufe, D. W. (1988). Recombinant human tumour necrosis factor administered as a 24-hour intravenous infusion. A phase I and pharmacologic study. *J. Natl. Cancer Inst.*, **80**, 1039–1044

122. Selby, P., Hobbs, S., Viner, C., Jackson, E., Jones, A., Newell, D., Calvert, A. H., McIwain, T., Fearon, K., Humphreys, J. and Shiga, T. (1987). Tumour necrosis factor in man: clinical and biological observations. *Br. J. Cancer*, **56**, 803–808

123. Fletcher Starnes, Jnr. H., Chapman, P. B., Jakubowski, A. A., Warren, R. S., Oettgen, H. F. and Gabrilove, J. L. (1988). In Bonavida, O., Gifford, G., Kirchner, H. and Old, L. J. (eds.) *Tumour Necrosis Factor/Cachectin and Related Cytokines*, pp. 177–182. (Basel: Karger)

124. Kist, A., Ho, Ad, Rath, U., Wiedenmann, B., Bauer, A., Schlick, E., Kirchner, H. and Mannel, D. N. (1988). Decrease of natural killer cell activity and monokine production in peripheral blood of patients treated with recombinant tumour necrosis factor. *Blood*, **72**, 344–348

125. Taguchi, T. (1987). Clinical studies of recombinant human tumour necrosis factor: In Bonavida, B., Clifford, G., Kirchner, H., Old, L. J. (eds.) *Tumour Necrosis/Cachectin and Related Cytokines*, pp. 196–204. (Basel: Karger)

126. Diehl, V., Pfreundschuh, M., Steinmetz, M. T. and Schaadt, M. (1987). Phase I studies of recombinant human tumour necrosis factor in patients with advanced cancer. In Bonavida, B., Clifford, G., Kirchner, H. and Old, L. J. (eds.) *Tumour Necrosis Factor and Related Cytokines*, pp. 183–188. (Basel: Karger)

127. Soma, G., Kitahara, N., Tsugi, Y., Kato, M., Oshima, H., Gatanga, T., Ihagawa, H., Noguchi, K., Tanake, Y. and Mizuno, D. (1987). Improvement of cytotoxicity of tumour necrosis factor by increase in basicity of its N-terminal region. *Biochem. Biophys. Res. Commun.*, **148**, 629–635

128. Sun, X. and Hsueh, W. (1987). Bowel necrosis induced by tumour necrosis factor in rats is mediated by platelet activating factor. *J. Clin. Invest.*, **53**, 45–53

129. Kriegler, M., Perez, C., Defay, K., Alber, I. and Lu, S. D. (1987). A novel form of TNF/cachectin is a cell surface cytotoxic transmembrane protein: Ramifications for the complex physiology of TNF. *Cell*, **53**, 45–53

130. Ruggiero, V. and Baglioni, C. (1987). Synergistic anti-proliferative activity of interleukin 1 and tumour necrosis factor. *J. Immunol.*, **138**, 661–663

131. McIntosh, J. K., Mule, J. J., Merino, M. J. and Rosenberg, S. A. (1989). Synergistic antitumour effects of immunotherapy with recombinant interleukin-2 and recombinant tumour necrosis factor alpha. *Cancer Res.*, **48**, 4011–4017

132. Bradley, T. R. and Metcalf, D. (1966). The growth of mouse bone marrow cells in vitro. *Aust. J. Exp. Biol. Sci.*, **4**, 287–300

133. Ichikawa, Y., Pluznik, D. H. and Sachs, L. (1966). In vitro control of the development of macrophage and granulocyte colonies. *Proc. Natl. Acad. Sci. USA*, **56**, 488–495

134. Moore, M. A. H. (1988). The use of haematopoietic growth factors and differentiation factors for bone marrow stimulation. In DeVita, J. R. V., Hellman, S. and Rosenberg, S. A. (eds.) *Important Advances in Oncology*, pp. 31–54. (Philadelphia: Lippincott)

135. Paul, W. E. and Ohara, J. (1987). B cell stimulatory factor 1 interleukin 4. *Annu. Rev. Immunol.*, **5**, 429–459

136. Campbell, H. D., Tucker, W. Q. J., Hort, Y., Martinson, M. E., Mayo, G., Clutterbuck, E. J., Sanderson, C. J. and Young, I. G. (1987). Molecular cloning, nucleotide sequence, and expression of the gene encoding human eosinophil differentiation factor (interleukin 5). *Proc. Natl. Acad. Sci. USA*, **84**, 6629–6633

137. Ikebuchi, K., Wong, G. G., Clark, S. C., Ihle, J. N., Hirai, Y. and Ogawa, M. (1987). Interleukin 6 enhancement of interleukin 3 dependent proliferation of multipotential hemopoietic progenitors. *Proc. Natl. Acad. Sci. USA*, **84**, 9035–9039

138. Poupart, P., Vandenabeele, P., Cayphas, S., Van Snick, J., Haegeman, G., Kruy, V., Fiers, W. and Content, J. (1987). B cell growth modulating and differentiating activity of recombinant human 26-kD protein. *EMBO J.*, **6**, 1219–1224

139. Lopez, A. F., To, L. B., Yang, G-C., Ganble, J. R., Shannon, M. F., Burns, G. F., Dyson, P. G., Juttner, C. A., Clark, S. and Vadas, M. A. (1987). Stimulation of proliferation, differentiation, and function of human cells by primate interleukin 3. *Proc. Natl. Acad. Sci. USA*, **84**, 2761–2765

140. Metcalf, D., Begley, C. G., Johnson, G. R., Nicola, N. A., Lopez, A. F. and Williamson, D. J. (1986). Effects of purified bacterially synthesized murine-csf (il-3) on hematopoiesis in normal adult mice. *Blood*, **68**, 46–57

141. Metcalf, D., Begley, C. G. and Nicola, N. A. (1985). The proliferative effects of human GM-CSF alpha and beta and murine G-CSF in microwell cultures of fractionated human marrow cells. *Leuk. Res.*, **9**, 521–527

142. Bruszewski, J., Lu, H., Ghen, K. K., Barendt, J., Platzer, E., Moore, M. A. S., Mertelsmann, R. and Welte, K. (1986). Recombinant human granulocyte colony-stimulating factor: Effects on normal and leukemic myeloid cells. *Science*, **232**, 61–65

143. Stanley, E. R., Guilbert, L. J., Tushinski, R. J. and Bartelmez, S. H. (1983). CSF-1 – A mononuclear phagocyte lineage-specific growth factor. *J. Cell. Biochem.*, **21**, 151–159

144. Nicola, N. A. (1987). Why do hemopoietic growth factor receptors interact with each other? *Immunol. Today*, **8**, 134–139

145. Dexter, T. M. and Spooncer, E. (1988). Growth and differentiation in the haematopoietic system. *Ann. Rev. Immunol.*, **4**, 423–441

146. Morstyn, G. and Burgess, A. W. (1988). Hemopoietic growth factors: A review. *Cancer Res.*, **48**, 5624–5637

147. Le Beau, M. M., Pettenati, M. J., Lemons, R. S., Diaz, M. O., Westbrook, C. A., Larson, R. A., Sherr, C. J. and Rowley, J. D. (1986). Assignment of the GM-CSF CSF-1 and FMS genes to human chromosome 5 provides evidence for linkage of a family of genes regulating hematopoiesis. *Cold Spring Harbor Symp. Quant. Biol.*, **51**, 899–909

148. Pettenati, M. J., Le Beau, M. M., Lemons, R. S., Shima, E. A., Kawasaki, E. S., Larson, R. A., Sherr, C. J., Diaz, M. O. and Rowley, J. D. (1987). Assignment of CSF-1 to 5Q33. 1. Evidence for clustering of gene regulating chromosome 5 in myeloid disorders. *Proc. Natl. Acad. Sci. USA*, **84**, 2970–2974

149. Sherr, C. J. (1988). The fms oncogene. *Biochim. Biophys. Acta*, **948**, 225–243

150. Young, D. C. and Griffin, J. D. (1986). Autocrine secretion of GM-CSF in acute myeloblastic leukemia. *Blood*, **68**, 1178–1181

151. Kaufman, B., Baer, M. R., Wong, G. A. O. and Preisler, H. D. (1988). Enhanced expression of the granulocyte-macrophage colony stimulating factor gene in acute myelocytic leukaemia cells following in vitro blast cell enrichment. *Blood*, **72**, 1329–1332

152. Ruff, M. R., Farrar, W. L. and Pert, C. B. (1986). Interferon g and granulocyte/macrophage colony-stimulating factor inhibit growth and induce antigens characteristic of myeloid differentiation in small-cell lung cancer cell lines. *Proc. Natl. Acad. Sci. USA*, **83**, 6613–6617

153. Ruff, M. R. and Pert, C. B. (1984). Small cell carcinoma of the lung: Macrophage specific antigens suggest haematopoietic cell origin. *Science*, **255**, 1034–1036

154. Vadas, M. A., Nicola, N. A. and Metcalf, D. (1983). Activation of antibody dependent cell mediated cytotoxicity of human neutrophils and eosinophils by separate colony stimulating factors. *J. Immunol.*, **130**, 795–799

155. Cannistra, S. A., Vellenga, E., Groshek, P., Rambaldi, A. and Griffin, J. D. (1988). Human granulocyte-monocyte colony-stimulating factor and interleukin 3 stimulate monocyte cytotoxicity through a tumour necrosis factor-dependent mechanism. *Blood*, **71**, 672–676

156. Sampson-Johannes, A. and Carlino, J. A. (1988). Enhancement of human monocyte tumoricidal activity by recombinant M-C8F. *J. Immunol.*, **141**, 3680–3686

157. Fabian, I., Kletter, Y. and Slavin, S. (1988). Therapeutic potential of recombinant granulocyte-macrophage colony stimulating factor and interleukin-3 in murine b-cell leukemia. *Blood*, **72**, 913–918

158. Malik, S. T. A., Hart, I. R., Martin, D. and Balkwill, F. R. (1989). Therapy of intraperitoneal ovarian cancer xenografts with liposome encapsulated MTP-PE and its potentiation by recombinant GM-CSF. (Submitted for publication)

159. Nicola, N., Metcalf, C. and Natsumoto, M. (1983). Purification of a factor inducing differentiation in murine myelomonocylic cells: Identification as granulocyte colony-stimulating factor G-CSF. *Biol. Chem.*, **258**, 9017–9024

160. Schlick, E. and Ruscetti, F. W. (1986). In vivo induction of terminal differentiation of malignant myelopoietic progenitor cells by CSF inducing biological response modifiers. *Blood*, **67**, 980–985

161. Vadhan-Raj, S., Keating, M., Lemaistre, A., Hittelman, W. N., McCredie, K., Trujillo, J. M., Broxmeyer, H. E., Henney, C. and Gutterman, J. U. (1987). Effects of recombinant granulocyte-macrophage colony stimulating factor in patients with myelodysplastic syndromes. *N. Engl. J. Med.*, **317**, 1545–1552

162. Vallenga, E., Young, D. C., Wagner, K., Wiper, D., Ostapovicz, D. and Griffin, J. D. (1987). The effects of GM-CSF and G-CSF in promoting growth of clonogenic cells in acute myelolastic leukemia. *Blood*, **69**, 1771–1776

163. Griffin, J. D., Young, D., Herrmann, F., Wiper, D., Wagner, K. and Sabbath, K. D. (1986). Effects of recombination human GM-CSF on proliferation of clonogenic cells in acute myeloblastic leukemia. *Blood*, **67**, 1448–1453

164. Broxmeyer, H. E., Williams, D. E. and Cooper, S. (1987). The influence in vivo of natural murine interleukin-3 on the proliferation of myeloid progenitor cells in mice recovering from sublethal doses of cyclophosphamide. *Leuk. Res.*, **11**, 201–205

165. Broxmeyer, H. E., Williams, D. E., Hangoc, G., Cooper, S., Gillis, S., Shadduck, R. K. and Bicknell, D. C. (1987). Synergistic myelopoietic actions in vivo after administration to mice of combinations of purified natural murine CSF. *Proc. Natl. Acad. Sci. USA*, **84**, 3871–3875

166. Welte, K., Bonilla, M. A., Gillio, A. P., Boone, T. C., Potter, G. K., Gabrilove, J. L., Moore, M. A. S., O'Reilly, R. J. and Souza, L. M. (1987). Recombinant human granulocyte colony-stimulating factor effects on hematopoiesis in normal and cyclophosphamide-treated primates. *J. Exp. Med.*, **165**, 941–948

167. Matsumoto, M., Matsubarg, S., Matsuno, T., Tamara, H., Hatlori, K., Nomura, H. and

Omo, M. (1987). Protective effect of human granulocyte colony stimulating factor (G-CSF) on microbial infection in mice with neutropenia. *Infect. Immunol.,* 55, 2715–2720

168. Bronchud, M. H., Scarffe, J. H., Thatcher, N., Crowther, D., Souza, L. M., Alton, N. K., Testa, N. G. and Dexter, T. M. (1987). Phase i/ii study of recombinant human granulocyte colony-stimulating factor in patients receiving intensive chemotherapy for small cell lung cancer. *Br. J. Cancer,* 56, 809–813

169. Morstyn, G., Souza, L. M., Keech, J., Sheridan, W., Campbell, L., Alton, Nk, Green, M. and Metcalf, D. (1988). Effect of granulocyte colony stimulating factor on neutropenia induced by cytotoxic chemotherapy. *Lancet,* 1, 667–671

170. Antman, K. S., Griffin, J. D., Elias, A., Socinski, M. A., Ryan, L., Cannistra, S. A., Oette, D., Whitley, M., Frei III, E. and Schnipper, L. E. (1988). Effect of recombinant human granulocyte-macrophage colony-stimulating factor on chemotherapy-induced myelo-suppression. *N. Engl. J. Med.,* 319, 593–598

171. Brandt, S. J., Peters, W. P., Atwater, S. K., Kurtzberg, J., Borowitz, M. J., Jones, R. B., Shpall, E. J., Bast, R., Gilbert, C. J. and Oette, D. H. (1988). Effect of recombinant human granulocyte-macrophage colony-stimulating factor on hematopoietic reconstitution after high-dose chemotherapy and autologous bone marrow transplantation. *N. Engl. J. Med.,* 318, 869–876

172. Donahue, R. E., Seehra, J., Norton, C., Turner, K., Metzger, M., Rock, B., Carbone, S., Seghal, R., Yang, Y. C., Garnick, M. and Clark, S. (1988). Haematologic effects of recombinant interleukin (IL-3) and granulocyte/macrophage colony stimulating factor (rhGM-CSF) in primates. *Proc. Am. Soc. Clin. Oncol.,* 7, 162

173. Gery, I., Gershon, R. K. and Waksman, B. H. (1972). Potentiation of the T lymphocyte response to mitogens. I. The responding cell. *J. Exp. Med.,* 136, 128–142

174. Auron, P. E., Webb, A. C., Rosemwaser, L. J., Mucci, S. F., Rich, A., Wolff, S. M. and Dinarello, C. A. (1984). Nucleotide sequence of human monocyte interleukin 1 precursor cDNA. *Proc. Natl. Acad. Sci. USA,* 81, 7907–7911

175. March, C. J., Mosley, B., Larsen, A., Cerretti, D. P., Braedt, G., Price, V., Gillis, S., Henney, C. S., Kronheim, S. R., Grabstein, K., Conlon, P. J. and Hopp, T. P. (1985). Cloning, sequence and expression of two distinct human interleukin 1 complementary DNA's. *Nature (London),* 315, 641–647

176. Gubler, U., Chua, A. O., Stern, A. S., Hellmann, C. P., Vitek, M. P., Dechiara, T. M., Benjamin, W. R., Collier, K. J., Dukovich, M., Familletti, P. C. and Fiedler-nagy, C. (1986). Recombinant human interleukin 1 alpha: Purification and biological characterisation. *J. Immunol.,* 136, 2492–2497

177. Kurt-Jones, E. A., Beller, D. I., Mizel, S. B.and Unanue, E. (1985). Identification of a membrane associated interleukin-1 in macrophages. *Proc. Natl. Acad. Sci. USA,* 82, 1204–1208

178. Dinarello, C. A., Cannon, J. G., Mier, J. W., Bernheim, H. A., Lopreste, G., Lynn, D. L., Love, R. N., Webb, A. C., Auron, P. E., Reuben, R. C., Rich, A., Wolff, S. M. and Putney, D. (1986). Multiple biological activities of human interleukin 1. *J. Clin. Invest.,* 77, 1734–1739

179. Oppenheim, J. J., Kovacs, E. J., Matsushima, K. and Durum, S. K. (1986). There is more than one interleukin 1. *Immunol. Today,* 7, 45–56

180. Le, J. and Vilcek, J. (1987). Tumor necrosis factor and interleukin 1: Cytokines with multiple overlapping biological activities. *Lab. Invest.,* 56, 234–248

181. Sims, J. E., March, C. J., Cosman, D., Widmer, M. B., Robson MacDonald, H., McHaham, C. J. and Grubin, C. E. (1988). cDNA expression cloning of the IL-1 receptor, a member of the immunoglobulin superfamily. *Science,* 241, 585–589

182. Bevilacqua, M. P., Pober, J. S., Majeau, G. R., Fiers, W., Cotran, R. S. and Gimbrone, N. A. Jnr. (1986). Recombinant tumor necrosis factor induces procoagulant activity in cultured human vascular endothelium: Characterisation and comparison with the actions of interleukin 1. *Proc. Natl. Acad. Sci. USA,* 83, 4533–4537

183. Pober, J. S., Gimbrone, M. A., Lapierre, L. A., Mendrick, D. L., Fiers, W., Rothlein, R. and Springer, T. A. (1986). Overlapping patterns of activation of human endothelial cells by interleukin 1, tumour necrosis factor, and immune interferon. *J. Immunol.,* 137, 1893–1896

184. Ramila, P. and Epstein, L. B. (1986). Tumour necrosis factor as an immunomodulator and mediator of monocyte cytotoxicity induced by itself, γ-interferon and interleukin-1. *Nature*

(London), **323**, 86–89

185. Holtmann, H. and Wallach, D. (1987). Downregulation of the receptors for tumour necrosis factor by interleukin 1 and 4-beta phorbol-12-myristate-13-acetate. *J. Immunol.*, **139**, 1161–1167

186. Cavender, D. E. and Edelbaum, D. (1987). Inhibition by IL-1 of endothelial cell activation induced by tumour necrosis factor or lymphotoxin. *J. Immunol.*, **141**, 3111–3116

187. Onozaki, K., Matsushima, K., Aggarwal, B. B. and Oppenheim, J. J. (1985). Human interleukin 1 is a cytocidal factor for several tumor cell lines. *J. Immunol.*, **135**, 3962–3968

188. Ruggiero, V. and Baglioni, C. (1987). Synergistic anti-proliferative activity of interleukin 1 and tumour necrosis factor. *J. Immunol.*, **138**, 661–663

189. Tsai, S. and Gaffney, E. V. (1986). Inhibition of cell proliferation by interleukin 1 derived from monocytic leukemia cells. *Cancer Res.*, **46**, 1471–1477

190. Tsai, S. C. J. and Gaffney, E. V. (1987). Modulation of cell proliferation by human recombinant interleukin-1 and immune interferon. *J. Natl. Cancer Inst.*, **79**, 77–81

191. Nakamura, S., Nakata, K., Kashmoto, S., Yoshida, H. and Yamada, M. (1986). Antitumour effect of recombinant human interleukin 1 alpha against murine syngeneic tumors. *J. Cancer Res.*, **77**, 767–773

192. Nakata, K., Kashimoto, S., Yoshida, H., Oku, T. and Nakamura, S. (1988). Augmented antitumor effect of recombinant human interleukin 1 alpha by indomethacin. *Cancer Res.*, **48**, 584–588

193. Braunschweiger, P. G., Johnson, C. S., Kumar, N., Ord, V. and Furmanski, P. (1988). Antitumour effects of recombinant human interleukin 1 alpha in RIF-1 and PANc 02 solid tumours. *Cancer Res.*, **48**, 6011–6016

194. Massague, J. (1987). The TGF-beta family of growth and differentiation factors. *Cell*, **49**, 437–438

195. Massague, J., Cheifetz, S., Ignotz, R. A. and Boyd, F. T. (1987). Multiple type beta transforming growth factors and their receptors. *J. Cell. Physiol. (Suppl.)*, **5**, 43–47

196. Balkwill, F. R. (1989). Transforming growth factors-β and related molecules. In *Cytokines in Cancer Therapy*, Chap. 7. (Oxford University Press)

197. Denynck, R., Goeddel, D. V., Ullrich, A., Gutterman, J. U., Williams, R. D., Bringman, T. S. and Berger, W. H. (1987). Synthesis of messenger RNAs for transforming growth factors alpha and beta and the epidermal growth factor receptor by human tumours. *Cancer Res.*, **47**, 707–712

198. Gerwin, B. I., Lechner, J. F., Reddel, R. R., Roberts, A. B., Robbins, K. C., Gabrielson, E. W. and Harris, C. C. (1987). Comparison of the production of transforming growth factor beta and platelet-derived growth factor by normal human mesothelial cells and meso-thelioma cell lines. *Cancer Res.*, **47**, 6180–6184

199. Knabbe, C., Lippman, M. E., Wakefield, L. M., Flanders, K. C., Kasid, A., Derynck, R. and Dickson, R. B. (1987). Evidence that transforming growth factor beta is a hormonally regulated negative growth factor in human breast cancer cells. *Cell*, **48**, 417–428

200. Kimchi, A., Wang, X-F., Weinberg, R. A., Cheifetz, S. and Massague, J. (1988). Absence of TGF-b receptors and growth inhibitory responses in retinoblastoma cells. *Science*, **240**, 196–199

201. Cate, R. L., Mattaliano, R. J., Hession, C., Tizard, R., Farber, N. M., Cheung, A., Ninta, E. G., Frey, A. Z., Gash, D. J., Chow, E. P., Fisher, R. A. and Bertonis, J. M. (1986). Isolation of the bovine and human genes for mullerian inhibiting substance and expression of the gene in animal cells. *Cell*, **45**, 685–698

202. Wrann, M., Bodmer, S., De Martin, R., Siepl, C., Hofer-Warbinek, R., Frei, K., Hofer, E. and Fontana, A. (1987). IFN inducible gene maps to a chromosomal band associated with a (4;11) translocation in acute leukaemia cells. *Proc. Natl. Acad. Sci. USA*, **6**, 1633–1636

203. Roberts, A. B., Sporn, M. B., Assoian, R. K., Smith, J. M., Roche, R. S., Wakefield, L. M., Heine, U. I., Liotta, L. A., Falanga, V., Kehrl, J. H. and Fauci, A. (1986). Transforming growth factor type beta: rapid induction fibrosis and angiogenesis in vivo and stimulation of collagen formation in vitro. *Proc. Natl. Acad. Sci. USA*, **83**, 4167–4171

204. Mustoe, T. A., Pierce, G. F., Thomason, A., Gramates, P., Sporn, M. B. and Deuel, T. F. (1987). Accelerated healing of incisional wounds in rats induced by transforming growth factor beta. *Science*, **257**, 1333–1336

205. Neta, R. and Oppenheim, J. J. (1988). Cytokines in therapy of radiation injury. *Blood*, **72**,

1093–1095
206. Smyth, M. J., Pieteresz, A. and McKenzie, I. F. C. (1988). Increased antitumour effect of immunoconjugates and tumour necrosis factor in vivo. *Cancer, Res.,* **48**, 3607–3612
207. Sato, K., Fujii, Y., Ono, M., Nomura, H. and Shizume, K. (1987). Production of interleukin 1a-like factor by a squamous cell carcinoma of the thyroid (T3M-5) derived from a patient with hypercalcaemia and leucocytosis. *Cancer Res.,* **47**, 6474–6480
208. Ramani, P. and Balkwill, F. (1987). Enhanced metastases of a mouse carcinoma after in vitro treatment with murine interferon gamma. *Int. J. Cancer,* **40**, 830–834

9
Targeted therapy: cell surface targets

R.H.J. BEGENT

INTRODUCTION

Many agents can kill cancer cells but are too toxic to normal tissues for effective treatment of common cancers. Targeted treatment, in which the therapeutic agent concentrates in the tumour relative to normal tissues, is an attractive means of overcoming this problem.

Targeted radionuclide therapy has been successful where a biochemical pathway specific to the tumour type can be targeted. Therapy of thyroid carcinoma with [131]iodine (^{131}I), and of neuroblastoma and phaeochromocytoma with ^{131}I-MIBG are illustrative. Targets of this type have not been found in common types of cancer but cell-surface antigens, which are abundant in tumours relative to normal tissues, have. Carcinoembryonic antigen (CEA) was the first with wide application in common epithelial malignancies, and monoclonal antibodies have been used to identify many more. This chapter will deal with targeting to these cell-surface antigens, the parameters determining the efficiency of such systems, the therapeutic agent to be delivered and therapeutic effects in animals and man.

HISTORY

Soon after the properties of antibodies were described by Behring and Kitasoto in 1890[1], it was appreciated that they might be used to discriminate between cancerous and normal tissues. Treatment of cancer with antibodies raised against human tumours was reported by Hericourt et al.[2]. They immunized dogs and donkeys with extracts of human carcinomas and sarcomas and gave repeated injections of the resulting antisera to the patients against whose tumours the antisera were raised. Responses were reported but treatment was curtailed by the development of an urticarial, erythematous rash and occasionally syncope after three or four injections. The treatment did not become established and development at that time would have been difficult because of the lack of methods to purify antibody and characterize tumour-associated antigens. It is interesting that reactions to repeated therapy, probably mediated by immunoglobulin G (IgG) and IgE, were identified as a limiting factor at this early stage.

In the 1950s, Pressman and Korngold[3] and Bale et al.[4] established the specificity of antibody targeting by showing that radiolabelled antibodies directed against transplantable animal tumours localized in the appropriate tumour to a greater extent than non-specific antibody. The antibodies used for these experiments were only partially purified so that much of the radiolabelled protein administered had no chance of binding to the target. Antibodies affinity purified on a column of the corresponding antigen were used by Mach and co-workers[5]. Human chorionic gonadotrophin (HCG) was the first human tumour-associated antigen successfully used as a target, in hamsters bearing xenografts of human choriocarcinoma in the cheek pouch[6]. Similar work with antibodies to carcinoembryonic antigen (CEA) showed that non-specific antibody did not localize in the human colon carcinoma xenografts to the same extent as antiCEA[5,7,8]. Monoclonal antibodies have now produced a host of antigen–antibody systems for tumour targeting[9] and raise the prospect of large-scale production of reproducible reagents. These have been extensively investigated in congenitally T cell-deficient nude mice bearing xenografts of human tumours, first employed for this purpose by Mach et al.[5].

In the early 1970s, attempts at γ camera imaging of human tumours with intravenous radiolabelled antibodies were unsuccessful, probably because the persistence of radiolabelled antibody in the blood and normal tissues obscured any specific localization in tumours. The subtraction technique used by Goldenberg et al.[10] overcame this problem for antibodies to CEA and was equally successful with antiHCG[11,12]. The distribution of antibody in blood and normal tissues was mimicked by obtaining an image of intravenously administered 99^m-technetium- (Tc-) labelled albumin and 99^m-pertechnetate. The image of Tc was then subtracted from that of the ^{131}iodine- (^{131}I-) labelled antibody to leave an image of specific localization of antibody in tumour.

The specificity of antibody localization in man has also been established by comparison with non-specific antibodies, and superior localization in tumour has been shown in a variety of tumour types and antibody–antigen systems[13,14] (for a review see reference 9).

ANTIBODIES AND THEIR TARGETING CHARACTERISTICS

The antibody molecule

IgG is the principal class to have been investigated. Its molecular weight of approximately 150 000 Da, glycosylation and charge give mouse monoclonal antibodies a halflife in the human circulation of about 48 h. Native human IgG has a longer halflife and genetically engineered chimeric human/mouse immunoglobulins, now coming into use, are probably intermediate[15]. F(ab')$_2$ is cleared more rapidly than intact antibody and Fab' faster still[13]. The persistence of antibody in the circulation means that it is available to pass through the endothelium for longer than conventional cytotoxic drugs which usually have a short halflife and are available for binding for a correspondingly short period. This must be set against the relatively poor diffusion of the larger Ig molecules through the endothelium. The percentage of the injected dose bound per gram of tumour in man is in the range 0.1–0.001%. This can give favourable tumour to normal tissue ratios though it has been argued that these may not be sufficient for effective therapy. For a review, see Dykes *et al.*[16].

Biodistribution

When an antibody is given intravenously, highest concentrations are generally found in the blood for the first few hours or days; however, some diffuses into normal and neoplastic tissues whether or not a specific antigen is present. If a specific reaction occurs between the antibody and a tumour-associated antigen, antibody is retained and may continue to accumulate over the next 8 h–7 days[17–18]. Concentrations of non-specific antibody are often as high as those of specific antibody for the first day or two but decline more rapidly. By contrast, specific and non-specific antibody are cleared relatively rapidly from normal tissues. Thus, the tumour to normal tissue ratio increases with time for specific antibodies but not for the non-specific.

Antibody targeted therapy of cancer requires that a favourable distribution of antibody be sustained in tumour relative to normal tissues. Suitable distributions have been shown in mice bearing xenografts of human tumours[17,19,20]. The factors influencing antibody distribution can be defined to some extent, and mathematical models have been used in conjunction with experimental data to attempt to understand the processes[21].

The principal factors determining the efficiency of tumour targeting are:

1. The concentration of antibody in tumour interstitial fluid (a measure of antibody available to bind to tumour-associated antigen);
2. The extent of binding;
3. Loss of antibody from the specific binding site;
4. The difference between the above factors in tumour and vulnerable normal tissues.

Interstitial fluid

The concentration gradient from blood into tumour or normal tissue affects the concentration of antibody in interstitial fluid. It is influenced by the rate of clearance of antibody from the circulation and from interstitial spaces.

Intact immunoglobulin clears relatively slowly from the blood and therefore maintains a favourable concentration gradient towards interstitial fluid of tumour or normal tissue. Smaller molecules, such as Fab' and, to a lesser extent, F(Ab')$_2$, clear more rapidly than intact IgG and attain lower concentration in the tumour[22]. Rapid clearance and low tumour concentration also occur with altered glycosylation of antibody[23], administration of a second antibody directed against the first[24,25] (see *Second antibody* below) and the presence of human antimouse antibody[26].

163

Blood flow and pressure

Agents which increase tumour perfusion, such as β adrenergic blocking agents, have been shown to increase tumour concentration of antibody[27]. Radiation and hyperthermia have also been shown to have this effect[28,29] though it is difficult to be sure that this is not also due to increased vascular permeability.

Permeability

Permeability of vascular endothelium for immunoglobulin molecules varies in different normal tissues according to the type of endothelium. Thus, in the mouse model of Covel[21], fenestrated epithelium of liver gives a permeability of more than 50 times that of gut which does not have this type of endothelium. The lung has an even higher permeability in this model, though it lacks fenestrated epithelium, and it is speculated that this is because of the large blood flow and extensive capillaries. Good data for the permeability of tumour vasculature are few but Gerlowski and Jain[30] studied permeability of 150 000 Da dextran in tumours and granulation tissue in a rabbit ear chamber system and showed good permeability for tumours relative to normal tissues. The large differences in permeability in different tissues reported by Covell[21] suggest that this will be an important parameter for successful targeting. Molecules smaller than intact immunoglobulin such as F(ab')₂ and Fab' are likely to permeate more effectively through the endothelium in contrast to their relatively poor performance in maintaining a concentration gradient between blood and interstitial fluid.

Penetration in tissues

Tissues with well organized structure and vasculature are likely to permit more orderly distribution of macromolecules like immunoglobulin than tumour where areas of hypoxia and necrosis are usually found. Multicellular spheroids of tumour cells grown in tissue culture have been used to investigate diffusion within tumours[31,32]. These suggest that smaller molecules such as Fab' and F(Ab')₂ penetrate further than intact immunoglobulin. Necrotic central areas of spheroids are not penetrated by any of the molecules. Penetration of molecules into spheroids is determined by diffusion whereas tissue perfusion *in vivo* is also driven by a pressure gradient from arteriole to venule which is responsible for a great part of the flux of molecules through tissues. There is evidence for the presence of high hydrostatic pressure and low intravenous pressure in tumour vasculature with arterial pressure similar to normal tissues. These factors appear to favour poor penetration of antibody within tumours compared with normal tissues (for review see Jain[33]). Variability in distribution within a tumour mass[34] is therefore not surprising. Uptake of antibody tends to be higher in tumours of less than 100 mg, in which these problems are likely to be less prominent[35].

Binding of antibody

This depends on interstitial fluid levels of antibody, which are predicted in the model of Covell *et al.*[21] to be less than those in plasma and to vary with each tissue. An estimate of interstitial fluid levels of antibody may be obtained by examination of lymph.

Specific reaction with antigen, either in tumour or normal tissues, will lead to retention and a tendency to reach concentrations above those in plasma. This will be influenced by the affinity of the antibody, though little experimental evidence of improved targeting with high-affinity antibodies has been reported. Genetically engineered modification of the hypervariable region[36] is an interesting way of modifying the antigen-binding region to optimize binding. Saturation of available antigen in tumour does not appear to be a problem in animal models over the concentration ranges in which it has been studied[25,37,38]. However, Leichner *et al.*[39] reported no advantage in increasing the administered dose of antiferritin antibodies in patients with hepatoma. Each antibody and tumour will probably need to be examined individually as regards the optimal dose.

Retention in tissues

Retention of antibody at the tumour after clearance from the circulation is essential for a good therapeutic ratio in targeting. There are very few data about the dynamic equilibrium between antibody in the interstitial fluid and that bound to tumour, nor about the catabolism of antibody in tumours. The latter appears to vary in different tissues, the liver and possibly the gut being important for intact antibody and the kidney for $F(Ab)'$ and $F(Ab)'_2$ fragments[21].

Figure 9.1 shows a simplified form of the relationship between some of the parameters defined above for blood, interstitial fluid and tumour. These were derived from measurements of tumour and blood activity in a patient studied by γ camera imaging. Similar considerations apply for normal tissues with the exception of specific antibody–antigen reactions. Data of this type need to be determined experimentally as far as possible for each antibody in man. The characteristics of the therapeutic modality targeted by the antibody need to be matched to the period of maximum specific tumour binding, before release of antibody from the tumour but after relative decline in antibody concentrations in normal tissues. The parameters can be influenced in various ways to obtain the best match.

Regulatory considerations

The safety, quality and efficacy of monoclonal antibodies have to be assured before they can be considered for use in man. As well as the usual considerations of purity, stability and activity, there has been concern about microbiological contamination, particularly with retroviruses in antibodies produced from cell lines grown in large-scale culture or in the form of ascites.

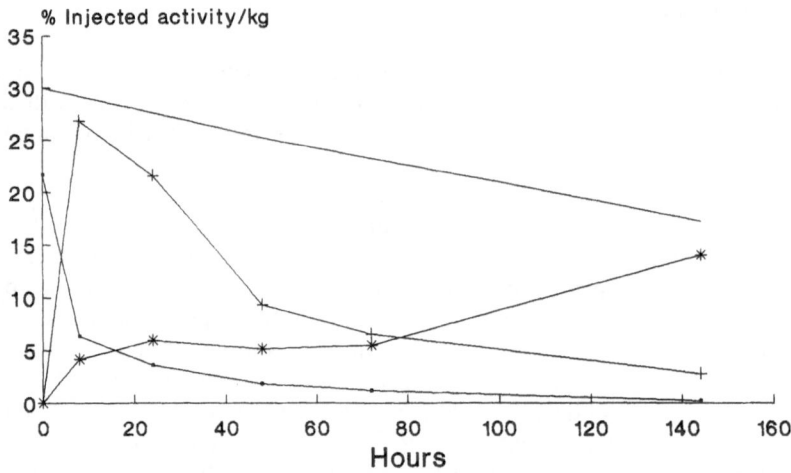

Figure 9.1 Graph showing the relationship of tumour and blood levels in a patient with particularly good tumour localization of ^{131}I-labelled antibody to CEA. Tumour activity was taken from γ camera imaging, blood from venous blood samples. Tumour to blood ratios are seen to rise up to 8 h and then to rise no further until 144 h. The activities given are corrected for physical decay of the isotope. The rate of decay of ^{131}I is shown
—■— blood; —+— tumour; —*— tumour: blood; — [131]I decay

Guidelines covering the whole of this area have been published by the Commission of the European Communities[40] and the Federal Drugs Administration of the USA. Chimeric antibodies produced from mouse and human immunoglobulin genes are also subject to other guidelines[41]. When monoclonal antibodies are produced in academic laboratories in smaller quantities than in industrial processes, less stringent guidelines have been accepted in order to facilitate clinical trials under the UK Department of Health doctors and dentists exemption scheme[42].

STRATEGIES FOR THERAPY

Natural effector mechanisms

It has been proposed that an antitumour effect can be produced by complement activation or antibody-dependent cell-mediated cytotoxicity. The concept of using the antibody–antigen reaction to initiate a cytotoxic cascade of the body's own natural effector mechanisms is attractive for its potential power if it can be manipulated precisely. Knowledge of the appropriate components of the immune system is growing rapidly but the subject is beyond the scope of this review. There is, however, optimism that specific activation of cytotoxic effector mechanisms at the site of antibody–antigen reaction in a tumour may give effective antitumour therapy.

Various targets and therapeutic strategies are being investigated. Anti-idiotype antibodies directed against the idiotype of the monoclonal immuno-globulin secreted by B cells have been used to treat B cell lymphomas[43-45].

This has the attraction that the target is theoretically truly tumour specific. Although sustained responses are reported, they seem to be exceptional and the mechanisms producing them are not understood.

The idea that human immunoglobulins may be more effective at activating natural effector mechanisms in man has been investigated. In one study, a chimeric antibody, having a rat immunoglobulin-derived hypervariable region directed against the human lymphoid cell antigen, CAMPATH-1, and human immunoglobulin-constant regions, has been produced by recombinant DNA technology. This produces antitumour effects in non-Hodgkin's lymphoma[15].

In an alternative approach, Koprowski et al.[46] have proposed that an antitumour effect observed against colon carcinoma in some patients given 17-1A antibody is mediated through the idiotypic network. This is based on the network hypothesis of Jerne[47] and uses idiotype determinants on antibodies as substitutes for conventional tumour antigens. Anti-idiotype antibodies (Ab2) directed against the binding region of the antitumour antibody (Ab1) are produced by the host. Ab2 has been classified by Jerne into the α type, which binds to an idiotype that is not close to the binding site, the γ type which binds close to the binding site so as to interfere with antigen binding, and the β type which binds directly to the antigen binding site. This β type is an internal image of the antigen and, if it is used for immunization, an antibody is produced which is directed against the antigen. Thus, monoclonal β Ab2 antibodies can be used to immunize against tumours or infections. Battacharia-Chatterjee et al.[48] have demonstrated production of Ab1, β Ab2 and Ab3 (anti-anti-idiotype) relating to a well-characterized human T cell leukaemia antigen. It is necessary to show the production of all the components of this system in man. Herlyn et al.[49] have treated patients suffering from colorectal cancer with polyclonal anti-idiotype antibodies against 17-1A mouse monoclonal antibody to colorectal carcinoma. Patients developed a humoral antitumour response and some improvements in tumour measurements were reported. The nature of the antibody response requires more precise characterization but the results are encouraging.

There is evidence that humoral responses may not be sufficient to eradicate more than a minimal tumour burden[50] and therapeutic strategies may be necessary which take this into account. Combination of idiotypic immunization and cyclophosphamide for treatment of murine lymphoma has been reported to be superior to either modality alone[51] and may be worthy of clinical trials. Combinations with cytokines to potentiate the response also merit investigation[52].

Radioimmunotherapy

Radioimmunotherapy, in which an α- or β-emitting radionuclide is linked to the antibody, has been investigated since the 1970s. The targeting efficiency can be monitored by following the distribution of radioactivity, and antitumour effect and normal tissue toxicity can be estimated by measurements of cumulative radiation dose. The resulting information is valuable for understanding other forms of antibody targeted therapy.

Table 9.1   Factors in radioimmunotherapy

Tumour
    Intrinsic radiosensitivy
    Potential doubling time
    Capacity to repair non-lethal radiation damage

Radionuclide
    Emission spectrum
    Physical halflife
    Ability to link to targeting agent

Biodistribution
    Macroscopic
    Microscopic

Table 9.1 lists the parameters on which radioimmunotherapy depends. The isotope does not have to be delivered to every cell. This may be a crucial advantage over other forms of antibody targeted therapy because of differences in antigen expression and variation in antibody penetration to different parts of the tumour. Antitumour activity can be achieved between one and a few hundred cell diameters away from the radiolabelled antibody molecule according to the path length and distribution of energy of the α- or β-emitting radionuclide used. This aspect has been reviewed by Humm[53]. The β emitters, [131]iodine and [90]yttrium, have been used in man. The α emitter, [211]astatine, has been shown to be effective in animal tumour models[54] and [212]bismuth in tissue culture[55].

Effective therapy requires that the temporal and anatomical considerations of the distribution of antibody, the radionuclide and the sensitivity of the tumour be matched.

Figure 9.1 illustrates the patterns of antibody and radionuclide distribution. The falling levels in the blood are associated with rising values in tumour and normal tissue interstitial fluid until equilibrium is reached. Interstitial fluid levels will then fall roughly in parallel with blood values. Specific binding to tumour and normal tissue will continue while there is antibody in the interstitial fluid and antigen is not saturated. Release of antibody through dynamic equilibrium and catabolism will eventually reduce tumour radionuclide levels. A favourable therapeutic ratio depends on exploiting the time when specific binding dominates over interstitial fluid levels of antibody, the latter being non-specific.

The halflife of antibody needs to be such that a substantial part of its energy is expended during the time of maximal specific tumour binding relative to normal tissue values. Experimental data in man to define this are sparse[18,56,57] but those available suggest that halflives of 3–14 days are likely to be optimal. The halflife of antibody in the circulation appears to be particularly important, for very different times of peak tumour concentration occur according to the rate of clearance from blood. The distribution of antibody shown in Figure 9.1 produced a partial response in the liver metastasis and is probably the least that is needed for effective therapy. These data can be used to estimate the effect of using radionuclides of different halflives on cumulative radiation dose to tumour and normal tissues and to assess antibody distribution in relation to therapy with modalities other than radiation.

The sensitivity of cells in different tumours may vary according to innate radiosensitivity, rate of cell division and rate of repair of radiation-induced damage. Sensitivity of tumour relative to normal tissues also varies and these factors have to be integrated into any formula for effective radioimmuno-therapy.

Animal studies

Delay in growth of xenografts of human carcinomas in experimental animals has been shown as a result of intravenously administered antibodies labelled with the β-emitting radionuclides, [131]iodine[16,19,20,58-66] and [90]yttrium[67]. The α emitter, [211]astatine, has also been effective in an animal lymphoma model[54].

Clinical studies

A series of over 100 patients with hepatoma have been treated with ^{131}I antibody to ferritin at Johns Hopkins Hospital[68]. 48% response with 7% complete remissions was reported but the effect of the ^{131}I antibody therapy cannot be assessed independently because external beam radiation and cyto-toxic drugs were also used in the protocol. The same group also reported 40% response in Hodgkin's disease treated only with ^{131}I antibody to ferritin. Clinically useful activity has also been shown in non-Hodgkin's lymphoma[69-71] in patients who were unresponsive to conventional therapy. [131]I antibody therapy has also been used to treat melanoma[72], colon carcinoma[18] and neuroblastoma[73]. Although responses are reported, it appears to be except-ional for these to be sustained. ^{90}Y-labelled antibody has been used for treatment of hepatoma, and radiation dose to tumour appears to be at a level capable of producing responses[74].

Radionuclides afford the opportunity to relate therapeutic effect and toxicity to the radiation dose administered to the tumour and normal tissues. [131]I is particularly convenient for this because the β emission responsible for most of the therapeutic effect is accompanied by a γ emission which can be counted in excised tissues or imaged by γ camera. γ camera imaging has yielded some serial measurements of radioactivity in tissues of patients receiving ^{131}I-labelled antibody[56,57,72]. However, observations were made at few time points and there were no data from the first 24 h when activity may be highest. The planar imaging method used[75] is reasonably accurate when there are no overlying tissues with significant levels of activity but is unsatis-factory for measuring activity in tumours or other organs lying deep in the body. Green et al.[76] have shown that this can be obviated so as to quantitate antibody distribution accurately by three-dimensional single-photon emission tomography with correction for Compton scatter. In this way, serial imaging can be used to give a graph of levels of radioactivity in tumour and normal

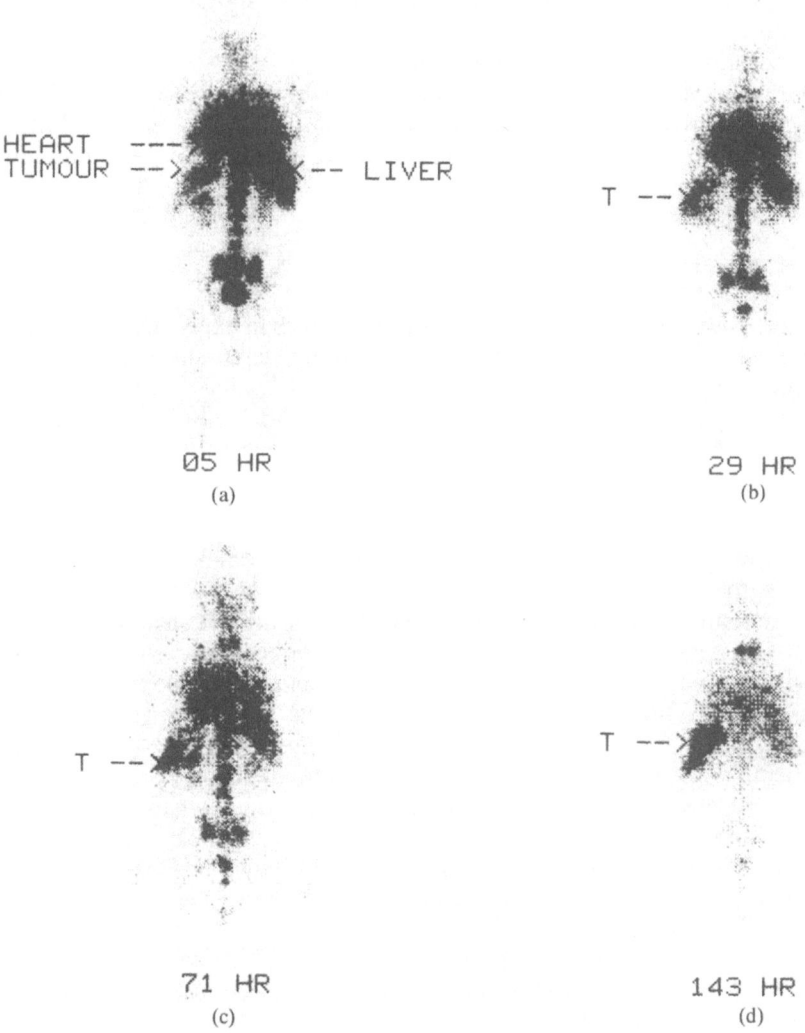

Figure 9.2 Posterior γ camera images showing the distribution of ^{131}I-labelled mouse monoclonal antibody to CEA in a patient with recurrent colon carcinoma: (a) 5 h after antibody administration activity is seen principally in the circulation; (b), (c) and (d) images at 29, 71 and 143 h show clearance from the circulation and normal tissues with retention in a tumour deposit (T) in the left upper abdomen

tissues. Cumulative radiation dose is then estimated by integration of the curves. A study of 16 patients treated for colorectal carcinoma at Charing Cross Hospital with ^{131}I-labelled antibody to CEA showed that maximum concentrations of radioactivity were found in tumour 8 h after administration.

Activity in tumour varied up to 9-fold in different patients. Higher levels were found on average in tumour than any other tissue. Liver, lung and blood were the other tissues in which antibody was concentrated relative to the rest of the body. Antibody cleared from all these tissues during 1 week. γ Camera images of a patient receiving ^{131}I-antibody to CEA are shown in Figure 9.2.

Measurements of cumulative radiation dose to tumour and normal tissues were made to assess the possibilities for effective therapy. The patient with the highest tumour activity had a β radiation dose to tumour of 5.1 cGy/mCi injected with a whole body dose of 0.25 cGy/mCi, a ratio of 20:1. Dykes *et al.*[16] have predicted that a ratio of 30:1 is needed for effective therapy, assuming that a whole body dose of 200 cGy is tolerable. By these criteria, effective therapy may be in range for some patients, particularly with repeated antibody administration as is now possible by use of cyclosporin A to prevent the human anti-antibody response[26]. For the majority, however, effective therapy would not appear practical with this antibody.

Bone marrow radiation is the dose-limiting toxicity with [131]I- and ^{90}Y-labelled antibody[56,72,74]. The data of Benua *et al.*[77] for ^{131}I therapy of thyroid cancer indicate that a radiation dose to blood of 200 cGy will produce myelosuppression from which recovery is predictable. This is probably applicable to radiolabelled-antibody therapy also. A higher bone marrow dose might be acceptable with appropriate facilities to support a myelo-suppressed patient. It is likely that recovery would be usual with 400 cGy to bone marrow and that even higher doses would be tolerable with autologous bone marrow transplantation.

In the best patient in the Charing Cross study, a tumour dose of 1020 cGy would be obtained for a blood dose of 200 cGy. Responses of cutaneous T cell lymphoma and B cell lymphoma have been reported with ^{131}I-labelled antibody therapy delivering a tumour dose estimated between 500–1000 cGy[69,70]. These responses are perhaps better than might be expected with external beam radiotherapy and may be the result of an underestimate of dose delivered to cancer cell nuclei.

Autoradiographic study of microscopic distribution of antibody within the tumour shows localization on and around tumour cells relative to stromal and necrotic areas of tumour as discussed previously[78-80]. The extent of the advantage produced by this factor is unknown. It may vary with different tumour types; the extensive stromal and mucinous areas common in colon carcinoma will separate cells to which antibody may bind specifically giving a lower apparent concentration of antibody than in a tumour of tightly packed tumour cells, such as hepatoma. This may explain the apparently higher tumour doses achieved in hepatoma by Order *et al.*[68].

Cytotoxic drugs

The extensive knowledge of the metabolism and toxicity of cytotoxic agents makes their investigation attractive to clinicians. Mathe *et al.*[81] began the study of cytotoxic drugs linked to antibodies by treating L1210 leukaemia cells with methotrexate coupled to antibody binding to the cells. Conjugates with many different drugs, including methotrexate, chlorambucil, adriamycin, daunorubicin, vindesine, α-amanitin, mitomycin C and neocarzinostatin, have all been shown to have activity *in vitro* or in animal tumour models[82,83].

The potency of cytotoxic drugs is low by comparison with toxins and attempts to deliver a large amount of drug on each antibody molecule can lead to loss of immunoreactivity of the antibody. Carrier molecules such as albumin and dextran (linked to the antibody) to which many drug molecules are coupled have been investigated[84]. It is uncertain whether they will persist in the circulation long enough to target satisfactorily in man. Internalization of the cytotoxic drug is also necessary and, as discussed above, immunoconjugates appear variable in the efficiency with which they cross the cell membrane. To these considerations must be added the ability of tumour cells to develop resistance to cytotoxic drugs. Nevertheless, any increase of therapeutic ratio of a cytotoxic drug by antibody targeting is likely to be useful in clinical practice. This is supported by a clinical trial with antibody to colorectal carcinoma linked to neocarzinostatin given via the hepatic artery to patients with liver metastases. Three of eight patients had a reduction of tumour volume on CT scan[85]. Favourable localization of the conjugate by comparison with normal colon was also demonstrated in this study.

Immunotoxins

Various toxins of plant and bacterial origin can be linked to antibodies to form immunotoxins[86]. In general, they act enzymatically once internalized into the tumour cell and are extremely potent. Ricin, found in beans of *Ricinus communis*, has been studied most extensively. The lectin B chain of ricin causes the molecule to bind non-specifically to many cell types, the molecule then being internalized for the A chain to have its cytotoxic effect. For antibody therapy, the isolated A chain can be linked to antibody or the linkage arranged so that the B chain is not active[87]. The conjugate will then localize specifically to tumours. The A chain catalytically inactivates the 60s ribosomal subunit of eukaryotic cells by modifying nucleoside residues of the 28s ribosomal RNA[88]. *In vitro* ricin A-antitumour antibody conjugates can be of the order of 10^3–10^4 times as toxic to tumour cells as ricin A chain alone[86]. This activity depends on internalization of ricin A chain and on its reaching the ribosomes once inside the cell. The rate and route of internalization have been shown to be important in the toxicity of immunotoxins[89]. Press *et al.*[90] have shown that, once internalized, inmunoconjugates may vary in effectiveness according to the epitope on the antigen molecule with which the targeting antibody reacts. Reaction with an epitope close to the cell membrane resulted in longer retention in the cell, slower metabolism and expulsion than when the antibody reacted with an epitope more distant from the cell membrane. In the latter case, the toxin is routed to lysosomes, degraded and expelled. These authors speculate that the difference may be because reaction with epitopes near the cell membrane facilitates incorporation of the immunotoxin into endosomal membranes which protect against proteolytic enzymes in lysosomes and facilitate delivery into the cytoplasm.

In studies *in vivo*, ricin A immunoconjugates initially suffered from rapid clearance from the circulation with poor tumour uptake. This has been shown to be caused by uptake of the immunoconjugate by Kupffer cells in the liver which bind mannose-terminating oligosaccharides of ricin A chain[91–93]. Deglycosylation of ricin A chain[92] and production of unglycosylated recombinant ricin A chain go some way to overcoming this problem.

Responses have been reported in one clinical study with ricin A chain linked to an antimelanoma antibody[94] but it is not yet established that these were mediated through the ricin A chain rather than natural effector mechanisms. A further study in colorectal cancer is also in progress[95]. Treatment of graft-versus-host disease with an immunotoxin directed against the CD5 antigen of T cells has had a beneficial effect in one reported patient[96], suggesting that targeting of immunoconjugates in another context is effective. These studies are with ricin A chain which is rapidly cleared because of its glycosylation (see above). Studies with deglycosylated or recombinant ricin A chain will be of interest and it is premature to make judgments of the efficacy or toxicity of immunotoxins.

LIMITATIONS TO THERAPY AND STRATEGIES TO OVERCOME THEM

Antibody targeted therapy is currently limited in man by three major factors. Either the therapeutic ratio is not high enough, or a therapeutic dose is not delivered to the target, or repeated therapy cannot be given. Much work is in progress to overcome these problems.

Improving the therapeutic ratio

Local therapy

Systemic toxicity of antibody-directed therapy can, in theory, be diminished and antitumour effect enhanced by giving the immunoconjugate into a body cavity to which the tumour is confined. Alternatively, the immunoconjugate can be given into the artery supplying localized tumour. The tumour is thus exposed to higher concentrations of immunoconjugate than it would be with intravenous administration. Systemic exposure should be similar or less and the therapeutic ratio therefore improved. Success depends on retention of immunoconjugate within the cavity targeted or area perfused. This is probably achieved when radiolabelled antibody is given into the cerebro-spinal fluid. Responses have been reported when patients with meningeal involvement by primary neural tumours and common epithelial malignancy were treated with intrathecal ^{131}I-labelled antibodies[97]. Intraperitoneal and intrapleural therapy of ovarian carcinoma with ^{131}I-labelled antibody has been reported to produce remissions in patients with disease of less than 2 cm diameter[98,99]. Ward *et al.*[100] only found this approach effective in controlling ascites. The benefit is limited by the fairly rapid diffusion of the antibody into the systemic circulation[99] so that myelosuppression is still the dose-limiting toxicity, as with intravenous radioimmunotherapy. Nevertheless, a therapeutic advantage is probably gained by this strategy for ovarian cancer confined to the peritoneal cavity. Intra-arterial therapy with radiolabelled antibody has been investigated for hepatic metastases of colorectal carcinoma via the hepatic artery and for brain glioma via the carotid artery[101]. This strategy has not been shown to be significantly superior to intravenous therapy, possibly because the slow clearance of antibody from the circulation means that most of the exposure of the tumour is to antibody which has recirculated rather than being on its first pass direct from the arterial catheter.

Second antibody

A second antibody directed against the primary (antitumour) antibody will accelerate the clearance of the latter from the circulation without causing a corresponding reduction in antibody localized within the tumour[24]. This has been shown to be effective in radioimmunotherapy[25]. Studies of cumulative radiation dose delivered by ^{131}I-labelled antibody in animal systems show, however, that the effective reduction of radiation dose to bone marrow, the most vulnerable tissue, is no more than 50%[17]. Findings are similar in studies in man[18].

Two phase systems

Natural effector mechanisms When antibodies bind to their specific antigen, they may change their conformation so as to activate systems such as the complement cascade or antibody-dependent cell-mediated cytotoxicity which destroy the antigen-bearing cell or organism. This confines the toxic action to the target site. Attempts to use antibodies simply as carriers of toxic agents may be too naive considering that the majority of antibody does not bind to tumour and is likely to be toxic to tissues through which it passes, or to be metabolized and excreted.

Prodrug activation Bagshawe *et al.*[102] have used an antitumour antibody linked to carboxypeptidase to localize to tumour. After waiting for clearance of this conjugate from the blood, a prodrug was given which is activated by carboxypeptidase to form a benzoic acid mustard. This is released at the tumour site and can eradicate xenografts of human choriocarcinoma in some nude mice. There is potential for production of other pairs of enzyme and prodrug. Systemic toxicity is minimized by generating the cytotoxic agent (which has a short halflife) at the tumour site.

Neutron capture therapy In neutron capture therapy, antitumour antibodies are labelled with boron. A tumour thus containing targeted boron will emit α particles when irradiated with thermal neutrons[103]. This approach is limited to tumours which are localized, and also by the limited availability of suitable neutron beam machines and by doubt about whether it would be possible to target enough boron.

Bispecific antibodies   Glennie *et al.*[104] constructed an F(ab')$_2$ in which one arm is directed against the tumour and the other against saporin, a ribosome inactivating toxin. This was investigated in an animal tumour model system and it was found that, although administration of antibody and saporin at separate sites had an antitumour effect, mixing saporin and the antibody before administration gave better results.

Therapeutic second antibody   A further approach advocated by Raso[105] and developed by Fodstad *et al.*[106] *in vitro* employs a second antibody (directed against the antitumour antibody) to carry abrin toxin, enhancing the efficiency of targeting in the manner of a double antibody immunoassay. This may be difficult to apply *in vivo* because of the need to eliminate nearly all the antitumour antibody from the blood and other normal tissues before giving the toxin-second antibody immunoconjugate.

Improving targeting to tumour cells

Antigen expression

In general, toxins and cytotoxic drugs must be internalized in the tumour cell to be effective. However, there is heterogeneity of antigen expression in most human tumours and it is very unlikely that all tumour cells will be targeted by the antibodies in use for common epithelial malignancies. Antibody-conjugated radionuclides and natural effector mechanisms will suffer less from this problem as 'bystander' cells, to which antibody has not bound, will also be affected. This is probably also true of prodrugs activated at the tumour site. Even so, Ceriani and Blank[66] have shown that a mixture of ^{131}I-labelled antibodies directed against different epitopes gives more effective radioimmunotherapy of xenografts of human colon carcinoma than single antibodies. Great variation between the efficiency of antibody localization in different patients is seen[13,18,79] and a system is needed to select one or more antibodies for individual patients.

Loss of antibody from tumour

Even though binding to tumour may be efficient, loss of bound activity appears to be substantial with radiolabelled antibodies. Techniques to prolong dwell time on tumours, such as concurrent administration of unconjugated antibody, have been described by Byers *et al.*[107].

Failure to achieve adequate antibody localization may also be due to poor access from the circulation, as discussed above.

Repeated therapy

When radiotherapy or chemotherapy eradicates cancer, it is almost always by repeated dose administration, each dose killing a proportion of the tumour cell population. It is highly likely that this will be the case with antibody targeted therapy, and the modest tumour responses seen with single-dose therapy to date are in keeping with this. However, repeated therapy is prevented by the formation of human antimouse antibody (HAMA) after one or more injections of mouse monoclonal antitumour antibody[45,72,108]. This causes hypersensitivity reactions and prevents antitumour antibody from localizing in the tumour. Various means of overcoming the problem have been investigated and a degree of success has already been achieved.

Immunosuppression

This approach is relevant both to suppression of the response to immunoglobulins as well as to immunogenic effector molecules, such as toxins[96] and enzymes linked to antibodies.

Cyclosporin A   The best results to date have been observed with this drug. Cyclosporin A is a powerful inhibitor of humoral immunity[109] and has been shown to prevent the antibody response to repeated injections of mouse monoclonal antibodies in rabbits[110]. A further study investigated the effect of cyclosporin A on the formation of HAMA in patients with CEA-producing tumours treated with repeated doses of ^{131}I-labelled mouse monoclonal antibody to CEA[26]. It was found that cyclosporin A permitted repeated therapy with antitumour monoclonal antibodies by suppressing HAMA formation. More antibody accumulated in the tumour with each dose and up to 4 times as many doses could usefully be given with cyclosporin A as without.

Cyclosporin A fails to suppress the secondary immune response[111] and is of no value once an anti-antibody response has developed. Concern that immunosuppression with cyclosporin A might accelerate tumour growth was not supported by the preliminary data reported by Ledermann *et al.*[26]

Cytotoxic drugs[112,113] have had limited success but it has been possible to induce tolerance to equine antilymphocyte globulin in some patients pretreated with cytotoxic immunosuppressive drugs and equine IgG that had been 'deaggregated' by ultracentrifugation[114]. Immunosuppression with large doses of cyclophosphamide has reduced the incidence of HAMA[113]. However, this is likely to lead to haematological toxicity which might compromise repeated therapy with immunoconjugates.

Modified immunoglobulin

F(ab')₂ fragments   These are less immunogenic than intact antibody[72] but human antimouse activity still occurs sufficiently frequently to prevent their repeated use.

Table 9.2 Comparison of methods of antibody targeted therapy

	Natural effector mechanism	Radionuclide	Cytotoxics	Toxin e.g. ricin	Two phase prodrug
Site of action	cell membrane	DNA	Cell division	Ribosomes	Cell division
Internalization necessary	No	No	Yes	Yes	No
Potency	++	+++	++	+++++	+++
Intrinsic resistance	No	Some	Yes	No	Some
Toxicity	Mild systemic	Bone marrow	?	?	?

Chimeric antibodies   Antibodies with low immunogenicity such as human–mouse hybrid antibodies or IgG with a mouse variable region and human constant region have been made[36,115,116]. It is unclear whether these antibodies would lead to the generation of an anti-idiotypic response. A clinical trial in patients with lymphoma[15] in whom no anti-antibody response was measurable does not resolve the problem because patients with lymphoma commonly fail to make anti-antibody responses[107,117]. This is thought to be a consequence of the immunosuppression which is a feature of lymphoma. Clinical trials in tumours not associated with immunosuppression are in progress and should resolve this issue.

Induction of tolerance   Anti-mouse antibodies are found less frequently in patients given an injection of a large dose of mouse antitumour antibody[118]. However, given weekly, this dose did not lead to tolerance[119]. The elimination of antigen-specific antibody forming cells by exposure to radiolabelled antigen has been achieved in mice[120] but not in patients, as treatment with large doses of radio-iodinated antitumour antibodies does not abolish the anti-antibody response[72] which is also detected in up to 60% of patients treated with the mouse anti-T cell antibody OKT3[121]. Wilkinson *et al.*[122] have coated antibodies with polyethylene glycol and shown that administration of these to mice renders them tolerant to subsequent administration of uncoated antibodies. Clinical trials are awaited.

CONCLUSIONS

There is now abundant evidence that antibodies can be targeted specifically to tumour cells. One of the greatest obstacles to using this for tumour eradication is the difficulty of targeting to sufficient tumour cells to eradicate the disease. The fact that most success has been in lymphoma may be because the antigens used as targets are present on a high proportion of tumour cells.

When fewer tumour cells bear the target antigen, strategies such as the use of β-emitting radionuclides which will kill 'bystander' cells may be effective: but improvement over the attempts at radiolabelled antibody therapy reported to date are needed. Toxicity to normal tissues through which radiolabelled antibody inevitably circulates is difficult to avoid altogether. However, much information about the macroscopic and microscopic distribution of antibodies is being obtained by monitoring radioactivity.

Natural effector mechanisms which are only activated when antibody reacts with its antigen should spare normal tissues. It remains to be seen whether this approach can be made sufficiently potent to eradicate established tumours, but the speed with which the relevant immune mechanisms are being elucidated suggests that progress can be expected.

Potency is a characteristic of targeted plant and bacterial toxins. If they can be internalized in a way which carries the toxin directly to its intracellular site of action in tumours whilst excretion through reticuloendothelial cells uses a different route which degrades them harmlessly, then their only drawback will be the need to target nearly all tumour cells. Prodrug activation at the tumour by antibody-targeted enzyme appears to have the potential to deal with all the problems. Activated drug is only produced at the tumour site if the system functions correctly. It can diffuse to non-antigen-bearing cells within the tumour mass and potent antitumour agents can be generated in the system.

A degree of patience is needed with the preclinical and clinical investigations of antibody targeted therapy. They all require that a number of different conditions be fulfilled for tumour killing to occur. This review has sought to define the more important of these. Progress is being made to an extent which justifies optimism about the eventual development of effective therapy of common malignancies.

Acknowledgements

The author is supported by the Cancer Research Campaign and is grateful to his colleagues in the Cancer Research Campaign Laboratories, Department of Medical Oncology, Charing Cross and Westminster Medical School with whom he has learnt about antibody targeting.

References

1. Macnalty, A. S. (1954). Emil Von Behring. *Br. Med. J.*, **1**, 668–670
2. Hericourt, J. and Richet, C. (1895). Traitement d'un cas de sarcome par la sérothérapie. *Hebd. C. R. Acad. Sci.*, **120**, 948–950
3. Pressman, D. and Korngold, L. (1953). The in vivo localisation of anti-Wagner osteogenic sarcoma antibodies. *Cancer*, **6**, 619
4. Bale, W. F., Spar, I. L., Goodland, R. L. and Woolfe, D. E. (1955). In vivo and in vitro studies of labeled antibodies against rat kidney and Walker carcinoma. *Proc. Soc. Exp. Biol. Med.*, **89**, 564–568
5. Mach, J-P., Carrel, S., Merenda, C., Sordat, B. and Cerottini, J-C. (1974). In vivo localisation of radiolabelled antibodies to carcinoembryonic antigen in human colon carcinoma grafted into nude mice. *Nature (London)*, **248**, 704–706
6. Quinones, J., Mizejarski, G. and Beierwaltes, W. H. (1971). Choriocarcinoma scanning

using radiolabelled antibodies to chorionic gonadotrophin. *J. Nucl. Med.*, **12**, 69–75

7. Primus, F. J., Wang, R. H., Goldenberg, D. M. and Hansen, H. J. (1973). Localisation of human GW-39 tumours in hamsters by radiolabelled heterospecific antibody to carcinoembryonic antigen. *Cancer Res.*, **37**, 2977–2982

8. Goldenberg, D. M., Preston, D. F., Primus, F. J. and Hanson, H. J. (1974). Photo-scan localisation of GW-39 tumours in hamsters using radiolabelled anticarcinoembryonic antigen immunoglobulin G. *Cancer Res.*, **34**, 1–9

9. Begent, R. H. J. (1985). Recent advances in tumour imaging: Use of radiolabelled antibodies. *Biochim. Biophys. Acta*, **780**, 151–166

10. Goldenberg, D. M., DeLand, F. H., Kim, E., Bennett, S., Primus, F. J., van Nagell, J. R., Estes, N., DeSimone, P. and Rayburn, P. (1978). Use of radiolabelled antibodies to carcinoembryonic antigen for the detection and localisation of diverse cancers by external photoscanning. *N. Engl. J. Med.*, **298**, 1384–1388

11. Begent, R. H. J., Searle, F., Stanway, G., Jewkes, R. F., Jones, B. E., Vernon, P. and Bagshawe, K. D. (1980). Radioimmunolocalisation of tumours by external scintigraphy after administration of 131I antibody to human chorionic gonadotrophin: preliminary communication. *J. R. Soc. Med.*, **73**, 624–630

12. Goldenberg, D. M., Kim, E. E., DeLand, F. H., Van Nagell, J. R. and Javadpour, N. (1980). Clinical radioimmunodetection of cancer with radioactive antibodies to human chorionic gonadotrophin. *Science*, **208**, 1284–1286

13. Mach, J-P., Carrel, S., Forni, M., Ritschard, J., Donath, A. and Alberto, P. (1980). Tumor localization of radiolabelled antibodies against carcinoembryonic antigen in patients with carcinoma. A critical evaluation. *N. Engl. J. Med.*, **303**, 5–10

14. Mach, J-P., Chatal, J. F., Lumbruso, J. D., Buchegger, F., Forni, M., Ritschard, J., Berche, C., Douillard, J. Y., Carrel, S., Herlyn, M., Steplewski, Z. and Koprowski, H. (1983). Tumour localisation in patients by radiolabelled monoclonal antibodies against colon carcinoma. *Cancer Res.*, **43**, 5593–5600

15. Hale, G., Dyer, M. J. S., Clark, M. R., Phillips, J. M., Marcus, R., Riechmann, L., Winter, G. and Waldmann, H. (1988). Remission induction in non-Hodgkin's lymphoma with reshaped human monoclonal antibody CAMPATH-1H. *Lancet*, **2**, 1394–1399

16. Dykes, P. W., Bradwell, A. R., Chapman, C. E. and Vaughan, A. T. M. (1987). Radioimmunotherapy of cancer: clinical studies and limiting factors. *Cancer Treat. Rev.*, **14**, 87–106

17. Pedley, R. B., Dale, R., Boden, J. A., Begent, R. H. J., Keep, P. A. and Green, A. J. (1989). The effect of second antibody clearance on the distribution and dosimetry of radiolabelled anti-CEA antibody in a human colonic tumour xenograft model. *Int. J. Cancer*, **43**, 713–718

18. Begent, R. H. J., Ledermann, J. A., Green, A. J., Bagshawe, K. D., Riggs, S. J., Searle, F., Keep, P. A., Adam, T., Dale, R. G. and Glaser, M. G. (1989). Antibody distribution and dosimetry in patients receiving radiolabelled antibody therapy for colorectal cancer. *Br. J. Cancer*, **60**, 406–412

19. Sharkey, R. M., Pykett, M. J., Siegal, J. A., Alger, E. A., Primus, F. J. and Goldenberg, D. M. (1987). Radioimmunotherapy of the GW-39 human colonic tumour xenograft with 131-I-labeled murine monoclonal antibody to carcinoembryonic antigen. *Cancer Res.*, **47**, 5672–5677

20. Buchegger, F., Vacca, A., Carrel, S., Schreyer, M. and Mach, J-P. (1988). Radioimmunotherapy of human colon carcinoma by 131-I-labelled monoclonal anti-CEA antibodies in a nude mouse model. *Int. J. Cancer*, **41**, 127–134

21. Covell, D. G., Barbet, J., Holton, O. D., Black, D. V., Parker, R. J. and Weinstein, J. N. (1986). Pharmacokinetics of monoclonal immunoglobulin G1, F(ab')$_2$ and Fab' in mice. *Cancer Res.*, **46**, 3969–3978

22. Harwood, P. J., Pedley, R. B., Boden, J. and Rogers, G. T. (1987). Significance of the circulatory clearance of tumour-localising IgG and F(ab')$_2$ for potential therapy studied in a CEA-producing xenograft model. *Tumor Biol.*, **8**, 19–25

23. Mattes, J. (1987). Biodistribution of antibodies after intraperitoneal or intravenous injection and effect of carbohydrate modifications. *J. Natl. Cancer Inst.*, **79**, 859–863

24. Begent, R. H. J., Keep, P. A., Green, A. J., Searle, F., Bagshawe, K. D., Jewkes, R. F., Jones, B. E., Barratt, G. M. and Ryman, B. E. (1982). Liposomally entrapped second antibody improves tumour imaging with radiolabelled (first) antitumour antibody. *Lancet*, **2**, 739–742

25. Begent, R. H. J., Bagshawe, K. D., Pedley, R. B., Searle, F., Ledermann, J. A., Green, A. J., Keep, P. A., Chester, K. A., Glaser, M. G. and Dale, R. G. (1987). Use of second antibody in radioimmunotherapy. *Natl. Cancer Inst. Monogr.*, **3**, 59–61

26. Ledermann, J. A., Begent, R. H. J., Bagshawe, K. D., Riggs, S. J., Searle, F., Glaser, M. G., Green, A. J. and Dale, R. G. (1988). Repeated antitumour antibody therapy in man with suppression of the host response by cyclosporin A. *Br. J. Cancer*, **58**, 654–657

27. Smyth, M. J., Pietersz, G. A. and Mckenzie, I. F. C. (1987). Use of vasoactive agents to increase tumour perfusion and the antitumour efficacy of drug-monoclonal antibody conjugates. *J. Natl. Cancer Inst.*, **79**, 1367–1373

28. Stickney, D. R., Gridley, D. S., Kirk, G. A. and Slater, J. M. (1987). Enhancement of monoclonal binding to melanoma with single dose radiation or hyperthermia. *Natl. Cancer Inst.*, **3**, 47–52

29. Msirikale, J. S., Klein, J. L., Schroeder, J. and Order, S. E. (1987). Radiation enhancement of radiolabelled antibody deposition in tumours. *Int. J. Radiat. Oncol. Biol. Phys.*, **13**, 1839

30. Gerlowski, L. E. and Jain, R. K. (1986). Microvascular permeability of normal and neoplastic tissues. *Microvasc. Res.*, **31**, 288–305

31. Sutherland, R., Buchegger, F., Schreyer, M., Vacca, A. and Mach, J-P. (1987). Penetration and binding of radiolabelled anti-carcinoembryonic antigen monoclonal antibodies and their antigen binding fragments in human colon multicellular tumor spheroids. *Cancer Res.*, **47**, 1627–1633

32. Kwok, C. S., Cole, S. E. and Liao, S-K. (1988). Uptake kinetics of monoclonal antibodies by human malignant melanoma multicell spheroids. *Cancer Res.*, **48**, 1856–1863

33. Jain, R. K. (1988). Determinants of tumour blood flow: a review. *Cancer Res.*, **48**, 2641–2658

34. Fand, I., Sharkey, R. M., Primus, F. J., Cohen, S. A. and Goldenberg, D. M. (1987). Relationship of antibody localisation and cell viability in a xenografted human cancer model as measured by whole body autoradiography. *Cancer Res.*, **47**, 2177–2183

35. Pedley, R. B., Bowden, J., Keep, P.A., Harwood, P. J., Green, A.J. and Rogers, G. T. (1987). Relationship between tumour size and uptake of radiolabelled anti-CEA in a colon tumour xenograft. *Eur. J. Nucl. Med.*, **13**, 197–202

36. Riechmann, L., Clark, M., Waldmann, H. and Winter, G. (1988). Reshaping human antibodies for therapy. *Nature (London)*, **332**, 323–327

37. Wahl, R. L., Liebert, M. and Wilson, B. S. (1986). The influence of monoclonal antibody dose on tumour uptake of radiolabeled antibody. *Cancer Drug Deliv.*, **3**, 243–249

38. Rogers, G. T., Pedley, R. B., Bowden, H., Harwood, P. J. and Bagshawe, K. D. (1986). Effect of dose escalation of a monoclonal anti-CEA IgG on tumour localisation and tissue distribution in nude mice xenografted with human colon carcinoma. *Cancer Immunol. Immunother.*, **23**, 107–112

39. Leichner, P. K., Klein, J. L., Siegelman, S. S., Ettinger, D. S. and Order, S. E. (1983). Dosimetry of 131-I-labelled antiferritin in hepatoma: specific activities in the tumour and liver. *Cancer Treat. Rep.*, **67**, 647–658

40. Committee for Proprietary Medicinal Products, Ad hoc Working Party on Biotechnology/Pharmacy (1988). Guidelines on the production and quality control of monoclonal antibodies of murine origin intended for use in man. *Tibtech*, **6**, G5–G8

41. Committee for Proprietary Medicinal Products, Ad hoc Working Party on Biotechnology/Pharmacy (1987). Guidelines on the production and quality control of medicinal products derived by recombinant DNA technology. *Tibtech*, **5**, G1–G4

42. (1986) Operation manual for control of production, preclinical toxicology and phase 1 trials of anti tumour antibodies and drug antibody conjugates. *Br. J. Cancer*, **54**, 557–568

43. Stevenson, G. T., Elliot, E. V. and Stevenson, F. K. (1977). Idiotypic determinants on the surface immunoglobulin of neoplastic lymphocytes: a therapeutic target. *Fed. Proc.*, **36**, 2268–2271

44. Stevenson, G. T. (1980). Preliminary experience in treating lymphocytic leukaemia with antibody to immunoglobulin idiotypes on the cell surface. *Br. J. Caner*, **42**, 495

45. Meeker, T. C., Lowder, J., Maloney, D. G., Miller, R. A., Thielmans, K., Warnke, R. and Levy, R. (1985). A clinical trial of anti-idiotype therapy for B cell malignancy. *Blood*, **65**, 1349–1363

46. Koprowski, H., Herlyn, D., Lubeck, M., DeFreitas, E. and Sears, H. F. (1984). Human anti-idiotype antibodies in cancer patients: Is modulation of the immune response beneficial

for the patient? *Proc. Natl. Acad. Sci. USA*, **81**, 216–219

47. Jerne, N. K. (1974). Towards a network theory of the immune system. *Ann. Inst. Pasteur Immunol.*, **15C**, 373

48. Battacharia-Chatterjee, M., Chatterjee, S. K., Vasile, S., Seon, B. K. and Kohler, H. (1988). Idiotypic vaccines against human T cell leukaemia. *J. Immunol.*, **141**, 1398–1403

49. Herlyn, D., Wettendorf, M., Schmoll, E., Iliopoulos, D., Schedel, I., Dreikhausen, U., Raab, R., Ross, A. H., Jaksche, H., Scriba, M. and Koprowski, H. (1987). Antiidiotype immunisation of cancer patients modulation of the immune response. *Proc. Natl. Acad. Sci. USA*, **84**, 8055–8059

50. George, A. J. T., Folkard, S. G., Hamblin, T. and Stevenson, F. K. (1988). Idiotypic vaccination as a treatment for B cell lymphoma. *J. Immunol.*, **141**, 2166–2174

51. Campbell, M. J., Esserman, L. and Levy, R. (1988). Immunotherapy of established murine B cell lymphoma; combination of idiotypic immunization and cyclophosphamide. *J. Immunol.*, **141**, 3227–3233

52. Matsui, M., Nakanishi, T., Nogouchi, T. and Ferrone, S. (1988). Synergistic in vitro and in vivo anti-tumour effect of daunomycin-anti-96-kDa melanoma-associated antigen monoclonal antibody CL 207 conjugate and recombinant IFN-gamma. *J. Immunol.*, **141**, 1410–1417

53. Humm, J. L. (1986). Dosimetric aspects of radiolabelled antibodies for tumour therapy. *J. Nucl. Med.*, **27**, 1490–1497

54. Harrison, A. and Royle, L. (1987). Efficacy of astatine-211-labelled monoclonal antibody in treatment of murine T cell lymphoma. *Natl. Cancer Inst. Monogr.*, **3**, 157–158

55. Kurtzman, S. H., Russo, A., Mitchell, J. B., DeGraff, W., Sindelar, W. F., Brechbiel, M. W., Gansow, O. A., Freidman, A. M., Hines, J. J., Gamson, J. and Atcher, R. W. (1988). 212-Bismuth linked to an antipancreatic carcinoma antibody: model for alpha-particle-emitter radiotherapy. *J. Natl. Cancer Inst.*, **80**, 449–452

56. Leichner, P. K., Klein, J. L., Garrison, J. B., Jenkins, R. E., Nickloff, E. L., Ettinger, D. S. and Order, S. E. (1981). Dosimetry of 131I-labelled anti-ferritin in hepatoma: a model for radioimmunoglobulin dosimetry. *Int. J. Radiat. Oncol. Biol. Phys.*, **7**, 323–333

57. Hammond, N. D., Moldofsky, P. J., Beardsley, M. R. and Mulhern, C. B. (1984). External imaging for quantitation of distribution of I-131 F(ab')2 fragments of monoclonal antibody in humans. *Med. Phys.*, **11**, 778–783

58. Ghose, T. and Guclu, A. (1974). Cure of a mouse lymphoma with radio-iodinated antibody. *Eur. J. Cancer*, **10**, 787–792

59. Zalcberg, J. R., Thompson, C. H., Lichtenstein, M. and McKenzie, F. C. (1984). Tumor immunotherapy in the mouse with the use of 131-I-labelled monoclonal antibodies. *J. Natl. Cancer Inst.*, **72**, 697–704

60. Jones, D. H., Goldman, A., Gordon, I., Pritchard, J., Gregory, B. J. and Kenshead, J. T. (1985). Therapeutic application of a radiolabelled monoclonal antibody in nude mice xenografted with human neuroblastoma: tumoricidal effects and distribution studies.

61. Lee, Y-S., Bullard, E., Zalutsky, M. R., Coleman, R. E., Wikstrand, C. J., Friedman, H. S., Colapinto, E. V. and Bigner, D. D. (1988). Therapeutic efficacy of antiglioma mesenchymal extracellular matrix 131-I-radiolabelled murine monoclonal antibody in a human glioma xenograft model. *Cancer Res.*, **48**, 559–566

62. Wakabayashi, S., Okamoto, S. and Taniguchi, M. (1984). Anti-tumour effects of radiolabelled syngeneic monoclonal anti-melanoma antibodies. *Gann*, **75**, 707–713

63. Chiou, R. K., Vessella, R. L., Limas, C., Shafer, R. B., Elson, M. K., Arfman, E. W. and Lange, P. H. (1988). Monoclonal antibody-targeted radiotherapy of renal cell carcinoma using a nude mouse model. *Cancer*, **61**, 1766–1775

64. Badger, C. C., Crohn, K. A., Shulman, H., Flourny, N. and Bernstein, I. D. (1986). Experimental radioimmunotherapy of murine lymphoma with 131I-labelled anti-T-cell antibodies. *Cancer Res.*, **46**, 6223

65. Etoh, T., Takahashi, H., Maie, M., Ohnuma, N. and Tanabe, M. (1988). Tumor imaging by antineuroblastoma monoclonal antibody and its application to treatment. *Cancer*, **62**, 1282–1286

66. Ceriani, R. L. and Blank, E. W. (1988). Experimental therapy of human breast tumours with 131I-labelled monoclonal antibodies prepared against the human milk fat globule. *Cancer Res.*, **48**, 4664–4672

67. Sharkey, R. M., Kaltovich, F. A., Shih, L. B., Fand, I., Govelitz, G. and Goldenberg, D. M.

(1988). Radioimmunotherapy of human colonic cancer xenografts with 90Y-labelled monoclonal antibodies to carcinoembryonic antigen. *Cancer Res.*, **48**, 3270–3275

68. Order, S. E., Stillwagon, G. B., Klein, J. L., Leichner, P. K., Siegelman, S. S., Fishman, E. K., Ettinger, D. S., Haulk, T., Kopher, K., Finney, K., Surdyke, M., Self, S. and Leibel, S. (1985). Iodine 131 antiferritin, a new treatment modality in hepatoma: A Radiation Oncology Group study. *J. Clin. Oncol.*, **3**, 1573–1582

69. Rosen, S. T., Zimmer, M., Goldman-Leikin, R., Gordon, L. I., Kazikiewicz, J. M., Kaplan, E. H., Variakojis, D., Marder, R. J., Dykewicz, M. S., Pierges, A., Silverstein, E. A., Roenigk, H. H. and Spies, S. M. (1987). Radioimmunodetection and radioimmunotherapy of cutaneous T cell lymphomas using an 131I-labelled monoclonal antibody: An Illinois cancer council study. *J. Clin. Oncol.*, **5**, 562–573

70. DeNardo, S. J., DeNardo, G. L., O'Grady, L. F., Levy, N. B., Mills, S. L., Macey, D. J., McGahan, J. P., Miller, C. H. and Epstein, A. L. (1988). Pilot studies of radioimmunotherapy of B cell lymphoma and leukaemia using I-131 Lym-1 monoclonal antibody. *Antibody Immunoconjugates Radiopharm.*, **1**, 17–33

71. Lenhard, R. E., Order, S. E., Sprungberg, J. J., Asbell, S. O. and Leibel, S. A. (1985). Isotopic immunoglobulin: A new systemic therapy for advanced Hodgkins disease. *J. Clin. Oncol.*, **3**, 1296–1300

72. Carrasquillo, J. A., Crohn, K. A., Beaumier, P., McGuffin, R. W., Brown, J. P., Hellstrom, K. E., Hellstrom, I. and Larson, S. M. (1984). Diagnosis of and therapy for solid tumours with radiolabelled antibodies and immune fragments. *Cancer Treat. Rep.*, **68**, 317–328

73. Lashford, L., Jones, D., Prichard, J., Gordon, I., Breatnach, F. and Kemshead, J. T. (1987). Therapeutic application of radiolabelled monoclonal antibody UJ13A in children with disseminated neuroblastoma. *Natl. Cancer Inst.*, **3**, 53–57

74. Leichner, P. K., Yang, N-C., Frenkel, T. L., Loudenslager, D. M., Hawkins, W. G., Klein, J. L. and Order, S. E. (1988). Dosimetry and treatment planning for 90Y-labelled antiferritin in hepatoma. *Int. J. Radiat. Oncol. Biol. Phys.*, **14**, 1033–1042

75. Thomas, S. R., Maxan, H. R. and Kereiaakes, J. C. (1976). In vivo quantitation of lesion radioactivity using external counting methods. *Med. Phys.*, **3**, 253–255

76. Green, A. J., Dewhurst, S. E., Begent, R. H. J., Bagshawe, K. D. and Riggs, S. J. (1990). Accurate quantitation of ^{131}I distribution by gamma camera imaging. *Eur. J. Nucl. Med.* (in press)

77. Benau, R. S., Cicale, N. R., Sonenberg, M. and Rawson, R. W. (1962). The relation of radioiodine dosimetry to results and complications in the treatment of metastatic thyroid cancer. *Am.J. Roentgenol.*, **87**, 171–182

78. Lewis, J. C. M., Bagshawe, K. D. and Keep, P. A. (1982). The distribution of parenterally administered antibody to CEA in colorectal xenografts. Preliminary findings. *Oncodev. Biol. Med.*, **3**, 161–168

79. Estaban, J. M., Colcher, D., Sugarbaker, P., Carrasquillo, J. A., Bryant, G., Thor, A., Reynolds, J. C., Larson, S. M. and Schlom, J. (1987). Quantitative and qualitative aspects of radiolocalization in colon cancer patients of intravenously administered MAb B72.3. *Int. J. Cancer*, **39**, 50–59

80. Begent, R. H. J., Keep, P. A., Searle, F., Green, A. J., Mitchell, H. D. C., Jones, B. E., Dent, J., Pendower, J. E. H., Parkins, R. A., Reynolds, K. W., Cooke, T. G., Allen Mersh, T. and Bagshawe, K. D. (1986). Radioimmunolocalisation and selection for surgery in recurrent colorectal cancer. *Br. J. Surg.*, **73**, 64–67

81. Mathe, G., Loc, T. B. and Bernard, J. (1958). Effet sur la leukaemie 1210 de la souris d'une combinason part diazotation d'amethopterine et de a-globulines de hamsters porteurs de cette leukaemie par heterograffe. *C. R. Acad. Sci. (D) Paris*, **246**, 1626–1628

82. Embleton, M. J. (1987). Drug-targeting by monoclonal antibodies. *Br. J. Cancer*, **55**, 227–231

83. Bourdon, M. A., Coleman, R. E. and Bigner, D. D. (1984). The potential of monoclonal antibodies as carriers of radiation and drugs for immunodetection and therapy of brain tumours. *Prog. Exp. Tumour Res.*, **28**, 79–101

84. Garnett, M. C. and Baldwin, R. W. (1986). An improved synthesis of a methotrexate-albumin-791T/36 monoclonal antibody conjugate cytotoxic to osteogenic sarcoma cell lines. *Cancer Res.*, **46**, 2407

85. Takahashi, T., Yamaguchi, T., Kitamura, K., Suzuyama, H., Honda, M., Yokota, T., Kotanagi, H., Takahashi, M. and Hashimoto, Y. (1988). Clinical application of monoclonal

antibody-drug conjugates for immunotargeting chemotherapy of colorectal carcinoma. *Cancer*, **61**, 881–888

86. Vitetta, E. S., Fulton, R. J., May, R. D., Till, M. and Uhr, J. W. (1987). Redesigning nature's poisons to create anti-tumor reagents. *Science*, **238**, 1098–1104

87. Thorpe, P. E. and Ross, W. C. J. (1982). The preparation and cytotoxic properties of antibody–toxin conjugates. *Immunol. Rev.*, **62**, 119

88. Endo, Y. and Tsurugi, K. (1987). RNA *N*-glycosidase activity of ricin A chain. *J. Biol. Chem.*, **262**, 8128–8130

89. Lambert, J., Senter, P., Yau-Young, A., Blatter, M. and Goldmacher, V. (1985). Purified immunotoxins that are reactive with human lymphoid cells. *J. Biol. Chem.*, **260**, 12035–12041

90. Press, O. W., Martin, P. J., Thorpe, P. E. and Vitetta, E. S. (1988). Ricin A-chain containing immunotoxins directed against different epitopes on the CD2 molecule differ in their ability to kill normal and malignant T cells. *J. Immunol.*, **141**, 4410–4417

91. Bourrie, B. J. P., Casellas, P., Blythman, H. E. and Jansen, R. K. (1986). Study on the plasma clearance of antibody-ricin A chain immunotoxins: Evidence for specific recognition sites on the A chain that mediate rapid clearance of the immunotoxin. *Eur. J. Biochem.*, **155**, 1

92. Blakey, D. C., Skillester, D. N., Price, R. J. and Thorpe, P. E. (1988). Uptake of native and deglycosylated ricin A chain immunotoxins by murine liver parenchymal and non-parenchymal cells in vitro and in vivo. *Biochem. Biophys. Acta*, **968**, 172

93. Byers, V. S., Pimm, M. V., Pawluczyk, I., Lee, H. M., Scannon, P. J. and Baldwin, R. W. (1987). Biodistribution of ricin toxin A-chain monoclonal antibody 791T/36 immunotoxins and the influence of hepatic blocking agents. *Cancer Res.*, **47**, 5277

94. Spitler, L. E., Rio, M., Khentigan, A. *et al.* (1987). Therapy of patients with malignant melanoma using a monoclonal antimelanoma antibody-ricin A chain immunotoxin. *Cancer Res.*, **47**, 1717–1723

95. Byers, V. S. and Baldwin, R. W. (1988). Therapeutic strategies with monoclonal antibodies and immunoconjugates. *Immunology*, **65**, 329–225

96. Kernan, N. A., Byers, V. S., Scannon, P. J., Mischak, R. P., Brockstein, J., Flomenberg, N., Dupont, B. and O'Reilly, R. J. (1988). Treatment of steroid-resistant graft-vs-host disease by in vivo administration of an anti-T-cell ricin A-chain immunotoxin. *J. Am. Med. Assoc.*, **259**, 3154–3157

97. Lashford, L. S., Davies, A. G., Richardson, R. B., Bourne, S. P., Bullimore, J. A., Eckert, H., Kemshead, J. T. and Coakham, H. B. (1988). A pilot study of 131I- monoclonal antibodies in the therapy of leptomeningeal tumors. *Cancer*, **61**, 857–868

98. Pectasides, D., Stewart, S., Courtney-Luck, N., Rampling, R., Munro, A. J., Krausz, T., Dhokia, B., Snook, D., Hooker, G., Durbin, H., Taylor-Papadimitiou, J., Bodmer, w. F. and Epenetos, A. A. (1986). Antibody-guided irradiation of malignant pleural and pericardial effusions. *Br. J. Cancer*, **53**, 727–732

99. Epentos, A. A., Monro, A. J., Stewart, S., Rampling, R., Lambert, H. E., McKenzie, C. G., Soutter, P., Rahemtulla, A., Hooker, G., Sivolapenko, G. B., Snook, D., Courtenay-Luck, N., Dhokia, B., Krausz, T. and Taylor-Papadimitriou, J. (1987). Antibody-guided irradiation of advanced ovarian cancer with intraperitoneally administered radiolabelled monoclonal antibodies. *J. Clin. Oncol.*, **5**, 1890–1899

100. Ward, B., Mather, S., Shephard, J., Crowther, M., Hawkins, L., Britton, K. and Slevin, M. L. (1988). The treatment of intraperitoneal malignant disease with monoclonal antibody guided 131I radiotherapy. *Br. J. Cancer*, **58**, 658–662

101. Epenetos, A. A., Courtenay-Luck, N., Pickering, D., Hooker, G., Durbin, H., Lavender, J. P. and Mckenzie, C. G. (1985). Antibody guided irradiation of brain glioma by arterial infusion of radioactive monoclonal antibody against epidermal growth factor receptor and blood group A antigen. *Br. Med. J.*, **290**, 1463–1466

102. Bagshawe, K. D., Springer, C. J., Searle, F., Antoniw, P., Sharma, S. K., Melton, R. G. and Sherwood, R. F. (1988). A cytotoxic agent can be generated selectively at cancer sites. *Br. J. Cancer*, **58**, 700–703

103. Mizusawa, E., Dahlman, H. L., Bennett, S. J., Goldenberg, D. M. and Hawthorne, M. F. (1982). Neutron-capture therapy of human cancer: in vitro results on the preparation of boron-labelled antibodies to carcinoembryonic antigen. *Proc. Natl. Acad. Sci. USA*, **79**, 3011–3014

104. Glennie, M. J., Brennand, D. M., Bryden, F., McBride, H. M., Stirpe, F., Worth, A. T. and Stevenson, G. T. (1988). Bispecific F(ab')2 antibody for the delivery of saporin in the treatment of lymphoma. *J. Immunol.*, **141**, 3662–3670

105. Raso, V. (1982). Antibody mediated delivery of toxic molecules to antigen bearing target cells. *Immunol. Rev.*, **62**, 93–117

106. Fodstad, O., Kvalheim, G. and Pihl, A. (1988). A new indirect approach to the therapeutic use of immunotoxins. *J. Natl. Cancer Inst.*, **80**, 439–443

107. Byers, V. S., Pawlucyzk, I., Berry, N., Durrant, L. Robins, R. A., Garnett, M. C., Price, M. R. and Baldwin, R. W. (1988). Potentiation of anti-carcinoembryonic antigen immunotoxin cytotoxicity by monoclonal antibodies reacting with co-expressed carcinoembryonic antigen epitopes. *J. Immunol.*, **140**, 4050–4055

108. Shawler, D. L., Bartholomew, R. M., Smith, L. M. and Dillman, R. O. (1985). Human immune response to multiple injections of murine monoclonal IgG. *J. Immunol.*, **135**, 1530–1535

109. Borel, J. F., Feurer, C., Gubler, H. U. and Stahelin, H. (1976). Biological effects of cyclosporin A: a new antilymphocytic agent. *Agents Actions*, **6**, 468

110. Ledermann, J. A., Begent, R. H. J. and Bagshawe, K. D. (1988). Cyclosporin A prevents the anti-murine antibody response to a monoclonal antitumour antibody in rabbits. *Br. J. Cancer*, **58**, 562–566

111. Lindsey, N. J., Harris, K. R., Norman, H. B., Smith, J. L., Lee, H. A. and Slapek, M. (1982). The effect of cyclosporin A on the primary and secondary immune responses in the rabbit. *Transplant. Proc.*, **12**, 252–555

112. Miller, R. A., Oseroff, A. R., Stratte, P. and Levy, R. (1983). Monoclonal antibody therapeutic trials in seven patients with T cell lymphoma. *Blood*, **62**, 988–995

113. Thistlethwaite, J. R., Cosimi, A. B., Delmomico, F. L., Rubin, R. H., Talkoff-Rubin, N., Nelson, P. W., Fang, L. and Russell, P. S. (1984). Evolving the use of OKT3 monoclonal antibody for the treatment of renal allogroft rejection. *Transplantation*, **38**, 695–701

114. Rossen, R. D., Butler, W. T., Nora, J. J. and Fernbach, D. J. (1971). Preventing antibody formation to anti-lymphocyte globulin in man. *J. Immunol.*, **106**, 11–19

115. Sun, L. K., Curtis, P., Rakowicz-Szulczynska, E., Ghrayeb, J., Chang, N., Morison, S. L. and Koprowski, H. (1987). Chimeric antibody with human constant regions and mouse variable regions directed against carcinoma associated antigen 17-1A. *Proc. Natl. Acad. Sci. USA*, **84**, 214–218

116. Beidler, C. B., Ludwig, J. R., Cardenas, J., Phelps, J., Papworth, C. G., Melcher, E., Sierzega, M., Myers, L. J., Unger, B. W., Fisher, M., Davd, G. S. and Johnson, M. J. (1988). Cloning and high level expression of a chimeric antibody with specificity for human carcinoembryonic antigen. *J. Immunol.*, **141**, 4053–4060

117. Schroff, R. W., Foon, K. A., Beatty, S. M., Oldham, R. K. and Morgan, A. C. (1985). Human anti-murine immunoglobulin responses in patients receiving monoclonal antibody therapy. *Cancer Res.*, **45**, 879–885

118. Sears, H. F., Herlyn, D., Steplewski, Z. and Koprowski, H. (1984). Effects of monoclonal antibody immunotherapy on patients with gastrointestinal carcinoma. *J. Biol. Respir. Med.*, **3**, 138–150

119. Saleh, M., Khazaehli, M., Peterson, R., Thompson, R., Carrano, R. and LoBuglio, A. (1986). Immune response to repeated large doses of mouse monoclonal antibody 17-1A. *Proc. Am. Soc. Clin. Oncol.*, **5**, 224

120. Ada, G. L. and Bryt, P. (1969). Specific inactivation of antigen reactive cells with 125-I-labelled antigen. *Nature (London)*, **222**, 1291–1292

121. Jaffers, G. J., Fuller, T. C., Cosimi, B., Russell, P. S., Winn, H. J. and Colvin, R. B. (1986). Monoclonal antibody therapy. Anti idiotypic and non-idiotypic antibodies to OKT3 arising despite intense immunosuppression. *Transplantation*, **41**, 572

122. Wilkinson, I., Jackson, C-J. C., Lang, G. M., Holford-Strevens, V. and Sehon, A. H. (1987). Tolerance induction in mice by conjugates of monoclonal immunoglobulins and monomethoxypolyethylene glycol: Transfer of tolerance by T cells and by T cell extracts. *J. Immunol.*, **139**, 326–331

10
Dietary intervention trials in subjects at high risk for breast cancer

N.F. BOYD, M. COUSINS AND V. MCGUIRE

INTRODUCTION

Rationale for breast cancer prevention studies

Breast cancer incidence and mortality vary widely around the world. The disease is approximately 7 times more common in women in Europe and North America than in women in Japan and other Asian countries[1]. International differences in disease rates are not due to inherited differences between populations, but rather to some environmental differences, because migrants who move from low-risk to high-risk countries acquire the breast cancer incidence of their adoptive country[2]. This change in risk may take two or more generations, as with Japanese migrants to The United States[3], or may take place more quickly, as it has with Polish migrants to the US and Italian migrants to Australia[4]. Further, breast cancer rates within some low-risk countries have changed substantially over time[2]. For example, increases in age-specific breast cancer incidence have been observed in Japan and Iceland, providing additional evidence that environmental factors can influence breast cancer risk. Although the identity of the environmental factors that influence breast cancer risk is currently unknown, there are reasons, discussed below, for believing that diet may be one of them.

Requirements for clinical trials of breast cancer prevention

Several conditions must be met before clinical trials of breast cancer prevention can be carried out. Because breast cancer is an uncommon event, for intervention trials to be feasible, it must be possible to select women at substantially increased risk for the disease, and it must be possible to identify an intervention believed to be capable of modifying risk. Further, subjects in the trial must comply with the intervention. Clearly, the more that is understood about mechanisms of disease causation, the easier it will be to identify high-risk subjects, to select strategies for preventive intervention and to assess the success of those interventions.

In this chapter, four issues relevant to intervention trials in women at high risk for breast cancer are considered. First, the evidence is reviewed that the parenchymal pattern of the breast on mammography can be used to identify women at increased risk of breast cancer. Next, the evidence is reviewed that dietary fat intake may influence breast cancer risk, and experience described with a clinical trial of dietary fat reduction in women with high-risk mammographic paterns. Finally, the evidence is discussed that plasma lipids are influenced by risk factors for breast cancer, including dietary fat, and may be biochemical markers of breast cancer risk.

THE IDENTIFICATION OF WOMEN AT INCREASED RISK FOR BREAST CANCER

Risk factors for breast cancer

There is an extensive literature describing factors that influence breast cancer risk[5-7]. In general, these factors do not define groups at substantially increased risk of breast cancer and do not suggest strategies that might be deployed to intervene and modify risk. In the past decade or so, attention has been directed to the possibility that the mammographic pattern of the breast might be susceptible to modification.

Mammographic dysplasia and breast cancer risk

It is widely recognized by radiologists that the appearance of the breast parenchyma seen on mammography varies between women. In 1976, Wolfe proposed a classification of the parenchymal pattern of the breast that appeared to distinguish women at different levels of risk of contracting breast cancer[8]. Wolfe's classification contained four categories designated N (where the breast parenchyma comprised only fat), DY (sheet-like or nodular densities in the parenchyma) and P1 and P2 (the appearance of 'prominent ducts'). Several other studies have now shown that the appearance of the breast parenchyma on mammography does provide information about breast cancer risk, and this work has been the subject of two recent reviews[9,10]. The mammographic appearance of densities referred to as DY or 'dysplasia' has been found by several workers to be associated with an increased risk of breast cancer, and this increase in risk appears to persist for years after the appearance is noted. The available evidence indicates that mammographic dysplasia is a risk factor for breast cancer that acts independently of other risk factors.

In our own previous work, we have found that radiologists can reliably identify mammographic dysplasia[11], and also that the relationship of mammographic dysplasia to breast cancer risk is strongly influenced by the age of the subjects studied, the source of subjects that are used as controls[12] and the proportion of the breast volume that is occupied by the radiological signs of dysplasia[13]. Further, as is described further below, the extensiveness of radiological dysplasia has been found to be associated with histological atypia on breast biopsy.

In previous work, we found that, in women aged less than 50, extensive mammographic dysplasia was strongly associated with breast cancer with odds ratios that varied from 4.9 to 7.4 according to radiologist, while, in older women, mammographic dysplasia was only weakly associated with breast cancer risk. Multivariate analysis showed that the association of mammographic dysplasia with breast cancer risk could not be explained by other known risk factors for the disease, indicating that it is an independent risk factor for breast cancer.

This association is very similar to that found by other workers who have used similar methods of quantitatively classifying dysplasia. Brisson et al.[14] found in a case control study that extensive mammographic dysplasia in women aged 25–44 was associated with breast cancer with an odds ratio of 7, and Wolfe et al.[15], using a planimeter to obtain a quantitative measure of the extent of mammographic density, found in a case control study that, in women under the age of 53, dysplasia in more than 75% of the breast volume was associated with breast cancer with an odds ratio of 7. Brisson et al. have also found, in a recently published study based upon a very large cohort of women, that the risk associated with mammographic density is greater in women aged less than 50 and persists for at least 9 years after the radiological appearance is first noted, but no attempt at quantitative classification of images had been made[16].

Relationship between histological and radiological indicators of breast cancer risk

The work of Wellings and Jensen[17,19,20] and of Page et al.[18] and of Dupont and Page[21] has established that some types of non-malignant lesions characterized by proliferation of the breast epithelium are associated with increased risk for the subsequent development of cancer. Their work has also developed criteria for the recognition of such lesions, and has defined histological, cytological and other features which influence the associated degree of risk of breast cancer.

Jensen, Rice and Wellings[19] and Wellings and Jensen[20], using a method of examining 2 mm thick sections of whole breast tissue with a subgross sampling technqiue and histological confirmation, showed that atypical lobules were found approximately 4 times more frequently in the breasts of women with breast cancer than in breasts taken from random autopsies, and drew attention to the similarity of these lesions to the hyperplastic alveolar nodule found in mice that has been directly shown by experiment to be premalignant.

These studies have also focused attention on the 'terminal ductal lobular unit' (TDLU), the hormonally responsive secretory unit of the breast, as the site where premalignant lesions are most likely to occur and the probable site of origin of breast cancer.

The relevance to risk of breast cancer of the method of grading atypia devised by Wellings and Jensen has been confirmed by the work of Dupont and Page[21] in a cohort study involving the follow up of more than 10 000 women who had undergone breast biopsies for benign disease. Using criteria for atypia that were similar to those used by Wellings and Jensen for 'severe atypia', Dupont and Page found a 5.3-fold increase in risk for those with atypia compared with somen of the same age with non-proliferative lesions. This risk rose to 11 fold if atypia were accompanied by a family history of breast cancer. Similar findings have been reported by other large studies that have used comparable methods of classification[22-24].

Several studies have now examined the association between these histological changes and the mammographic appearances whose association with breast cancer risk was discussed above. Wellings and Wolfe[25], using the method of histological classification described by Wellings and Jensen, reported an association between the higher risk histological grades and the P2 and DY mammographic patterns in a series of 143 patients.

Bright et el.[26] compared xeroradiographic and histological findings in women with benign breast disease and reported associations between mammographic dysplasia and extralobular fibrosis and epithelial hyperplasia, but did not grade the epithelium.

Fisher and co-workers[27] compared the histology and radiology of breast from women with cancer and fibrocystic disease and found no association between epithelial change and mammographic appearance. The selection as a comparison group of women with fibrocystic disease may, however, have led to a falsely negative conclusion. Further, the mammographic classification was based on specimen radiology, which may not be comparable to whole breast radiology.

Moskowitz et al.[28] found no association between epithelial hyperplasia and mammographic pattern in women having breast biopsies as a result of attending a screening centre. However, no method of grading was employed, and, indeed, no explicit mention of pathology review is made in the report.

Urbanski et al.[29] examined the association between the extent of mammographic dysplasia and ductal prominence in the mammogram and histological patterns in the terminal duct lobular unit (TDLU). Surgical biopsies from a consecutive series of women aged 50 or less were reviewed and classified, without knowledge of mammographic pattern, according to the grade of the epithelium in the TDLU. Mammograms from the same subjects were independently classified according to the extent of the radiological signs of dysplasia and ductal prominence. Histological grade and the extent of mammographic dysplasia were found to be significantly associated and atypia in the TDLU was found more frequently in those with extensive mammographic dysplasia. No association was found between the severity of dysplasia and ductal prominence.

These results add to evidence that extensive mammographic dysplasia in women aged less than 50 is a risk factor for breast cancer and provide a biological basis for that association. These results do not indicate, however, that histological changes in the TDLU are responsible for the radiological densities with which they are associated.

RATIONALE FOR THE SELECTION OF DIETARY FAT AS AN INTERVENTION

Animal evidence

Animal experiments showing that dietary fat intake influences mammary carcinogenesis have been the subject of several recent reviews[30,31]. Increasing dietary intake of fat is associated with an increase in the number of animals that develop tumours, an increase in the number of tumours that develop per animal and, in experiments involving carcinogens, a reduction in the latent interval before the appearance of tumours. The effects of dietary fat intake on mammary carcinogenesis have been demonstrated in several rodent models involving spontaneous, carcinogen-induced and hormone-induced tumours. The effects of dietary fat on mammary carcinogenesis appear to be greater with unsaturated than with saturated fatty acids. However, some long chain unsaturated fatty acids, such as eicosapentanoic acid, may inhibit carcinogenesis. Dietary fat appears to act at the promotional stage of carcinogenesis and the demonstrated effects of high-fat diets include an increase in the size of transplanted mammary tumours. Some studies have suggested that high-fat diets may also have an influence on tumour initiation.

The mechanism by which high-fat diets influence mammary carcinogenesis is not well understood. Although an effect of dietary fat on the secretion of some hormones, such as oestrogen and prolactin, has been suggested, experimental evidence indicates that such changes cannot explain the effects of dietary fat on the development of mammary tumours. There is some evidence indicating that dietary fat may influence the proliferative activity and responsiveness to mammotropic hormones of mammary epithelial cells[32].

Although animal experiments clearly show that dietary fat intake influences mammary carcinogenesis, it is, at present, unknown to what extent these data apply to humans. In the following section, the evidence concerning dietary fat intake and breast cancer risk in women is considered.

Human evidence

In contrast to animal evidence, human evidence concerning a relationship between dietary fat intake and breast cancer risk is inconsistent. A recent review of this evidence identified 45 reports published in English that addressed this relationship, including 4 cohort studies, 14 case control studies, and 27 correlational studies of varous designs[33]. Only 1 of the 4 cohort studies examined total fat intake in relation to cancer risk and found no association[34]. Two of the 3 cohort studies that examined the relationship between breast cancer risk and meat intake found significant levels of association[35,36].

Only 1 of the 8 case control studies that examined total fat intake in relation to cancer risk found a significant association[37]. Seven other case control studies showed significant associations between specific fat-containing foods and risk of breast cancer[38-50]. One case control study, that of Miller, has recently been reanalysed by Howe[51] using nutrient data from both 24 h recall and diet history from the previous 6 months. Using linear regression analysis, saturated fat was found to be significantly associated with risk of breast cancer, with risk rising in a linear manner with increasing consumption of saturated fat. Analysis of the data separately for premenopausal and postmenopausal women showed the effects of saturated fat to be confined to premenopausal women, among whom there was a more than 5-fold difference in risk between the highest and lowest levels of fat intake.

All of the international and time trend studies that formally tested the association found a significant relationship between total *per capita* fat consumption and breast cancer risk, as did 4 of the 6 national correlational studies that examined this association.

Strong study designs (cohort and case control studies) have therefore failed to demonstrate consistently an association between fat consumption and breast cancer risk, although several investigators have found such an association within certain subgroups of patients or with specific sources of dietary fat. Correlational studies, designs that are generally regarded as being more susceptible to uncontrollable bias or confounding than are cohort or case control studies, have more consistently shown associations between fat intake and breast cancer risk.

It follows from the foregoing discussion of consistency that the association between dietary fat consumption and breast cancer risk is strong only in international correlation studies. The relationship is weaker in correlation studies carried out within countries and is either weak or absent in cohort and case control studies. A particularly important feature of all such studies is the range of fat intake observed in the populations observed.

Epidemiological investigation of the role of fat in breast cancer differs from most other aetiological studies in that there is no group available that has not had some exposure to the agent under study. Investigators are therefore only able to examine the risk of breast cancer in relation to the extent of exposure, as assessed by the quantity of fat ingested. If, in cohort and case control studies, populations are examined whose fat intake is systematically less variable than the variation in fat consumption between countries, then the associations found between fat intake and breast cancer risk will be weaker than those found in international correlation studies, if they can be identified at all.

The potential effects of this methodologic limitation are illustrated in Figure 10.1. In this figure, the variability in fat intake which was seen in the most rigorous cohort study reported to date, that of Willett[34] which examined the relationship between fat intake and breast cancer incidence, is contrasted with that seen in the only international correlation study which provided data on both fat intake and breast cancer incidence, that of Gray *et al.*[52]. Breast cancer incidence and *per capita* fat intake in the 22 countries included in Gray's correlation study were plotted and the least squares regression line fitted to the data. The scale on the abscissa showing percentage calories as fat was fitted by establishing two points, 39% of calories from fat from Willett's

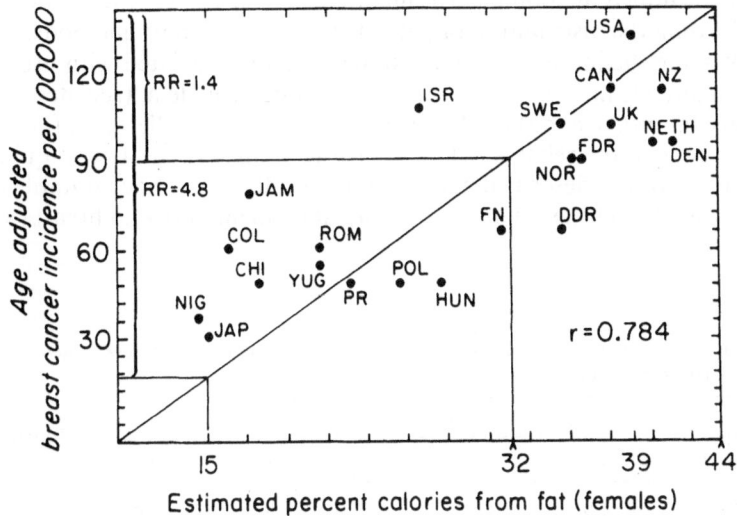

Figure 10.1 Estimate of the breast cancer risk detectable within the Western population in association with dietary fat. CAN=Canada; CHI=Chile; COL=Columbia; DDR=German Democratic Republic; DEN=Denmark; FDR=Federal Republic of Germany; FN=Finland; HUN=Hungary; ISR=Israel; JAM=Jamaica; JAP=Japan; NETH=The Netherlands; NIG=Nigeria; NOR=Norway; NZ=New Zealand; POL=Poland; PR=Puerto Rico; ROM=Romania; SWE=Sweden; UK=United Kingdom; USA=United States; YUG=Yugoslavia [Reprinted with permission from *Journal of the National Cancer Institute*]

data for the USA, and 15% of calories from fat for Japan from the data provided by Kagawa[53]. A linear scale was then constructed between these points.

As shown in Figure 10.1, the approximately 5-fold international variation observed in breast cancer incidence is strongly associated with differences in estimated fat consumption ($r=0.78$). To estimate the differences in cancer incidence that might be found in association with fat intake within a country, if the international data indeed do indicate a causal association, we have projected onto the regression line the range in fat intake reported in Willett's cohort study. Fat intake varied from 32% of calories (mean of lowest quintile) to 44% of calories (mean of highest quintile). As shown in the figure, this range of fat intake would be expected to be associated with relatively small differences in cancer incidence and the ratio of the risks in the highest and lowest quintiles would be approximately 1.4. This risk ratio would be even smaller if other methodologic limitations existed, such as measurement error.

The influence of measurement error on the largest relative risk of breast cancer that is likely to be detected in association with dietary fat can be estimated from data provided by Willett *et al.* The questionnaire used by Willett to collect dietary information from the nurses cohort was a semi-quantitative method of retrospective enquiry. This method of enquiry had been validated by comparing fat consumption as determined by questionnaire

191

and as determined by food records maintained over 7 days[54]. Data were then given showing the distribution of patients according to both methods.

To examine the influence of measurement error associated with use of the questionnaire we have assumed that diet records provide a 'true' description of dietary fat intake and that, if they were used to collect dietary information from the cohort, the relative risk of 1.4 between highest and lowest quintiles, whose derivation is described above, would be identified. Each quintile of fat intake would then be asociated with a 10% increment in risk of breast cancer.

Table 10.1 Estimates of the effects of error in dietary measurement on the assessment of breast cancer risk (from Willett *et al.*[34])

Quintile of diet questionnaire	Diet record quintiles					Apparent risk
	1	*2*	*3*	*4*	*5*	
'True' RR	1.0	1.1	1.2	1.3	1.4	
Lowest	53	14	12	18	3	1.115
Highest	3	12	21	32	33	1.292
Apparent RR						1.159

Data from Table 1 of Willett[34] give the distribution of subjects in the highest and lowest quintiles of fat intake according to the questionnaire classified according to fat intake as assessed by diet records. In Table 10.1, we estimated the effects of such misclassification on the cancer risk association with the highest and lowest quintiles of fat intake as determined by questionnaire. Misclassification will reduce the apparent difference in risk between the upper and lower quintiles compared with the 'true' difference in risk, so that a true difference of 1.4 will appear to be only 1.16. It is likely that other sources of error, such as the error in measurement associated with the diet records themselves, will further reduce the detectable risk.

We conclude from this review of the evidence that further study of the relationship between dietary fat and breast cancer risk is required before dietary recommendations can be made concerning this disease. In particular, intervention studies, which expand the range of fat intake within the population studied, are capable of overcoming the constraint placed upon observational epidemiology by the narrow range of fat intake that occurs spontaneously in the population. Intervention studies are therefore more likely than observational studies to generate the information required to determine whether dietary fat intake is causally related to breast cancer risk, and whether a population at high risk for breast cancer can reduce its risk by reducing dietary fat consumption. If breast cancer risk could be shown to be reduced by reducing dietary fat intake, this would constitute the strongest available evidence that dietary fat was relevant to breast cancer risk in humans.

DIETARY FAT REDUCTION IN WOMEN WITH MAMMOGRAPHIC DYSPLASIA: FEASIBILITY AND EARLY OUTCOMES

Information about the relationship of mammographic dysplasia to breast cancer risk, together with epidemiological and animal experimental data suggesting a relationship between dietary fat consumption and breast cancer risk, prompted us to examine the relationship of mammographic dysplasia to dietary fat. We reasoned that, if the high fat content that is typical of the 'Western' diet is causally related to breast cancer, then it is also likely to be related to changes in the breast that are associated with cancer risk. Alterations in nutrition to provide a diet more characteristic of parts of the world where breast cancer risk is low could then be expected to reverse these changes.

To examine this question, we have carried out a randomized controlled trial of dietary fat reduction in patients with mammographic dysplasia. The initial goals of this study were to determine whether it was feasible to carry out a trial of dietary fat reduction in this group of patients, to assess compliance with a reduced-fat diet, and to assess the effect of dietary change on the radiological appearances of mammographic dysplasia after 1 year of dietary change. In addition, we noted the frequency of histological changes found in patients who had surgical biopsy of the breast after entering this trial[55].

Two hundred and ninety-five women with mammographically demonstrated breast dysplasia were recruited from the Breast Diagnostic Clinic at Women's College Hospital, and randomly allocated to receive one of two types of dietary advice. A group of controls was given general advice about maintaining a healthy diet according to Canada's Food Guide but subjects were not counselled to change the composition of their diets. The average fat intake of this group was 35% of calories. A second group of subjects was given advice and education about reducing dietary fat intake to 15% of total calories. In both groups, breast dysplasia was assessed mammographically one year after randomization, and the appearances compared with those present at the time of randomization.

The principles of the dietary intervention involved the preparation of an individualized dietary prescription, based on a careful assessment of each subject's eating habits at entry to the study, in which fat was substituted by the isocaloric exchange of complex carbohydrate. Subjects were encouraged to introduce these dietary principles into their diet as soon as possible, and to adopt the new diet fully within 4 weeks. In addition, we provided several dietary aids that included dietetic scales, a food guide containing the subject's individualized meal pattern, daily food allowance, and additional information, such as exchange lists for fat, cereals, fruit and vegetables, an extensive shoppers guide, suggestions for eating away from home, and approximately 200 low-fat high-carbohydrate recipes.

After randomization, subjects in the intervention group were seen once every month for 12 months, and those in the control group every 4 months for 12 months. At each visit, both groups provided a record of food eaten on 3 randomly selected days. The principal method of assessing compliance was the nutrient analysis of food records. In addition, serum cholesterol was measured in all patients at randomization and at intervals afterwards corresponding to the collection of food records. Further, duplicate meals for a 24-hour period were collected from a subset of subjects 6 or 12 months after entry and chemically analysed.

To date, 295 subjects have entered the study and 227 have completed at least one year of the study. Their mean age was 43 years, and 76% were premenopausal. Ten per cent of the subjects had a first-degree relative with breast cancer. Subjects in the intervention and control groups were similar with respect to risk factors for breast cancer.

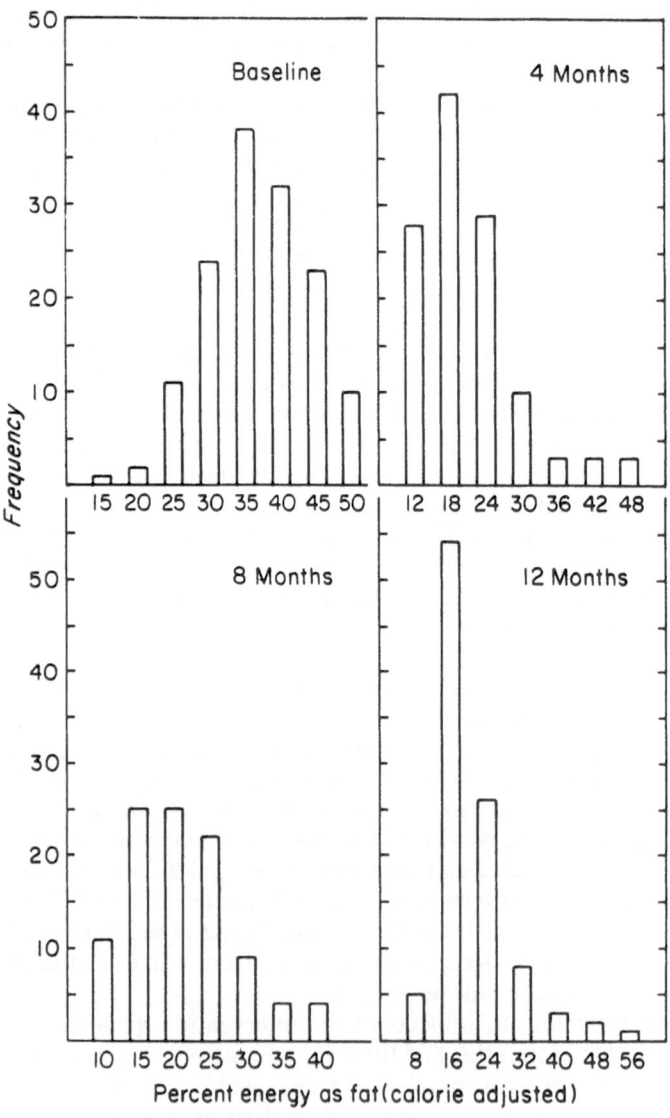

Figure 10.2 Dietary fat intake in intervention group according to nutrient analysis of food records and time from randomization

The intake of dietary fat, as assessed by the nutrient analysis of food records at baseline, 4, 8, and 12 months after randomization is shown in Figure 10.2. The intake of dietary fat in the control group, in terms of the proportion of calories derived from fat, remained stable over the 12 months of observation. Four months after randomization, the dietary fat intake of the intervention group fell from a mean of 36% of calories at baseline to a mean of 21%. From 4 months to 12 months after randomization, approximately 60% of the intervention group had an intake of dietary fat that fell within 5% of the target of 15% of calories, and approximately 80% had an intake within 10% of this target. Protein intake was unchanged and the mean percentage of calories from carbohydrate rose from 43% to 56%. The reduction in total fat intake in the intervention group was due to a reduction in both saturated and polyunsaturated fat and the ratio of these sources of fat did not change over the course of 12 months. Intake of dietary cholesterol also fell in the intervention group. The increase in carbohydrate consumption was attributable to increased intake of starch and other complex carbohydrate without any significant increase in sucrose consumption.

Statistical comparison of fat and carbohydrate intake between invervention and control groups after randomization were highly significant ($p<0.0001$) at all intervals after randomization. The changes in dietary fat consumption indicated in the food records were supported by a quantitative relationship between nutrient intake and changes in serum cholesterol. Further, duplicates of all food consumed during one 24-hour period were collected from 57 volunteer subjects, 29 from the intervention group and 28 from the control group, at either 6 or 12 months after randomization, and the food samples were homogenized and chemically analysed. Chemical analysis of fat showed that the intervention group consumed an average of 27 g/day (18% of calories) and that the control group consumed an average of 47 g/day (31% of calories)[56].

Subjects were examined by mammography before entry and again after completing 1 year in the trial. Pairs of mammographic images were then compared independently by two radiologists without knowledge of the dietary group to which subjects belonged or of the sequence in which films had been taken. No statistically significant differences were found between the groups in either the extent or density of mammographic dysplasia.

Twenty-eight patients have had a surgical biopsy of the breast since entering this study and slides were collected from these subjects and reviewed. Sixteen biopsies have been performed on women randomized to the control group. Five showed invasive cancer, and 2 atypical hyperplasia. The remainder showed either proliferation without atypia or non-proliferative changes. Twelve biopsies have been performed on subjects randomized to the intervention group. Two showed invasive cancer, 2 *in situ* carcinoma, and 2 atypical hyperplasia. None showed proliferative change without atypia and 6 showed non-proliferative changes. The development of 7 cancers in this group of subjects is 3.89 times the number expected (95% confidence interval 1.85–8.16) based upon age-specific person years of follow up for the Ontario population.

While carrying out this clinical trial of dietary fat reduction in patients with mammographic dysplasia, we noted that patients with cyclical mastopathy at entry frequently experienced striking relief of symptoms after reduction of dietary fat. Similar findings have been reported by Rose *et al.* in an uncontrolled study[57]. We therefore carried out a second trial whose purpose was to test the hypothesis that symptoms of cyclical mastopathy are relieved by a reduction in dietary fat accompanied by an increase in complex carbohydrate[58]. Twenty-one patients with severe and persistent cyclical mastopathy were recruited and randomly allocated to a dietary intervention of the same type as described above. The target of 15% of calories was again used in the intervention group.

Total fat intake in the intervention group fell from a mean of 34% of calories to a mean of approximately 21% of calories, which was maintained for 6 months. Carbohydrate consumption increased in the intervention group from 47% of calories at baseline of 60% of calories. No changes were observed in the intake of alcohol, caffeine, or α-tocopherol.

Changes in the severity of breast swelling and tenderness during the course of the study are shown in Figure 10.3. Results are expressed as the difference in severity scores recorded in the diaries between the postmenstrual (day 7) and premenstrual (2 days before the onset of menstruation) phases of the cycle, the absence of a difference indicating an absence of cyclical changes in these symptoms.

As Figure 10.3 shows, there was, in the intervention group, a striking reduction in the severity of cyclical breast swelling and tenderness over the course of 6 months. Statistical assessment by analysis of variance of these changes in the 18 patients for whom complete data were available gave p values of 0.0399 [$F(3,14) = 3.63$] for breast swelling and 0.0001 [$F(3,14) = 18.37$] for breast tenderness. These changes in self-reported symptom severity were similar to those found by a physician who interviewed these subjects.

Details of the biochemical changes noted in this trial have been given elsewhere[58]. Plasma levels of oestrone, oestradiol and progesterone were similar in both groups throughout the study. Levels of sex hormone-binding globulin and prolactin did not differ significantly between the groups at any time.

Serum cholesterol did not differ signficantly between the groups at any time but statistically significant changes within the intervention did occur that were close to those predicted. Changes in consumption of total energy ($r = 0.76; p = 0.02$), total fat ($r = 0.69; p = 0.04$), saturated fat ($r = 0.65; p = 0.06$), polyunsaturated fat ($r = 0.68; p = 0.04$), protein ($r = 0.90; p = 0.0009$) and dietary cholesterol ($r = 0.75; p = 0.02$) were all significantly correlated with change in the severity of the symptom of breast tenderness at 6 months.

None of the hormonal measurements (oestrone, oestradiol, progesterone, prolactin or sex hormone-binding globulin) showed evidence of an association with change in symptoms but change in serum cholesterol did show an association that was of borderline statistical significance ($r = 0.69, p = 0.06$).

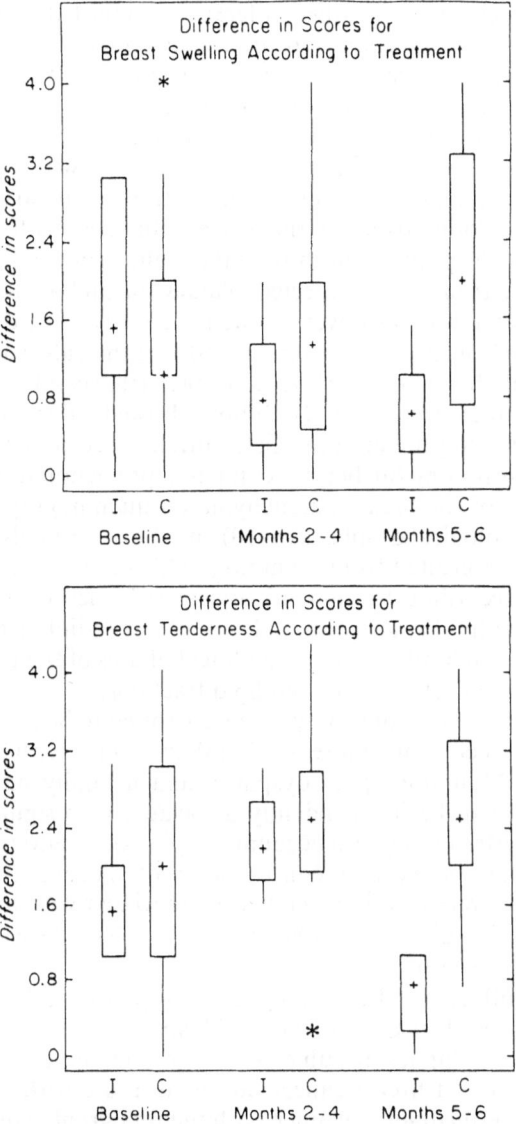

Figure 10.3 Changes in breast tenderness and swelling associated with dietary intervention. Data are shown as 'box plots' in which the mean is shown as a cross, the interquartile range as a box, and the range (estimated as a multiple of the interquartile range) as lines extending from the box. Data points lying outside the estimated range are shown as asterisks [Reprinted from *Lancet* with the permission of the Editor]

PLASMA LIPIDS AS POSSIBLE MARKERS OF BREAST CANCER RISK

The risk of breast cancer associated with mammographic dysplasia discussed above provides an opportunity to identify factors which influence risk of breast cancer. Biochemical or other differences found between women with and without this mammographic appearance may provide information about the causes of the radiological change and of the associated cancer risk.

The possibility that mammographic dysplasia might be associated with distinctive biochemical changes was raised during earlier work in which we measured plasma lipids and lipoproteins in women with mammographic dysplasia who were taking part in a clinical trial of dietary fat reduction described above. Comparison of the values obtained with age- and sex-specific values for the population showed that values for total cholesterol did not differ notably from those expected. Values for high-density lipoprotein cholesterol (HDLC) were, however, skewed markedly toward the upper end of the distribution for the population, and 50% of the values fell at or above the 75th percentile for women of the same age. Triglycerides (TG) and low-density lipoprotein cholesterol (LDLC) both showed a distribution that was skewed towards the lower end of the distribution expected in the population.

To examine this finding further, we compared premenopausal women with different patterns of the breast parenchyma on mammography. One group had extensive radiological dysplasia (n=30) and the other no dysplasia (n=16). Both groups were recruited from mammographic units in the same way and then compared according to epidemiological risk factors, anthropometric measures, nutrient intake, and plasma levels of oestradiol, progesterone and prolactin obtained in both follicular and luteal phases of the menstrual cycle, as well as total plasma cholesterol and lipid fractions.

Women with mammographic dysplasia were found to be leaner, more often nulliparous, and to consume more alcohol than women without these radiological changes. Mammographic dysplasia and a family history of breast cancer were found to be independently associated with significantly higher levels of HDLC after taking into account the possible confounding effects of per cent body fat, parity and consumption of alcohol and dietary fat. Triglyceride levels were also independently associated with a family history of breast cancer. No differences were found in plasma levels of oestradiol, progesterone or prolactin[59].

The separate influences of mammographic dysplasia and a family history of breast cancer on HDLC and TG are illustrated in Figure 10.4. Plasma levels of HDLC were highest in subjects with both mammographic dysplasia and a family history of breast cancer, lowest in those with neither of these attributes, and intermediate in women with mammographic dysplasia but no family history. TG levels were also influenced by both of these variables but in the opposite direction.

These findings suggest that the mammographic densities referred to as dysplasia are associated with an alteration in lipid metabolism. It is of interest, therefore, that several treatments for benign breast disease also influence plasma lipids. In particular, danazol, which has been shown to reverse the radiological appearance of dysplasia[60], has been reported[61-63] to lower plasma levels of HDLC by about 40%.

Examination of the relationship of HDLC to other epidemiological features of breast cancer shows several additional points of similarity. Adult women in Western society have higher plasma levels of HDLC than men and

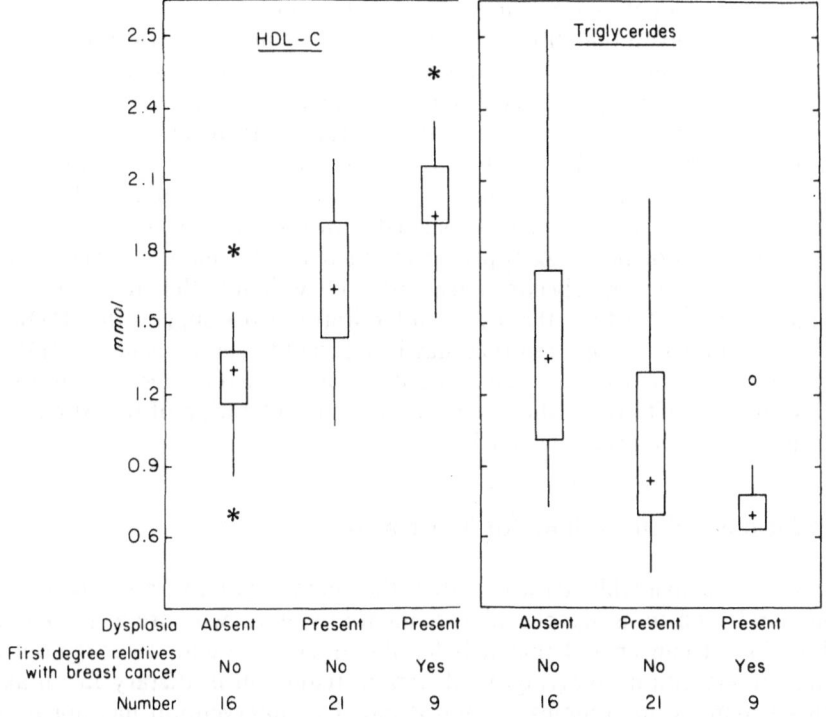

Figure 10.4 Plasma levels of high-density lipoprotein cholesterol and triglycerides according to the presence or absence of mammographic dysplasia or a family history of breast cancer. Data are shown as 'box plots'; for explanation, see legend to Figure 10.3 [Reprinted from *British Journal of Cancer* with the permission of the Editor]

this difference is influenced by female sex hormones[64]. Puberty in females is associated with higher levels of plasma HDLC than in males[65].

Measurements of HDLC levels in different countries show that, in general, HDLC levels are higher in women in countries where the risk of breast cancer is also high. Belgian women, who are at greater risk of breast cancer, have substantially higher levels of HDLC than either Chinese or Korean women[66]. Female migrants to Israel of European or North American origin have higher levels of HDLC and a greater risk of breast cancer than migrants from Asia or Africa and the Israeli-born Jews had intermediate levels[67]. In addition, Finnish women have higher levels of HDLC than Japanese women[68].

Child bearing is known to reduce breast cancer risk and a recent large cohort study conducted in Belgium showed that HDLC levels are lower in parous than nulliparous women and that HDLC levels are approximately 40% lower after pregnancy than before[69].

Several studies, including the one described above, have shown that a reduced-fat diet reduces HDLC and raises TG levels in healthy premenopausal women[70-74]. The influence of dietary fat reduction on HDLC levels differed according to the type of fat changed, and a reduction in both polyunsaturated and saturated fat appears to be required to lower HDLC levels. Observational surveys show that HDLC level is associated with dietary practices and suggest that differences in diet are responsible for the differences in HDLC level found between countries that were referred to above[75,76].

Alcohol consumption has been found consistently to increase risk of breast cancer[77] and there is an abundant literature showing that alcohol consumption raises HDLC levels[78]. Body weight appears to exert different effects on breast cancer risk before and after the menopause. Risk of premenopausal breast cancer is associated with normal or lean body type[79], whereas postmenopausal risk appears to be increased by obesity[80]. HDLC has been found to be negatively correlated with body weight both before and after the menopause[81]. Further, the results of laboratory work suggest that HDLC possesses biological properties that may be relevant to carcinogenesis. HDLC has been shown to promote the growth of tumours in serum-free cell culture[82] and to interact with oestradiol to promote the proliferation of breast cancer cell lines grown in serum-free medium[83].

Conclusions and suggestions for future work

The evidence available indicates that the mammographic appearance of density referred to as 'dysplasia' does identify women who are at increased risk of breast cancer and that it is feasible in such patients to carry out a dietary intervention involving a substantial reduction in dietary fat intake with an increase in complex carbohydrate. This intervention has not been shown to change the appearance of the breast parenchyma but does result in striking symptom relief in women with severe cyclical breast tenderness and swelling. It now appears possible to study the effects of longer periods of dietary change on the mammographic appearance of the breast and, in a substantially larger number of subjects, on breast cancer incidence.

The biochemical changes found to be associated with mammographic dysplasia suggest that plasma lipids, particularly HDLC, may be a marker of breast cancer risk and that plasma levels of HDLC are influenced by a number of other risk factors for breast cancer, including dietary fat.

Interest in the relationship of HDLC to disease has to date been concerned primarily with its protective role in coronary heart disease. The results shown here, as well as data in the literature, suggest that further investigation of the role of HDLC in relation to breast cancer risk is warranted. The association of plasma lipid levels with other risk factors for breast cancer should be examined, including studies of the association with familial risk for the disease and the association of lipid levels with histological changes that confer increased risk. A large-scale dietary intervention study in women with mammographic dysplasia would allow examination of the effect of a dietary change which will lower HDLC levels on breast cancer risk. Although HDLC levels and coronary heart disease are negatively correlated within countries, they are positively correlated between countries[84]. Dietary fat reduction would therefore be expected to lower heart disease risk even though HDLC levels are reduced. For example, the 'prudent diet' currently recommended by the American Heart Association has been shown to lower HDLC levels[85].

The influence of a low-fat high-carbohydrate diet on symptoms of cyclical mastopathy suggests that fat has short-term physiological effects on the breast. These effects should be more precisely characterized, in view of the evidence that dietary fat and premenstrual breast symptoms may be related to breast cancer risk[86,87]. The development of physical methods of characterizing breast tissue would obviously help considerably in characterizing these effects and magnetic resonance imaging is now being assessed from this point of view.

References

1. Doll, R. and Peto, R. (1981). *The Causes of Cancer: Quantitative Estimates of Avoidable Risks of Cancer in the United States.* (Oxford: Oxford University Press)
2. Buell, P. (1974). Changing incidence of breast cancer in Japanese-American women. *J. Natl. Cancer Inst.*, **51**, 1479–1483
3. Kmet, J. (1970). The role of migrant populations in studies of selected cancers. *J. Chronic Dis.*, **23**, 305–324
4. Haenzel, W. (1970). Studies of migrant populations. *J. Chronic Dis.*, **23**, 289–231
5. Kelsey, J. L. (1979). A review of the epidemiology of human breast cancer. Epidemiologic Reviews. (Eds). Johns Hopkins University School of Hygiene and Public Health i: 74–109
6. Kelsey, J. L. and Barkowitz, G. S. (1988). Breast cancer epidemiology. *Cancer Res.*, **48**, 5615
7. Macmahon, B., Cole, P. and Brown, J. (1973). Etiology of human breast cancer: a review. *J. Natl. Cancer Inst.*, **50**, 21–42
8. Wolfe, J. N. (1976). Risk for breast cancer development determined by mammographic parenchymal pattern. *Cancer*, **37**, 2486
9. Saftlas, A. F. and Szklo, M. Mammographic parenchymal patterns and breast cancer risk. *In Epidemiologic Reviews* 1987. Szklo, M., Gordis, L., Gregg, M. B. and Levine, M. M. (eds.) Johns Hopkins University School of Hygiene and Public Health.
10. Goodwin, P. J. and Boyd, N. F. (1988). Mammographic parenchymal pattern and breast cancer risk: A critical appraisal of the evidence. *Am.J. Epidemiol.*, **127**, 1097–1108
11. Boyd, N. F., Wolfson, C., Moskowitz, M., Carlile, T., Petitclerc, C., Ferri, H., Fishell, E., Gregorie, A., Kiernan, M., Longley, J., Simor, I. and Miller, A. B. (1986). Observer variation in the classification of mammographic parenchymal patterns with breast cancer. *J. Chron. Dis.*, **39**, 465–472
13. Boyd, N. F., O'Sullivan, B., Campbell, J. E., Fishell, E., Simor, I., Cooke, G. and Germanson, T. (1982). Mammographic signs as risk factors for breast cancer. *Br. J. Cancer*, **45**, 185–193
14. Brisson, J., Merletti, F., Sadowski, N. L. *et al.* (1982). Mammographic parenchymal patterns of the breast and breast cancer risk. *Am. J. Epidemiol.*, **115(3)**, 428–437
15. Wolfe, J. N., Saftlas, A. F. and Salane, M. (1987). Mammographic parenchymal patterns and quantitative evaluation of mammographic densities: A case control study. *Am. J. Roentgenol.*, **148**, 1087–1092
16. Brisson, J., Morrison, A. S. and Khalid, H. (1988). Mammographic parenchymal features and breast cancer in the breast cancer detection demonstration project. *J. Natl. Cancer Inst.*, **80**, 1534–1539
17. Wellings, S. R., Jensen, H. M. and Marcum, R. G. (1975). An atlas of the subgross pathology of the human breast with special reference to possible precancerous lesions. *J. Natl. Cancer Inst.*, **55**, 231
18. Page, D. L., Vander Zwaag, R., Rogers, L. W. *et al.*, (1978). Relation between component parts of fibrocystic disease complex and breast cancer. *J. Natl. Cancer Inst.*, **61**, 1055–1063
19. Jensen, H. M., Rice, J. and Wellings, S. R. (1976). Precancerous lesions in the human breast. *Science*, **191**, 295–297
20. Wellings, S. R. and Jensen, H. M. (1973). On the origin and progression of ductal carcinoma of the human breast. *J. Natl. Cancer Inst.*, **50**, 1111–1118
21. Dupont, W. D. and Page, D. L. (1984). Risk factors for breast cancer in women with

proliferative breast disease. *N. Engl. J. Med.*, **312**, 146

22. Kodlin, D., Winger, E. E., Morgenstern, N. L. and Chen, U. (1977). Chronic mastopathy and breast cancer: a follow up study. *Cancer*, **39**, 2603–2607
23. Davis, H. H., Simons, M. and Davis, J. B. (1964). Cystic disease of the breast: relationship to carcinoma. *Cancer*, **17**, 957–978
24. Hutchinson, W. B., Thomas, D. B., Hamlin, W. B., Roth, G. J., Peterson, A. V. and Williams, B. (1980). Risk of breast cancer in women with benign breast disease. *J. Natl. Cancer Inst.*, **65**, 13–20
25. Wellings, S. R. and Wolfe, J. N. (1978). Correlative studies of the histologic and radiographic appearance of the breast parenchyma. *Radiology*, **129**, 299
26. Bright, R. A., Morrison, A. S., Brisson, J., Burstein, N. A., Sadowsky, N. S., Kopans, D. B. and Myer, J. E. (1988). Relationship between mammographic and histologic features of breast tissue in women with benign biopsies. *Cancer*, **61**, 266–271
27. Fisher, E. R., Paleker, A., Kim, W. S. and Redmond, C. (1978). The histopathology of mammographic patterns. *Am. J. Clin. Pathol.*, **69**, 421
28. Moskowitz, M., Gartside, P. and McLaughlin, C. (1980). Mammographic patterns as markers for high risk benign breast disease and incidence cancers. *Radiology*, **134**, 293–295
29. Urbanski, S., Jensen, H. M., Cooke, G., McFarlane, D., Shannon, P., Kruikov, V. and Boyd, N. F. (1988). The association of histological and radiological indicators of breast cancer risk. *Br. J. Cancer*, **58**, 474–479
30. Welsch, C. W. (1986). Interrelationships between dietary fat and endocrine processes in mammary gland tumorigenesis. In Ip, C., Birt, D. F., Rogers, A. E., Mettlin, C. (Eds.) *Dietary Fat and Cancer Progress in Clinical and Biological Research*, **222**, 623–654
31. Rogers, A. E. and Lee, S. Y. Chemically induced mammary gland tumors in rats: modulation by dietary fat. *ibid*, 255–282
32. Welsch, C. W., DeHoog, J. V., O'Conner, D. H. and Sheffield, L. G. (1985). Influence of dietary fat levels on development and hormone responsiveness of the mouse mammary gland. *Cancer Res.*, **45**,6147–6154
33. Goodwin, P. and Boyd, N. F. (1987). A critical appraisal of the evidence that dietary fat intake is related to breast cancer risk in humans. *J. Natl. Cancer Inst.*, **79**, 473–485
34. Willett, W. C., Stampfer, M. J., Colditz, G. A. *et al.* (1987). Dietary fat and the risk of breast cancer. *N. Engl. J. Med.*, **316**, 22–28
35. Hirayama, T. (1978). Epidemiology of breast cancer with special reference to the role of diet. *Prevent. Med.*, **7**, 173–195
36. Phillips, R. L. and Snowdon, D. A. (1983). Association of meat and coffee use with cancers of the large bowel, breast, and prostate among Seventh-Day Adventists: Preliminary results. *Cancer Res.*, **43** (Suppl.), 2403s–2408s
37. Sarin, R., Tandon, R. K., Paul, S. *et al.* (1985). Diet, body fat and plasma lipids in breast cancer. *Indian J. Med. Res.*, **81**, 493–498
38. Phillips, R. L. (1975). Role of life-style and dietary habits in risk of cancer among Seventh-Day Adventists. *Cancer Res.*, **35**, 3513–3522
39. Nomura, A., Henderson, B. E. and Lee, J. (1978). Breast cancer and diet among the Japanese in Hawaii. *Am. J. Clin. Nutr.*, **31**, 2020–2025
40. Miller, A. B., Kelly, A., Choi, N. W. *et al.* (1978). A study of diet and breast cancer. *Am. J. Epidemiol.*, **107**, 499–509
41. Lubin, J. H., Burns, P. E., Blot, W. J. *et al.* (1981). Dietary factors and breast cancer risk. *Int. J. Cancer*, **28**, 685–689
42. Graham, S., Marshall, J., Mettlin, C. *et al.* (1982). Diet in the epidemiology of breast cancer. *Am. J. Epidemiol.*, **116**, 68–75
43. Hislop, T. C., Coldman, A. J., Elwood, J. M. *et al.* (1986). Childhood and recent eating patterns and risk of breast cancer. *Cancer Detect. Prevent.*, **9**, 47–58
44. Katsouyanni, K., Trichopoulos, D., Boyle, P. *et al.* (1986). Diet and breast cancer: A case-control study in Greece. *Int. J. Cancer*, **38**, 815–820
45. Kolonel, L. N., Nomura, A. M., Hinds, M. W. *et al.* (1983). Role of diet in cancer incidence in Hawaii. *Cancer Res.*, **43** (Suppl.), 2397s–2402s
46. Talamini, R., La Vecchia, C., Decarli, A. *et al.* (1984). Social factors, diet and breast cancer in a northern Italian population. *Br. J. Cancer*, **49**, 723–729
47. Zemla, B. (1984). The role of selected dietary elements in breast cancer risk among native and migrant populations in Poland. *Nutr. Cancer*, **6**, 187–195

48. Nomura, A. M., Hirohata, T., Kolonel, L. N. *et al.* (1985). Breast cancer in Caucasian and Japanese women in Hawaii. *Natl. Cancer Inst. Monogr.*, **69**, 191–196
49. Hirohata, T., Shigematsu, T., Nomura, A. M. *et al.* (1985). Occurrence of breast cancer in relation to diet and reproductive history: A case-control study in Fukuoka, Japan. *Natl. Cancer Inst. Monogr.*, **69**, 187–190
50. Lubin, F., Wax, Y. and Modan, B. (1986). Role of fat, animal protein, and dietary fiber in breast cancer etiology: A case-control study. *J. Natl. Cancer Inst.*, **77**, 605–612
51. Howe, G. R. (1985). The use of polytomous dual response data to increase power in case-control studies: An application to the association between dietary fat and breast cancer. *J. Chronic Dis.*, **38**, 663–670
52. Gray, G. E., Pike, M. C. and Henderson, B. E. (1979). Breast-cancer incidence and mortality rates in different countries in relation to known risk factors and dietary practices. *Br. J. Cancer*, **39**, 1–7
53. Kagawa, Y. (1978). Impact of Westernization on the nutrition of Japanese: Changes in physique, cancer, longevity and centenarians. *Prevent. Med.*, **7**, 205–217
54. Willett, W. C., Sampson, L., Stampfer, M. I. *et al.* (1985). Reproducibility and validity of a semiquantitative food frequency questionnaire. *Am. J. Epidemiol.*, **122**, 51–65
55. Boyd, N. F., Cousins, M., Beaton, M., Fishell, E., Wright, B., Fish, E., Kriukov, V., Lockwood, G., Trichler, D., Hanna, W. and Page, D. L. (1988). Clinical trial of low fat, high carbohydrate diet in subjects with mammographic dysplasia: report of early outcomes. *J. Natl. Cancer Inst.*, **80**, 1244–1248
56. Lee-Han, H., Cousins, M., Beaton, M. *et al.* (1988). Compliance in a randomized clinical trial of dietary fat reduction in patients with breast dysplasia. *Am. J. Clin. Nutr.*, **48**, 575–586
57. Rose, D. P., Boyar, A., Haley, N., Cohen, L., Lahti, H. and Strong, L. E. (1985). Low fat diet in fibrocystic disease of the breast with cyclical mastalgia: a feasibility study. *Am. J. Clin. Nutr.*, **42**, 856
58. Boyd, N. F., McGuire, V., Shannon, P., Cousins, M., Kriukov, V., Mahoney, L., Fish, E., Lickley, L., Lockwood, G. and Trichler, D. (1988). The effect of a low fat high carbohydrate diet on symptoms of cyclical mastopathy. *Lancet*, **2**, 128–132
59. Boyd, N. F., McGuire, V., Fishell, E., Kruikov, V., Lockwood, G. and Trichler, D. (In press). Plasma lipids in premenopausal women with mammographic dysplasia. *Br. J. Cancer*
60. Asch, R. M. and Greenblatt, R. B. (1977). The use of an impeded androgen–Danazol–in the management of benign breast disorders. *Am. J. Obstet. Gynecol.,* **129**, 130
61. Luciano, A. A., Hauser, K. S. and Sherman, B. M. (1983). Effects of Danazol on plasma lipid and lipoprotein levels in normal women. *Atherosclerosis*, **43**, 133–137
62. Schewepe, K. W. and Assmann, G. (1984). Changes of plasma lipids and lipoprotein levels during Danazol treatment for endometriosis. *Horm. Metab. Res.*, **16**, 593–597
63. Fahraeus, L., Larsson-Cohn, U. Ljungberg, S. and Wallentin, L., (1984). Profound alterations of lipoprotein metabolism during danazol treatment for endometriosis. *Fertil. Steril.*, **42**, 52–57
64. Lipid Research Clinics Program Epidemiology Committee (1979). Plasma lipid distribution in selected North American populations. *Circulation*, **60**, 427–439
65. Srinivasan, S. R., Sundaram, G. S., Williamson, G. D., Webber, L. S. and Berenson, G. S. (1985). Serum lipoproteins and endogenous sex hormones in early life: Observations in children with different lipoprotein profiles. *Metabolism*, **34**(9), 861–867
66. Kesteloot, H., Huang, D. X., Claes, J. *et al.*, (1985). Serum lipids in the People's Republic of China: Comparison of western and eastern populations. *Arteriosclerosis*, **5**, 427–433
67. Halfton, S. T., Rifkind, B. M., Harlap, S. *et al.* (1980). Plasma lipids and lipoproteins in adult Jews of different origins: The Jerusalem Lipid Research Clinic Prevalence Study. *Isr. J. Med. Sci.*, **18**, 1113–1120
68. Punnonen, R., Jokela, H., Kudo, R., Punnonen, K., Pyykko, K. and Pystynen, P. (1987). Serum lipids in Finnish and Japanese postmenopausal women. *Atherosclerosis*, **68**, 241–247
69. van Stiphout, W. A. H., Hofman, A. and de Bruijn, A. M. (1987). Serum lipids in young women before, during and after pregnancy. *Am. J. Epidemiol.*, **126**, 922–928
70. Jones, D. Y., Judd, J. T., Taylor, P. R., Campbell, W. S. and Nair, P. P. (1987). Influence of caloric contribution and saturation of dietary fat on plasma lipids in premenopausal women. *Am. J. Clin. Nutr.*, **45**, 1451–1456
71. Kuusi, T., Ehnholm, C., Huttunen, J. K., Kostainen, E. *et al.* (1985). Concentration and composition of serum lipoproteins during a low fat diet at two levels of polyunsaturated fat.

J. Lipid Res., **26**, 360–367

72. Brussaard, J. H., Dallinga-Thie, G., Groot, P. H. E. and Katan, M. B. (1980). Effects of amount and type of dietary fat on serum lipids, lipoproteins and apoproteins in man. *Atherosclerosis*, **36**, 515

73. Ehnholm, C., Huttenen, J. K., Pietinen, P., Leino, U., Mutanen, M., Kostianen, E., Pikkarainen, J., Dougherty, R., Iacono, J. and Puska, P. (1982). Effect of diet on serum lipoproteins in a population with a high risk of coronary heart disease. *N. Engl. J. Med.*, **207**, 850–855

74. Shepherd, J., Packard, C. J., Patsch, J. F., Gotto, A. M. and Taunton, O. D. (1978). Effects of dietary polyunsaturated and saturated fat on the properties of high density lipoproteins and the metabolism of apoprotein A1. *J. Clin. Invest.*, **61**, 1582–1592

75. Sacks, F. M., Castelli, W. P., Donner, A. and Kass, E. H. (1975). Plasma lipids and lipoproteins in vegetarians and controls. *N. Engl. J. Med.*, **292**, 1148–1151

76. Tamir, D., Edelstein, P., Reshef, A., Halfon, S. and Palti, H. (1987). Serum cholesterol (total, low density lipoprotein cholesterol, and high density lipoprotein cholesterol) triglyceride levels and fat consumption among Jerusalem Arab and Jewish schoolchildren. *Prevent. Med.*, **16**, 752–760

77. Graham, S. (1987). Alcohol and breast cancer risk, Editorial. *N. Engl. J. Med.*, **316**, 1211–1212

78. Williams, P. T., Krauss, R. M., Wood, P. D., Albers, J. J., Dreon, D. and Ellsworth, N. (1985). Association of diet and alcohol intake with high density lipoprotein subclasses. *Metabolism*, **34**, 524–530

79. Willet, W. C., Browne, M. L., Bain, C. *et al.* (1985). Relative weight and risk of breast cancer among premenopausal women. *Am. J. Epidemiol.*, **122**, 731–740

80. de Waard, F., Cornelius, J. P., Aoki, K. and Yoshida, M. (1977). Breast cancer incidence according to weight and height in two cities of the Netherlands and in Aichi prefecture, Japan. *Cancer*, **40**, 1269–1275

81. Heiss, G., Johnson, N. J., Reiland, S. *et al.* (1980). The epidemiology of plasma high density lipoprotein cholesterol levels. The lipid research clinics program prevalence study. *Circulation*, **62** (Suppl. IV), 116–136

82. Gospodarowicz, D., Lui, G-M. and Gonzalez, R. (1984). High density lipoproteins and the proliferation of human tumour cells maintained on extracellular matrix-coated dishes and exposed to defined medium. *Cancer Res.*, **42**, 3704–3713

83. Jozan, S., Faye, J. C., Tourmier, J. F. *et al.* (1985). Interaction of estradiol and high density lipoproteins on proliferation of the human breast cancer cell line MCF-7 adapted to grow in serum free conditions. *Biochem. Biophys. Res. Commun.*, **133**, 105–112

84. Miller, N. E. (1987). Lipoprotein metabolism. *Clin. Endocrinol. Metab.*, **1**, 603–622

85. Kohlmeier, M., Striker, G. and Schlierf, G. (1988). Influences of "normal" and "prudent" diets on biliary and serum lipids in healthy women. *Am. J. Clin. Nutr.*, **42**, 1201–1205

86. Wynder, E. L., MacCornack, F. A. and Stellman, S. D. (1978). The epidemiology of breast cancer in 785 United States Caucasian women. *Cancer*, **41**, 2341–2354

87. Kaplan, S. D. and Acheson, R. M. (1966). A single etiological hypothesis for breast cancer. *J. Chron. Dis.*, **19**, 1221–1230

Index

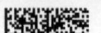